HYPERTENSION MEDICINE

CURRENT ◊ CLINICAL ◊ PRACTICE

HYPERTENSION MEDICINE

Edited by

MICHAEL A. WEBER, MD

State University of New York
Downstate College of Medicine
Brooklyn, New York

Foreword by

NORMAN K. HOLLENBERG, MD, PhD

Brigham and Women's Hospital, Boston, MA

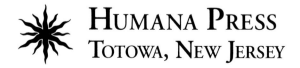 HUMANA PRESS
TOTOWA, NEW JERSEY

Dedication
To my wife, Sandra

FOREWORD

This is an outstanding book. We live in an age where a declaration of conflict of interest is expected. Let me confess that Dr. Weber and I are long-standing friends who have worked together on many occasions, in fact, we worked together on a major project the week that the pages of this book arrived. Clearly, I would have had a problem if this book was less than excellent, but it is not.

Hypertension is a major medical problem, almost certainly the most common chronic disease in the urban world. With the exception of pediatrics, at least 20–25% of patients seen in any practitioner's office—whether they practice general medicine or a subspecialty—have hypertension as part of their medical story. Over the past 30 years, the management of hypertension has moved from a formulaic approach that experts tried to apply to everyone, to highly individualized management. This is a field that is evolving quickly, not only in the area of pathogenic insight, but also in the areas of blood-pressure control, which measures should receive priority, and identification of patient subsets in whom special goals or approaches to therapy are appropriate. We have a wide range of choices, and clearly want to use the available approaches to their best advantage.

Each chapter in this book has been written by an authority in the field. Equally important, or perhaps more important, is the remarkably focused chapter headings. In most books, what would have been a single subject is addressed in three chapters, as one example. The first of this triad focuses on the concepts involved in setting targets when starting hypertension treatment. The next chapter focuses on choosing the first agent. The third chapter in the triad focuses on managing an inadequate response to the first agent. Why does this strategy work so well, which it does? The answer, I believe, lies in the focus. Because the author has only that specific topic to address, it is addressed in adequate detail. These are, after all, the truly important questions. Samuel Goldwyn is reputed to have said "Never make predictions, especially about the future." To close this Foreword, I am going to make a prediction. This is going to be a very successful publication. There is something in it for everyone who sees patients, and it is well-informed, thoughtfully organized, well written, and judicious in the selection of emphasis and of detail.

Norman K. Hollenberg, MD, PhD
Brigham and Woman's Hospital, Boston, MA

PREFACE

Hypertension Medicine is intended to be read by clinicians and to be helpful in a practical and immediate fashion. I have chosen topics that should cover common questions and emerging areas of interest. It always seems logical to explore in depth the basic sciences and epidemiology that provide the underpinnings of our knowledge of hypertension practice. But I have tried to avoid this temptation, using only the background necessary to explain or amplify clinical ideas.

We have emphasized brevity. I have asked our authors to minimize references and to prepare chapters short enough to be read comfortably at one sitting. We have sought an informal tone, as though the writer and the reader are having a collegial conversation. I have also asked the authors not to shy away from controversy or personal opinions; candor is vital when sharing clinical information and new concepts with colleagues.

The first section of *Hypertension Medicine* deals with the relevant background to hypertension: why we diagnose it, and why in most patients we now believe it should be treated aggressively. We then consider some of the major underlying mechanisms of hypertension, particularly those that help explain our approaches to treatment. The next section focuses on techniques for evaluating patients before treatment, bearing in mind that so many hypertensive patients have concomitant conditions like lipid disorders and diabetes mellitus, and often already have evidence of cardiovascular and renal changes. The final section deals with treatment. The discussion of antihypertensive drugs is relatively short. Rather, our major emphasis is in dealing with practical issues of management: how to select treatment to optimize results in difficult-to-treat hypertensive patients, and how to deal with major concomitant problems.

I am grateful to my many colleagues who were willing to share their expert knowledge and contribute chapters to this book. I also thank my distinguished friend Norman Hollenberg for agreeing to write a foreword, and my office coordinator Jeanne Minsky who worked so effectively with the authors and the dedicated editorial staff at Humana Press in bringing this project together.

Michael A. Weber, MD

CONTENTS

CONTRIBUTORS

PHILIP A. ATKIN, BPHARM, PhD • *Department of Clinical Pharmacology, Royal North Shore Hospital, St. Leonards, New South Wales, Australia*

HENRY R. BLACK, MD • *Chairman, Department of Preventive Medicine, Rush–Presbyterian St. Luke's Medical Center, Chicago, IL*

JON D. BLUMENFELD, MD • *Associate Professor of Medicine, Weill Medical College of Cornell University, and Associate Attending in Medicine, Division of Hypertension and The Cardiovascular Center, New York Presbyterian Hospital, New York, NY*

DAVID A. CALHOUN, MD • *Vascular Biology and Hypertension Program, Department of Medicine, University of Alabama at Birmingham, Birmingham, AL*

HAL L. CHADOW, MD • *Assistant Director, Division of Cardiology, The Brookdale University Hospital and Medical Center, and Assistant Professor of Medicine, SUNY Health Science Center, Brooklyn, NY*

VINCENT DEQUATTRO, MD • *Professor of Medicine and Director, Hypertension Diagnostic Laboratory, Division of Cardiology, University of Southern California, Los Angeles, CA*

JAYANT DEY, MD • *Section on Hypertensive Diseases, Department of Internal Medicine, Ochsner Clinic and Alton Ochsner Medical Foundation, New Orleans, LA*

ZHANBIN FENG, MD • *Section on Hypertensive Diseases, Department of Internal Medicine, Ochsner Clinic and Alton Ochsner Medical Foundation, New Orleans, LA*

JOHN M. FLACK, MD, MPH • *Associate Chairman, Department of Internal Medicine, Director, Cardiovascular Epidemiology and Clinical Applications Program, and Professor of Medicine and Community Medicine, Wayne State University School of Medicine, Detroit, MI*

STANLEY S. FRANKLIN, MD • *Clinical Professor of Medicine, Heart Disease Prevention Program, University of California, Irvine, CA*

HARALAMBOS GAVRAS, MD • *Hypertension and Atherosclerosis Section, Department of Medicine, Boston University School of Medicine, Boston, MA*

IRENE GAVRAS, MD • *Hypertension and Atherosclerosis Section, Department of Medicine, Boston University School of Medicine, Boston, MA*

THOMAS D. GILES, MD • *Section of Cardiology, Department of Medicine, LSU School of Medicine, New Orleans, LA*

CARLENE M. GRIM, BSN, MSN, SpDN • *President, Shared Care Research and Education, Torrance, CA*

CLARENCE E. GRIM, BS, MS, MD • *Professor of Cardiovascular Medicine, Medical College of Wisconsin, Milwaukee, WI*

EHUD GROSSMAN, MD • *Internal Medicine D, The Chaim Sheba Medical Center, Tel-Hashomer, Israel*

W. DALLAS HALL, MD, MACP • *Emeritus Professor of Medicine, Emory University School of Medicine, Atlanta, GA*

MARK HOUSTON, MD, FACP • *Associate Clinical Professor of Medicine, Vanderbilt University Medical Center, Director, Hypertension Institute, Saint Thomas Medical Group, St. Thomas Hospital, Nashville, TN*

JOSEPH L. IZZO, JR., MD • *Professor of Medicine, Pharmacology, and Toxicology, and Chief, Division of Clinical Pharmacology, School of Medicine and Biomedical Sciences, State University of New York at Buffalo, Buffalo, NY*

STEVO JULIUS, MD • *Division of Hypertension, Department of Internal Medicine, University of Michigan Medical School, Ann Arbor, MI*

LENA KILANDER, MD, PhD • *Department of Public Health and Caring Sciences/ Geriatrics, Uppsala, Sweden*

LAWRENCE R. KRAKOFF, MD • *Chief of Medicine, Englewood Hospital and Medical Center, Englewood, NJ and Professor of Medicine, Mount Sinai School of Medicine, New York, NY*

ELLIS R. LEVIN, MD • *Professor of Medicine and Pharmacology, University of California, Irvine, and Chief, Endocrinology and Metabolism, Long Beach Veterans Affairs Medical Center, Long Beach, CA*

GEORGE A. MANSOOR, MD • *Assistant Professor of Medicine, Division of Hypertension and Clinical Pharmacology, Department of Medicine, University of Connecticut School of Medicine, Farmington, CT*

G. E. MCVEIGH, MD, PhD • *Department of Therapeutics and Pharmacology, The Queen's University of Belfast, Belfast, Northern Ireland*

FRANZ H. MESSERLI, MD • *Section on Hypertensive Diseases, Department of Internal Medicine, Ochsner Clinic and Alton Ochsner Medical Foundation, New Orleans, LA*

JOEL M. NEUTEL, MD • *Orange County Heart Institute and Research Center, Orange, CA*

SUZANNE OPARIL, MD • *Vascular Biology and Hypertension Program, Department of Medicine, University of Alabama at Birmingham, Birmingham, AL*

ROBERT A. PHILLIPS, MD, PhD, FACC • *Hypertension Section, Mount Sinai Medical Center, New York, NY*

THOMAS G. PICKERING, MD • *Cardiovascular Center, Department of Medicine, The New York Presbyterian Hospital–Cornell University Medical College, New York, NY*

JEROME G. PORUSH, MD • *Director of Nephrology, Nephrology Division, The Brookdale University Hospital and Medical Center, Brooklyn, NY*

L. MICHAEL PRISANT, MD, FACC, FACP • *Professor of Medicine, Hypertension Unit, Section of Cardiology, Medical College of Georgia, Augusta, GA*

C. VENKATA S. RAM, MD • *Texas Blood Pressure Institute, University of Texas Southwestern Medical Center, Dallas, TX*

IRA W. REISER, MD • *Nephrology Division, The Brookdale University Hospital and Medical Center, Brooklyn, NY*

DOMENIC A. SICA, MD • *Professor of Medicine and Pharmacology, Chairman, Clinical Pharmacology and Hypertension, and Director, University Ambulatory Research, Medical College of Virginia of Virginia Commonwealth University, Richmond, VA*

DAVID H. G. SMITH, MD • *Orange County Heart Institute and Research Center, Orange, CA*

DILEK K. SOWERS, MD, FACEP • *Bon Secours Emergency Department, Bon Secours Hospital, Grosse Pointe, MI*

JAMES R. SOWERS, MD • *Professor of Medicine and Physiology, and Chief, Endocrinology, Diabetes, and Hypertension, SUNY Health Science Center at Brooklyn, Brooklyn, NY*

KURT M. R. SOWERS, MD • *Division of Endocrinology, Diabetes, and Hypertension, SUNY Health Science Center at Brooklyn, Brooklyn, NY*

SAMUEL SPITALEWITZ, MD • *Brookdale University Hospital and Medical Center, Brooklyn, NY*

GORDON S. STOKES, MD, FRACP • *Hypertension Unit, Department of Cardiology, Royal North Shore Hospital, St. Leonards, New South Wales, Australia*

JOEL A. STROM, MD • *Director, Division of Cardiology, The Brookdale University Hospital and Medical Center, and Professor of Medicine, SUNY Health Science Center, Brooklyn, NY*

TUDOR VAGAONESCU, MD, PhD • *Hypertension Section, Mount Sinai Medical Center, New York, NY*

DONALD G. VIDT, MD • *Senior Physician, Department of Nephrology/Hypertension, Cleveland Clinic Foundation, Cleveland, OH and Professor of Internal Medicine, Ohio State University, Columbus, OH*

MICHAEL A. WEBER, MD • *State University of New York, Downstate Medical Center, Brooklyn, New York*

MYRON H. WEINBERGER, MD • *Director, Hypertension Research Center, Indiana University School of Medicine, Indianapolis, IN*

MATTHEW R. WEIR, MD • *Division of Nephrology and Clinical Research Unit, Department of Medicine, University of Maryland School of Medicine, Baltimore, MD*

WILLIAM B. WHITE, MD • *Chief, Division of Hypertension and Clinical Pharmacology, Department of Medicine, University of Connecticut School of Medicine, Farmington, CT*

LI LAN YOON, MD • *Department of Therapeutics and Pharmacology, The Queen's University of Belfast, Belfast, Northern Ireland*

I BACKGROUND ISSUES IN HYPERTENSION

1

Studies Justifying the Use of Treatment to Prevent Cardiovascular Events

Henry R. Black, MD

CONTENTS

We are now in the era of "evidence-based medicine." Although expert opinion and the results of nonrandomized trials and observational studies may provide guidance for us to make therapeutic decisions, it is generally agreed that the most reliable evidence is that obtained from large, prospective, well-controlled long-term clinical trials designed to evaluate clinical outcomes, not simply intermediate or surrogate end points. Fortunately, for those of us treating hypertension, such data are available and have been for decades *(1)*.

From: *Hypertension Medicine*
Edited by: M. A. Weber © Humana Press Inc., Totowa, NJ

Table 1-1
Trials Addressing Whether Treating Diastolic Hypertension in
Younger Persons Reduces Morbidity and Mortality

Study	Date published
Veterans Administration Cooperative Study	1967, 1970
United States Public Health Services Study (USPHS)	1977
Australian Therapeutic Trials in Mild Hypertension	1982
Medical Research Council Trial (MRC)	1985

Numerous clinical trials have been done to evaluate the value of treating hypertension *(1)*. Some of the published trials have addressed whether patients with high blood pressure (BP) should be treated *(2–6)*, some have looked at how aggressively they should be treated *(7,8)*, and others have asked what classes of drug or drugs we should use to treat our hypertensive patients *(9–13)*. Are there really important differences between classes of antihypertensives or is the only important thing that BP be lowered? Finally, many clinical trials in hypertension are in progress *(14–16)*. It is hoped that these studies will answer the many remaining questions. Pathophysiologic constructs are interesting but can be misleading. Epidemiologic analyses provide hypotheses for us to test. Only clinical trials done in people can confidently guide our treatment decisions and tell us how best to treat our patients.

WHETHER TO TREAT YOUNGER PERSONS
WITH DIASTOLIC HYPERTENSION

Table 1-1 lists the important trials that addressed the most basic question: Will reducing BP also reduce morbidity and mortality in hypertensives? The first of these trials, the Veterans Administration Cooperative Study (VA) trial, began in 1964. By 1967 in only 143 subjects and after only 18 mo of follow-up, this study showed a clear benefit of active treatment for those with diastolic blood pressure (DBP) between 115 and 129 mmHg *(2)*. Treatment with a combination of a diuretic, vasodilator, and sympatholytic (reserpine) dramatically reduced hypertension-related mortal and morbid events (27 vs 2, respectively) compared to treatment with a placebo. In 1970, after an average of approx 3.3 yr of observation, the VA study also demonstrated the benefit of treating hypertensive patients with an entry DBP of 90–114 mmHg *(3)*. Most of this benefit was evident in those with a DBP between 105 and 114 mmHg and in those with a comorbid condition and/or end organ damage, namely those with the highest absolute risk (17).

Over the next 15 yr, several other studies confirmed and extended those findings *(4–6)*. These included the United States Public Health Service Study *(4)* and the Australian Therapeutic Trial in Mild Hypertension *(5)*. In both, diuretics were the initial active therapy. In the Medical Research Council (MRC) trial, which enrolled 17,354 participants with a DBP between 95 and 109 mmHg, half of the volunteers were randomized to receive placebo and half to active therapy, of which 50% got a diuretic and 50% a β-blocker as initial treatment *(6)*. These studies, together with the VA trial, clearly showed that treating diastolic hypertension reduces strokes by approx 40%, but neither individually nor in the aggregate could they show a statistically significant reduction in myocardial infarction (MI) or coronary artery disease (CAD) events.

WHETHER TO TREAT OLDER PERSONS WITH HYPERTENSION

Although the benefit of treating younger hypertensive patients (≤69 yr) was proven by the mid-1980s, many still doubted whether there would be benefit in older persons, with diastolic, systolic and diastolic or isolated systolic hypertension. Although there were substantial numbers of participants over 60 yr in the VA Cooperative Study, in the Australian trial *(18)* and in the MRC study *(6)*, no one older than 69 yr at entry was eligible to participate.

In the 1980s and 1990s, the issue of whether to treat older persons was settled (Table 1-2). The first group of trials entered older subjects with diastolic hypertension. These included the European Working Party in the Elderly (EWPHE) published in 1985 *(19)*, then the Swedish Trial of Old Patients (STOP-Hypertension) in 1991 *(20)*, and finally the Medical Research Council—Elderly (MRC-E) Study published in 1992 *(21)*. The MRC-E trial also enrolled older persons with isolated systolic hypertension, who made up 43% of their cohort. These trials

Table 1-2
Trials Addressing Whether to Treat Older Persons with Hypertension

Study	Date published
European Working Party in the Elderly (EWPHE)	1985
Systolic Hypertension in the Elderly Program (SHEP)	1991
Swedish Trial of Old Patients (STOP-Hypertension)	1991
Medical Research Council Trial—Elderly (MRC-E)	1992
Systolic Hypertension in Europe (Syst-EUR)	1997

Table 1-3
Effects of Therapy in Older Patients with Hypertension
(% Relative Risk Reduction)[a]

	Australian trial	EWPHE	STOP-Hyper-tension	MRC	HDFP	SHEP	Syst-EUR
Stroke	33	36	47	25	44	33	42
CAD	18	20	13	19	15	27	26
CHF	NP	22	51	NP	NP	55	29
All CVD	31	29	40	17	16	32	31

[a]CHF, congestive heart failure; CVD, cardiovascular disease; NP, not provided.

clearly showed the benefit of treating older individuals with elevated DBP (≥90 mmHg). The benefit achieved was even greater than that seen in younger hypertensive patients (22). Table 1-3 shows that there is consistent reduction in stroke and CAD and heart failure, even though none of these studies used an angiotensin-converting enzyme (ACE) inhibitor.

EWPHE began treatment with a diuretic, and in both STOP and MRC-E, volunteers got either diuretics or β-blockers as initial therapy (19). The MRC-E trial, to the surprise of many, clearly demonstrated the superiority of diuretics compared to β-blockers, perhaps because diuretics were much more effective at reducing systolic blood pressure (SBP) (21). β-Blockers in the MRC-E trial were, in fact, no better than placebo. It is for this reason that the National High Blood Pressure Working Group on Hypertension in the Elderly (23) and the Sixth Joint National Committee on the Prevention, Detection, Evaluation and Treatment of High Blood Pressure (JNC VI) (24) did not recommend β-blockers as initial treatment for hypertension in older persons.

Table 1-4
Trials Addressing What Our Goal for Antihypertensive Therapy Should Be

Study	Date published
Hypertension Detection and Follow-up Program (HDFP)	1979
Hypertension Optimal Treatment (HOT)	1998
United Kingdom Prospective Diabetics Study (UKPDS)	1998

Two other studies, the Systolic Hypertension in the Elderly Program (SHEP) *(25)* and the Systolic Hypertension in Europe (Syst-EUR) *(26),* addressed the issue of whether treating older persons with isolated systolic hypertension (SBP ≥ 160 mmHg with DBP <90 mmHg in SHEP and <95 mmHg in Syst-EUR) would also confer benefit. SHEP, whose main results were published in 1991, began treatment with a low dose of chlorthalidone (12.5 mg), increasing it to 25 mg and then adding atenolol (25–50 mg) or reserpine (0.05–0.10 mg) if needed, to reach the BP goal. Syst-EUR, published in 1997, used different classes of agents to lower BP. The initial treatment was a moderately long-acting calcium antagonist (nitrendipine), followed by the ACE inhibitor enalapril, and, finally, the diuretic hydrochlorothiazide.

Both studies had similar results (Table 1-3) and unequivocally showed the value of treating older persons with isolated systolic hypertension. The benefit was evident within slightly more than 2 yr in Syst-EUR and by 4.5 yr in SHEP, meaning than an older individual with those BPs whose life expectancy is presumably at least that long would benefit from treatment and should receive therapy.

WHAT OUR GOAL SHOULD BE FOR
ANTIHYPERTENSIVE THERAPY

There have been two clinical trials in hypertension that have directly addressed the question of whether we would reduce hypertension-related morbidity and mortality by more aggressive compared with less aggressive antihypertensive therapy *(7,8)* (Table 1-4). The first of these was the Hypertension Detection and Follow-up Program (HDFP) *(7).* This trial was begun in 1972 in the United States and was completed in 1979. The investigators reflected the American, but not the European or Australian, view that it was not ethical after the VA trial was completed to do a placebo-controlled study in hypertensive patients with an elevated DBP. Therefore, HDFP compared the results of treating hypertensive patients to a goal (<90 mmHg if entry DBP was >100 mmHg or a 10 mmHg reduction if entry DBP was 90–99 mmHg) vs usual care. Rather than having a placebo as the control, HDFP compared a group called Stepped Care (SC) that was treated with active medication (a diuretic followed by methyldopa, hydralazine, and guanethidine, if needed), and treated to that goal, with a control group whose members were cared for by their primary physicians and treated however vigorously their physicians deemed necessary, the so-called referred care (RC) group. The SC group really should have been called Special Care because these individuals were seen very frequently and received care and surveillance for many problems other than hypertension. The RC group should have been called Routine Care because these individuals were seen only at the HDFP clinical centers twice in the 5 yr and were otherwise treated per their physicians' routine. The participants in RC actually received similar medication but fewer were treated and those who received treatment were certainly less aggressively managed. At the end of the trial, the participants in the SC group had their DBP lowered to an average of 83 mmHg compared with an average of 89 mmHg in the RC group. All-cause mortality, the primary end point in HDFP, as well as cardiovascular mortality were both statistically significantly reduced in the SC vs RC group. The benefit was seen in all demographic groups except for white women, whose absolute risk was very low. HDFP did not enroll enough white women to be able to show benefit in these relatively low-risk individuals.

The second study looking at the DBP goal of therapy was the Hypertension Optimal Treatment (HOT) study, completed in 1998 (8). HOT was specifically designed to determine whether hypertensive patients ages 50–80 with elevated DBP (100–115 mmHg at baseline) would do better if DBP was lowered to <80 mmHg, vs <85 vs <90 mmHg. HOT was done in a Prospective Randomized Open Label Blinded Evaluation design. In such trials, the drug administered is known to investigators and participants but all end points are evaluated by a committee blinded to the drug actually used or, in this case, the BP goal. All subjects received a dihydropyridine calcium antagonist started at a low dose (5 mg of felodipine) followed by either an ACE inhibitor or β-blocker at low dose, if more therapy was needed to achieve the predetermined goal. The investigator decided which class of drug to add. If the goal was still not reached, further increases in the dose of felodipine to 10 mg (step 3) and then increased doses of the second drug were mandated (step 4). Finally, a diuretic or other therapy was added (step 5) to achieve the study goal. The cohort enrolled was very large (nearly 19,000) and the follow-up was planned to be approx 2–2.5 yr (40,000 participant-yr). The study was extended to an average follow-up of 3.7 yr (71,000 participant yr) when the event rate in all groups was substantially less than predicted. These participants were practically immortal.

The main result in HOT was disappointing to some because there was no difference in the rates of study end points between these groups. The optimal BP was calculated to be 138/83 mmHg, a strikingly similar finding to that of the HDFP. There was no evidence of an on-treatment DBP under which the event rate rose (i.e., there was no J-point ascertained). In the 1501 subjects with type 2 diabetes, there was a highly statistically significant trend ($p < 0.001$) for reduced cardiovascular (CV) events when DBP was lowered to <80 mmHg. This finding supports the concept that the lower the achieved DBP the better, especially in those with a high absolute risk for events.

In my view, HOT should not be viewed as a failed study. More than 90% of the cohort, primarily recruited from private practices in 26 countries, had their DBP reduced to <90 mmHg and were able to maintain that level for several years. In fact, more than 50% of those randomized to be treated to a DBP of <80 mmHg achieved this very aggressive goal. The treatment used was conventional and simple to implement. Ordinary doctors treating ordinary patients with ordinary medicines achieved the study BP goals and did so without causing harm. To accomplish this level of success, combination therapy was usually necessary. Only about one third of those who were to be treated to <90 mmHg got to that level with a single agent, and only 26% treated to <80 mmHg reached it with monotherapy. HOT taught us that practitioners can achieve very aggressive goals, but it often takes multiple drugs to reach those goals. Doctors given goals can achieve them. Although HOT did not clearly discover a DBP level that was too low, it did show that the subjects treated aggressively did not have more adverse reactions. If anything, the group randomized to and treated to <80 mmHg had an improvement in quality of life and cognitive function, especially when compared with those that were resistant to therapy (27).

A more recently published trial, the United Kingdom Prospective Diabetes Study (UKPDS) (28), confirmed the substantial benefit of more aggressive compared with less aggressive antihypertensive therapy in type 2 diabetics. In UKPDS, the goal and achieved BP in the control group were both much higher than in HOT, but the same level of comparative benefit was achieved.

WHICH DRUGS OR DRUG REGIMEN TO USE TO TREAT HYPERTENSION

Because the value of treating hypertension is no longer in question, the most important remaining issue is how to do it. Although lifestyle modification can be effective in some hypertensive patients, no clinical trial data exist that have shown that a nonpharmacologic regimen will reduce morbidity and mortality (29,30). Lifestyle modification, especially weight loss and sodium restriction, will reduce BP modestly in many patients in the short term (31). Few studies have shown that even those who can adhere to a diet and achieve BP reduction will maintain that benefit for more than 18–24 mo. In fact, in the only clinical trial that ever compared morbidity and mortality in those treated with lifestyle modifications alone vs those treated with lifestyle modification and pharmacologic agents—the Treatment of Mild Hypertension Study (TOMHS)—showed that the combination of drugs and lifestyle regimen reduced events statistically significantly better than successful lifestyle modification alone (12). Nonetheless, weight loss, physical activity, moderation of alcohol and salt intake, and attempts to reduce and cope with stress should all be strongly and unambiguously recommended to hypertensive patients (24). The clinician and the patient, however, should know that for the overwhelming majority of those treated to lower BP and prevent cardiovascular events, pharmacologic agents will be required.

The majority of the clinical trials done recently have addressed the issue of which drugs to use (9–13,20,21,28) (Table 1-5). For the most part, these studies have focused on which drug to begin therapy, ignoring, perhaps, the fact that most hypertensives will require more than one agent to reach a patient's goal.

The first major studies that compared initial therapy addressed whether regimens beginning with diuretics were as good as those beginning with β-blockers (6,9,10,21). With the exception of older hypertensive patients, in whom diuretics are clearly superior (21), there is no evidence that either class of agents prevents cardiovascular events better than the other (13).

Table 1-5
Trials Addressing Which Drug or Drug Regimen to
Use to Treat Hypertension

Study	Date published
Medical Research Council (MRC)	1985
International Prospective Primary Prevention Study in Hypertension (IPPPSH)	1985
Heart Attack Primary Prevention in Hypertension Trial (HAPPHY)	1987
Medical Research Council—Elderly (MRC-E)	1992
Treatment of Mild Hypertension Study (TOMHS)	1993
VA Cooperative Study of Monotherapy	1993

Unfortunately, there are still no definitive comparative studies of either the older class of antihypertensives appropriate for monotherapy (diuretics and β-blockers) compared to the newer classes (calcium antagonists, ACE inhibitors, α-blockers, α/β-blockers or angiotensin receptor blockers) or of the newer classes to each other. Only the TOMHS and Veterans Administration Study of Monotherapy have attempted to do this, and neither trial was large enough to be able to define differences in event reduction or even differences in antihypertensive efficacy except in some subgroups (11,12). For example, older (≥60 yr) African American men had greater BP reduction with diuretics and calcium antagonists than with other classes of drugs in the Veterans Administration Study of Monotherapy. This differential BP response, however, was not evident in whites or African American men under 60 yr. Small and occasionally statistically but not clinically significant differences in clinical or metabolic adverse reactions were noted, but these differences were not important enough to provide the solid evidence necessary to make firm therapeutic recommendations (32–34). There is no difference in the benefits achieved in men and women, especially in older persons or those at risk (35).

WHICH DRUGS TO USE IN SUBGROUPS OF HYPERTENSIVE PATIENTS

Although clinical trials done specifically in hypertensive patients were unable to allow us to make broad evidence-based recommendations, other trials were quite helpful in delineating special subgroups

Table 1-6
Trials Addressing Which Drugs to Use in Subgroups
of Hypertensive Patients

Study	Date published
β-Blocker Heart Attack Trial (BHAT)	1982
Studies of Left Ventricular Dysfunction (SOLVD)	1992
Survival and Ventricular Enlargement (SAVE)	1992
Captopril Study in Type 1 Diabetics	1993

of hypertensive patients for whom certain classes of agents would be preferred or even the drugs of choices *(36–39)*. The data on which such recommendations are based came from clinical trials that were not planned to be studies of drug treatment in hypertensive patients but came rather from studies done in subgroups of patients with complications or risk factors commonly encountered in hypertensive patients and in which the drugs employed are also used to reduce BP (Table 1-6). For example, ACE inhibitors should be part of the regimen for hypertensive type 1 diabetics with proteinuria *(36)*. β-Blockers should be given after MI *(37)*. Diuretics and ACE inhibitors and possibly β-blockers should be given to hypertensive patients with heart failure *(38)*. Hypertensive patients who survive an anterior wall MI and have a reduced ejection fraction should have an ACE inhibitor included in the regimen *(38)*. These recommendations can be made with assurance because clinical trials (the Captopril Diabetes Study *(36)*, β-Blocker Heart Attack Trial *(37)*, Survival and Ventricular Enlargement *(38)*, Studies of Left Ventricular Dysfunction *(39)*, and many others) demonstrated that those agents reduced events. These studies were the basis of the "compelling indications" recommendations by JNC VI to use these classes of drugs in those subgroups of hypertension *(24)*.

There are also many other clinical situations in which the choice of antihypertensive therapy should be selected or avoided because of a comorbid condition or risk factor present in a particular patient *(24)* (Table 1-7). In these situations, there either has not been or more likely never will be a clinical trial that provides the level of evidence some clinicians require. Any reasonable clinician, however, would likely treat such an individual according to the suggestions made by JNC VI. The presence of benign prostatic hypertrophy in a hypertensive patient who needs drug therapy, e.g., would be a good reason to include an α-blocker in the regimen, because this class of drugs improves symptoms in men with this problem. Even if diuretics are the drugs of choice

Table 1-7
Considerations for Individual Antihypertensive Drug Therapy[a]

Indication	Drug Therapy
Compelling Indications Unless Contraindicated	
Diabetes mellitus (type 1) with proteinuria	ACE I
Heart failure	ACE I, diuretics
Isolated systolic hypertension (older patients)	Diuretics (preferred), CA (long-acting DHP)
Myocardial infarction	β-Blockers (non-ISA), ACE I (with systolic dysfunction)
May Have Favorable Effects on Comorbid Conditions	
Angina	β-Blockers, CA
Atrial tachycardia and fibillation	β-Blockers, CA (non-DHP)
Cyclosporine-induced hypertension (caution with the dose of cyclosporine)	CA
Diabetes mellitus (types 1 and 2) with proteinuria	ACE I (preferred), CA
Diabetes mellitus (type 2)	Low-dose diuretics
Dyslipidemia	α-Blockers
Essential tremor	β-Blockers (non-CS)
Heart failure	Carvedilol, losartan
Hyperthyroidism	β-Blockers
Migraine	β-Blockers (non-CS), CA (non-DHP)
Myocardial infarction	Diltiazem, verapamil
Osteoporosis	Thiazides
Preoperative hypertension	β-Blockers
Prostatism (BPH)	α-Blockers
Renal insufficiency (caution in renovascular hypertension and creatinine >3 mg/dL)	ACE I
May Have Unfavorable Effects on Comorbid Conditions	
Bronchospastic disease	β-Blockers
Depression	β-Blockers, central α-agonists, reserpine
Diabetes mellitus (types 1 and 2)	β-Blockers, high-dose diuretics
Dyslipidemia	β-Blockers (non-ISA), diuretics (high-dose)
Gout	Diuretics

Continued

Table 1-7 *Continued*

Indication	Drug Therapy
May Have Unfavorable Effects on Comorbid Conditions	
2° or 3° heart block	β-Blockers, CA (non-DHP)
Heart failure	β-Blockers (except carvedilol), CA (except amlodipine, felodipine)
Liver disease	Labetalol, methyldopa
Peripheral vascular disease	β-Blockers
Pregnancy	ACE I, angiotensin II receptor blockers
Renal insufficiency	Potassium-sparing agents
Renovascular disease	ACE I, angiotensin II receptor blockers

*a*Modified from ref. 24. ACE I, angiotensin-converting enzyme inhibitors; BPH, benign prostatic hyperplasia; CA, calcium antagonists; DHP, dihydropyridine; ISA, intrin sympathomimetic activity; MI, myocardial infarction; and non-CS, noncardioselective.

in older persons, elderly hypertensive patients with gout should almost surely be treated with some other class of agents.

Sometimes comorbid conditions may influence the choice of initial therapy, based not on the likelihood of improvement in symptoms or worsening of a comorbid condition, but because of other clinical factors. Diuretics, e.g., will increase bone mass and may prevent osteoporotic fractures *(40)*. Thus, diuretics would be a good choice in a hypertensive patient who has or was at risk of having osteoporosis.

The issue in two particularly important subgroups, the elderly and type 2 diabetes, is less clear. Although β-blockers and diuretics may have adverse metabolic effects (raising triglycerides, lowering high-density lipoprotein cholesterol and worsening glucose tolerance), *(32–34)* the SHEP study *(41)* demonstrated clear benefit in the subgroup with type 2 diabetes. In Syst-EUR, in which the regimen began with a dihydropyridine followed by an ACE inhibitor and a diuretic, the subgroup with type 2 diabetes also did particularly well. Perhaps the key point is that both of these studies show the clear benefit of lowering BP in hypertensive patients with a high absolute risk. In 1994, the National High Blood Pressure Working Group on Diabetes included ACE inhibitors, α-blockers, α/β-blockers, calcium antagonists, and diuretics all as appropriate choices for initial therapy in diabetes *(42)*. Now the group would probably add angiotensin receptor blockers to that list.

In the elderly the choice is also complex. As discussed, diuretics are clearly better than β-blockers but data from Syst-EUR *(26)* clearly

Table 1-8
Some Clinical Trials Currently in Progress

Study	Date due to be completed
Rationale and Design for the Antihypertensive and Lipid Lowering Treatment to Prevent Heart Attack Trial (ALLHAT)	2002
Rationale and Design for the Controlled Onset Verapamil Investigation of Cardiovascular Endpoints (CONVINCE) Trial	2002
Valsartan Antihypertensive Long-Term Use Evaluation (VALUE)	2003

showed the benefits of treatment with a moderately long-acting dihydro-pyridine as well. Here, too, in this other high-risk group, effective lowering of BP is perhaps more important than exactly how it is done.

WHAT CLINICAL TRIALS CURRENTLY IN PROGRESS WILL TELL US

More than 30 large randomized clinical trials in hypertension are currently in progress *(14)* (Table 1-8). The largest (42,500 have been recruited), the Antihypertensive Lipid Lowering Trial to Prevent Heart Attack (ALLHAT), is comparing an ACE inhibitor, an α-blocker, and a dihydropyridine calcium antagonist to a diuretic in hypertensive patients over age 55 who have another cardiovascular risk factor or target organ damage *(15)*. MI is the primary end point. This study, which has more than 15,000 type 2 diabetics, will tell us whether any of these classes of agents should be preferentially used in that subgroup. The Controlled Onset Cardiovascular Verapamil Trial of Cardiovascular Endpoints will compare older drugs (diuretics and β-blockers) to a nondihydropyridine calcium antagonist (verapamil as Covera HS), a preparation designed to be released in a similar fashion to the chronobiology of BP and heart rate *(16)*.

A number of studies will look at hypertensive diabetes with protein-uria, other studies will enroll hypertensive patients with life ventricular hypertrophy, and some studies are assessing the value of combined antihypertensive and lipid lowering therapy (ALLHAT and others) and/ or other therapies (folic acid and vitamin E) to prevent cardiovascular events in hypertensives *(14)*. Finally, a study is currently being planned to determine whether treating older hypertensive patients with stage 1 systolic hypertension (SBP 140–159/<90 mmHg) will reduce morbidity and mortality as was proven for stage 2 to 3 isolated systolic hypertension (>160 mmHg/<90 mmHg), in SHEP and Syst-Eur.

CONCLUSION

In the more than three decades since the completion of the first clinical trial in hypertension, the VA trial, the value of treating hypertension is now solidly based on hard and unassailable evidence. Although these trials may not truly mimic what the practitioner deals with on a daily basis, practitioners treating patients with high BP can be reasonably certain that much of what they are doing is evidence based, if they apply the lessons we have learned from clinical trials:

1. Rely on lifestyle modification to lower BP modestly and make hypertension patients more responsive to treatment but not necessarily to prevent morbidity and mortality.
2. Begin treatment in hypertensive adults under the age of 60 with diuretics or β-blockers unless they have a comorbid condition or another clinical feature, which alters that choice.
3. Begin treatment in older hypertensive patients with either diuretics or a dihydropyridine calcium antagonist, especially if they have stage 2 to 3 isolated systolic hypertension.
4. Plan to treat to a DBP of <85 mmHg and even lower (<80 mmHg) in diabetics. The goal for SBP is probably <140 mmHg in nondiabetics and <130 mmHg in diabetics.
5. Plan to need more than one drug for the majority of hypertensive patients and inform them that this may be the case.
6. Keep informed of the results of the many trials in progress and be willing to change practice if the data are compelling. If they are not, stay with what is known to be effective.

REFERENCES

1. Gueyffier F, Froment A, Gouton M (1996) New meta-analysis of treatment trials of hypertension: improving the estimate of therapeutic benefit. *J Hum Hypertens* 10:1–8.
2. Veterans Administration Cooperative Study Group on Antihypertensive Agents (1969) Effects of treatment on morbidity in hypertension: results in patients with

diastolic blood pressures averaging 115 through 129 mm Hg. *JAMA* 202:1028–1034.

3. Veterans Administration Cooperative Study Group on Antihypertensive Agents (1970) Effects of treatment on morbidity in hypertension. II. Results in patients with diastolic blood pressure averaging 90 through 114 mm Hg. *JAMA* 213:1143.

4. U.S. Public Health Service Hospitals Cooperative Study Group, Smith WM (1977) Treatment of mild hypertension: results of a ten-year intervention trial. *Circ Res* 40(Suppl 1):98–105.

5. Management Committee of the Australian Therapeutic Trial in Mild Hypertension (1982) Untreated mild hypertension. *Lancet* 185–191.

6. Medical Research Council Working Party on Mild Hypertension (1985) MRC trial of treatment of mild hypertension: principle results. *Br Med J* 201:97–104.

7. Hypertension Detection and Follow-up Program Cooperative Group (1979) Five-year findings of the Hypertension Detection and Follow-up Program. *JAMA* 242:2561–2571.

8. Hansson L, Zanchetti A, Carruthers SG, et al. (1998) Effects of intensive blood-pressure lowering and low-dose aspirin in patients with hypertension: principal results of the Hypertension Optimal Treatment (HOT) randomized trial. *Lancet* 351:1755–1762.

9. Wilhelmsen L, Berglund G, Elmfeldt D, et al. (1987) β-Blockers versus diuretics in hypertensive men: main results of the HAPPHY trial. *J Hypertens* 5:561–572.

10. The IPPPSH Collaborative Group (1985) Cardiovascular risk and risk factors in a randomized trial of treatment based on the β-blocker oxprenolol: the International Prospective Study Primary Prevention Study in Hypertension (IPPPSH). *J Hypertens* 3:379–392.

11. Materson BJ, Reda DJ, Cushman WC, et al., for the Department of Veterans Affairs Cooperative Study Group on Antihypertensive Agents (1993) Single-drug therapy for hypertension in men: a comparison of six antihypertensive agents with placebo. *N Engl J Med* 328:914–921.

12. Neaton JD, Grimm RH Jr, Prineas RJ, et al., for the Treatment of Mild Hypertension Study Research Group (1993) Treatment of Mild Hypertension Study: final results. *JAMA* 270:713–724.

13. Psaty BM, Smith NL, Siscovick DS, et al. (1997) Health outcomes associated with antihypertensive therapies used as first-line agents: a systematic review and meta-analysis. *JAMA* 277:739–745.

14. World Health Organization—International Society of Hypertension Blood Pressure Lowering Treatment Trialists' Collaboration (1998) Protocol for prospective collaborative overviews of major randomized trials of blood-pressure-lowering treatments. *J Hypertens* 16:127–137.

15. Davis BR, Cutler JA, Gordon DJ, et al. (1996) Rationale and design for the Antihypertensive and Lipid Lowering Treatment to Prevent Heart Attack Trial (ALLHAT). *Am J Hypertens* 9:342–360.

16. Black HR, Elliott WJ, Neaton JD, et al. (1998) Rationale and design for the Controlled Onset Verapamil Investigation of Cardiovascular Endpoints (CONVINCE) Trial. *Contr Clin Trials* 19:370–390.

17. Veterans Administration Cooperative Study Group on Antihypertensive Agents (1972) Effects of Treatment on Morbidity in Hypertension. III. Influence of age, diastolic pressure, and prior cardiovascular disease; further analysis of side effects. XLV:991–1004.

18. Management Committee (1981) Treatment of mild hypertension in the elderly. *Med J Aust* 2:398–402.

19. Amery A, Birkenhäger WH, Brixko P, Bulpitt C, Clement D, Deruyttere M, De Schaepdryver A, Dollery C, Fagard R, Forette F, Forte J, Hamdy R, Henry JF, Joossens JV, Leonetti G, Lund-Johansen P, O'Malley K, Petrie J, Strasser T, Tuomilehto J, Williams B (1985) Mortality and morbidity results from the European Working Party on High Blood Pressure in the Elderly trial. *Lancet* 1:1349–1354.

20. Dahlöf B, Lindholm LH, Hansson L, Scherstén B, Ekbom T, Wester PO (1991) Morbidity and mortality in the Swedish Trial in Old Patients with Hypertension (STOP-Hypertension). *Lancet* 338:1281–1285.

21. MRC Working Party (1992) Medical Research Council trial of treatment of hypertension in older adults: principal results. *Br Med J* 304:405–412.

22. Lever AF, Ramsay LE (1995) Treatment of hypertension in the elderly. *J Hypertens* 13:571–579.

23. National High Blood Pressure Education Program Working Group (1994) National High Blood Pressure Education Program working group report on hypertension in the elderly. *Hypertens* 23:275–285.

24. The Sixth Report of the Joint National Committee on Prevention, Detection, Evaluation, and Treatment of High Blood Pressure (1997) *Arch Intern Med* 158:2413–2446.

25. SHEP Cooperative Research Group (1991) Prevention of stroke by antihypertensive drug treatment in older persons with isolated systolic hypertension: final results of the Systolic Hypertension in the Elderly Program (SHEP). *JAMA* 265:3255–3264.

26. Staessen JA, Fagard R, Thijs L, et al., for the Systolic Hypertension—Europe (Syst-Eur) Trial Investigators (1997) Morbidity and mortality in the placebo-controlled European Trial on Isolated Systolic Hypertension in the Elderly. *Lancet* 350:757–764.

27. Wiklund I, Halling K, Ryden-Bergsten T, et al. (1997) Does lowering the blood pressure improve the mood? Quality-of-life results from the Hypertension Optimal Treatment (HOT) Study. *Blood Pressure* 6:357–364.

28. UK Prospective Diabetes Study Group (1998) Tight blood pressure control and risk of macrovascular and microvascular complications in type 2 diabetes: UKPDS 38. *Br Med J* 317:703–713.

29. Trials of Hypertension Prevention Collaborative Research Group (1997) Effects of weight loss and sodium reduction intervention on blood pressure and hypertension incidence in overweight people with high-normal blood pressure: the Trials of Hypertension Prevention phase II. *Arch Intern Med* 157:657–667.

30. Appel LJ, Moore TJ, Obarzanek E, et al., for the DASH Collaborative Research Group (1997) A clinical trial of the effects of dietary patterns on blood pressure. *N Engl J Med* 336:1117–1124.

31. Cutler JA, Follmann D, Allender PS (1997) Randomized trials of sodium reduction: an overview. *Am J Clin Nutr* 65 (Suppl):643S–651S.

32. Black HR (1991) Metabolic considerations in the choice of therapy for the hypertensive patient. *Am Heart J* 121:707–715.

33. Kasiske BL, Ma JZ, Kalil RSN, Louis TA (1995) Effects of antihypertensive therapy on serum lipids. *Ann Intern Med* 122:133–141.

34. Lind L, Pollare T, Berne C, Lithell H (1994) Long-term metabolic effects of antihypertensive drugs. *Am Heart J* 128:1177–1183.

35. Guyiffer F, Boutitie F, Boissel JP, et al. for the INDANA Investigators (1997) Effect of antihypertensive drug treatment on cardiovascular outcomes in women and men: a meta-analysis of individual patient data from randomized, controlled trials. *Ann Intern Med* 126:761–767.

36. Lewis EJ, Hunsicker LG, Bain RP, Rohde RD, for the Collaborative Study Group (1993) The effect of angiotensin-converting-enzyme inhibition on diabetic nephropathy. *N Engl J Med* 329:1456–1462.

37. β-Blocker Heart Attack Research Group (1982) A randomized trial of propranolol in patients with acute myocardial infarction: mortality results. *JAMA* 247:1707–1714.

38. SOLVD Investigators (1991) Effect of enalapril on survival in patients with reduced left ventricular ejection fractions and congestive heart failure. *N Engl J Med* 325:293–302.

39. Pfeffer MA, Braunwald E, Moyé LA, et al., for the SAVE Investigators (1992) Effect of captopril on mortality and morbidity in patients with left ventricular dysfunction after myocardial infarction: results of the Survival and Ventricular Enlargement Trials. *N Engl J Med* 327:669–677.

40. Morton DJ, Barrett-Connor EL, Edelstein SL (1994) Thiazides and bone mineral density in elderly men and women. *A J Epi* 139(11):1107–1115.

41. Curb JD, Pressel SL, Cutler JA, et al., for the Systolic Hypertension in the Elderly Program Cooperative Research Group (1996) Effect of diuretic-based antihypertensive treatment on cardiovascular disease risk in older diabetic patients with isolated systolic hypertension. *JAMA* 276:1886–1892.

42. National High Blood Pressure Education Program Working Group (1994) National High Blood Pressure Education Program working group report on hyper-tension in diabetes. *Hypertension* 23:145–158.

2

Effects of Aging on Blood Pressure

Vincent DeQuattro, MD

High blood pressure (BP) (hypertension) is the leading cause of death by way of the cardiovascular consequences of heart attack and stroke. High BP is related in part to aging, especially in our industrial civilization. In certain "unacculturated" societies (such as that of the Yanamamo Indians) BP does not rise with age. People of this South American tribe are short-lived in general, and the lack of effects of aging on their BP may be related in part to their agrarian lifestyle and also the high potassium and low sodium diet of the hunter-gatherer.

DEMOGRAPHY

In the United States, the prevalence of patients with high BP increases every year, since half of the people over age 65 have hypertension *(1)*.

From: *Hypertension Medicine*
Edited by: M. A. Weber © Humana Press Inc., Totowa, NJ

Currently, 12–15% of the adult population is in the age >65 yr group, and 20% is ages 45–64 yr. The median age is at its highest point since the U.S. census began to track it more than 160 yr ago. One American in 8.7 is over age 65. There are more Americans older than 65 than there are ones younger than 25. By the year 2030, the age >65 yr group will double in number to one in four, or 65 million Americans. By the year 2040, 20% of the population will be over age 65, and another 20% will be in the age 45–64 group *(2)*. Therefore, as the average age increases, and if the relationship of age with high BP continues, an increasing proportion of Americans will have hypertension. How important is this?

Hypertension contributes to the leading costs in health care. Currently, an American physician devotes 40% of his or her hospital time to adults above age 65. Ninety-seven percent of older adults use more than one drug per day, and 30% use more than five drugs per day. Hospitalized older adults receive an average of 10 different drugs. The expenses of senior care will consume 75% of the total health care dollar by the year 2030. Can the aging vascular disease relationship be altered?

The Framingham Study identified aging and high BP as the predominant risk factors for coronary heart disease. Although the hypertensive patient at age 30 has a very low risk of having a cardiovascular event, by age 65 his or her risk for stroke or heart attack will have increased fourfold over that of a person with normal BP. BP increases with age for both African Americans and Caucasians. Using the figure of 160/95 mmHg, the prevalence of hypertension over age 65 is 60% among African Americans and 44% among Caucasians. For 140/90 mmHg, 75% of African American patients and 60% of Caucasian patients have elevated BP.

SYSTOLIC HYPERTENSION

The prevalence of isolated systolic hypertension (>160 mmHg) increases with aging with 5% in the age 60–69 group, 10% in the age 70–79 group, and 16% in the age >80 group. The magnitude of systolic blood pressure (SBP) correlates even more closely with stroke, heart failure, coronary heart disease, left ventricular mass, and renal failure compared to diastolic blood pressure. Hypertension surpasses cigarette smoking, obesity, or family history and rivals cholesterol and diabetes as a risk factor for cardiovascular disease in the aging population. What are the changes associated with aging that lead to higher BP and increased cardiovascular risk?

False BP elevation is associated with aging as well. The so-called Osler maneuver is an evaluation of the peripheral pulse, which assists the physician in determining whether the resistance of the blood vessel walls is elevated compared to the pressure within the vessel. This resistance is related to the structural changes in the vessel wall with age. This maneuver palpates the radial pulse while the cuff occludes the artery in the upper arm. If the artery can be felt, it is said to be a positive test.

ALTERED CARDIOVASCULAR FUNCTIONS WITH AGE: CAUSES OF HYPERTENSION

Cardiovascular functions that change with aging, increased peripheral vascular resistance and arterial rigidity, are in concert with reduced cardiac output, cardiac and stroke index, baroreceptor sensitivity, and β-adrenoreceptor sensitivity *(3)*. Aging often affects renal function adversely and may lead to reductions in glomerular filtration rate, renal blood flow, and plasma renin activity, and these combined with increased plasma volume contribute to the rise in BP *(4)*. With aging there may be reductions in brain metabolism, nerve conduction velocity, basal metabolic rate, vital capacity, and maximal breathing capacity, which serve to raise BP. The effects of aging on the kidney are reductions in renal mass and renal tubular and arteriolar intimal function leading to elevated BP, along with increased glomerular sclerosis. Amazingly, perhaps, approximately one third of older patients have no loss of renal blood flow, renal mass, or creatinine clearance, whereas for most, there is a 30–50% reduction in renal cortical mass, blood flow, creatinine and free water clearance, and a heightened tendency to conserve sodium. Other physiologic changes occurring with aging have effects on BP regulation; the normal drop in BP after meals *(5)* (related in part to a shifting of blood flow to the splanchnic circulation) is more pronounced in the older patient. This may be related to baroreceptor hyporesponsiveness in some patients. Therefore, drugs taken at mealtime may result in more BP reduction than at other times because of the added orthostatic effects of eating.

Every year hypertension via aging leads to end-stage renal disease and enormous monetary costs, as well as suffering. In the 1990s, $2.8 billion was spent on the treatment of renal disease per year. Hypertension-induced nephrosclerosis accounts for 25% of end-stage renal disease in the United States, and African Americans are proportionately at a higher risk of 4:1. What are some other pathologic alterations in the aging person that result in higher BP?

ALTERED ARTERIAL COMPLIANCE OF AGING: GENESIS

Along with the age-related reductions already discussed are several that reduce arterial compliance and enhance responsiveness to sympathetic neural stimuli (6,7). There is a tendency toward expanded plasma volume, although renovascular resistance is higher and renal blood flow is reduced. Simultaneously this results in lower plasma renin levels and cardiac output related to the increased vascular resistance. The aging process compromises sympathetic neural function; β-receptors are downregulated, and reflexively, perhaps, higher levels of α-mediated neural tone (8) increase peripheral vascular resistance and raise pulse pressure.

The compliance (the elastic recoil) of the great vessels is reduced with age and, in part, is a result of the elevated BP. Neurohumoral imbalance affects both the smooth muscle of the blood vessel and the impaired endothelium, and increased collagen is laid down replacing elastin. Along with increased apoptosis and cell death, the result is reduced arterial compliance. A surfeit of angiotensin II synthesis explains, in part, raised norepinephrine and endothelin release and concomitantly reduced release of prostacyclin and nitric oxide. Because of the drop in compliance, the reflected wave is heightened, the change in pressure after the initial peak or shoulder is enhanced, and systolic pressure rises and diastolic pressure lowers. The resultant heightened "pulse pressure" is predictive of both functional capacity of the patient in terms of the arterial blood flow reserve for exercising limb muscles and future cardiovascular morbid events (9).

ADDITIONAL MEDICAL CONCERNS IN SENIOR HYPERTENSIVE PATIENTS

Unfortunately, with aging there are concurrent ailments such as degenerative joint disease, diabetes mellitus, congestive heart failure, angina, and cerebrovascular disease, which further complicate the hypertensive process and its therapy in the aging patient. Atherosclerotic obstruction of the renal vessels may superimpose renovascular hypertension in the aging person. Therefore, it is necessary to examine the senior patient carefully for renal and carotid bruits, and other vascular changes. The risks of cardiovascular complications—fatal and nonfatal coronary vascular events, strokes, renal disease, left ventricular hypertrophy, diminished cardiac output and arterial compliance, and increased peripheral vascular resistance—are all related to the rise in BP with aging. Thus, the prevalence of coronary heart diseases increases with age: of hypertensive patients >60 yr 44% have coronary artery disease, compared with 31% for those <40 yr. Concomitantly, the incidence of insulin resistance and type II diabetes increases with age. Some standard antihypertensives may interfere with the management of the diabetic patient. Thiazide diuretics and β-receptor blockers may affect glucose tolerance adversely, and β-blockers may mask the symptoms of hypoglycemia after insulin therapy.

THERAPEUTIC CONCERNS IN SENIOR HYPERTENSIVE PATIENTS

There are several important considerations in the pharmacokinetics of therapy in hypertensive seniors; drug clearance and thus half-life are prolonged. Drug absorption is generally unchanged, but distribution is altered secondarily to reduced body water and lean body mass, as well as to increased body fat. Hepatic elimination is reduced as liver mass declines, and thus so does metabolic clearance. Hepatic blood flow declines 40–45% by age 65, and liver microsomal enzyme activity is reduced.

β-Receptor blocker therapy may not be as effective as using diuretic or the low-dose combination of the two in the older hypertensive patient, perhaps owing to lower patient compliance because of real or imagined side effects. A minority of studies suggest that there is a reduction in the efficacy of angiotensin-converting enzyme inhibitor on BP control in the older patient, and others suggest that the calcium channel blockers are more effective in the older patient, especially those with low renin activity. Atenolol was not as effective as the calcium channel blocker verapamil in reducing both BP and left ventricular mass in a study of elderly patients with high BP.

Evidence from "outcome" trials of more than 20,000 elderly hypertensive patients demonstrated the benefits of BP control (10). The myth of "100 plus year age" as a marker for an acceptable SBP has been replaced by "less than 140 less than 90." These studies demonstrated that BP reductions of 12 mmHg systolic and 4–6 mmHg diastolic in seniors are associated with reductions of coronary mortality of 25% and stroke mortality of 45% *(10,11)*. Thus, the relationship of aging to BP is a two-way street: rising BP may be fatal for the senior, and lowering it is potentially life saving. Patients should have BP lowered to the range of 130–140 systolic, and to 80–90 diastolic. In diabetic patients, the goal should be <85 diastolic, and <130 systolic *(12)*. Although BP rises with age, antihypertensive therapy has been shown to reduce morbidity and mortality significantly in patients older than age 80 as well as those younger than age 80. Current trends in treating hypertensive seniors breathe optimism. Fortunately, the proportion of hypertensive patients on therapy is increasing with age, with 47% on therapy in the age 65–74 group, compared with 41% in the age 55–64 group.

REFERENCES

1. Tjoa HI, Kaplan NM (1990) Treatment of hypertension in the elderly. *JAMA* 264:1015–1018.
2. Burt VL, Whelton P, Roccella EJ, et al. (1995) Prevalence of hypertension in the US adult population: results from the Third National Health and Nutrition Examination Survey 1988–1991. *Hypertension* 25:305–313.
3. Wei JY (1992) Age and the cardiovascular system. *N Engl J Med* 327(24):1735–1739.
4. Frocht A, Fillit H (1984) *Am J Geriatr Soc* 32:28–43.
5. Vaitkevicius PV, Esserwein DM, Maynard AK, et al. (1991) Frequency and importance of postprandial blood pressure reduction in elderly nursing-home patients. *Ann Intern Med* 115(11):865–870.
6. Lakka TA, Salonen R, Kaplan GA, Salonen JT (1999) Blood pressure and the progression of carotid atherosclerosis in middle-aged men. *Hypertension* 34:51–56.
7. Ishikawa K, Ohta T, Zhang J, et al. (1999) Influence of age and gender on exercise training-induced blood pressure reduction in systemic hypertension. *Am J Cardiol* 84:192–196.
8. de Ortiz HK, DeQuattro V, Schoentgen S, Stephanian E (1982) Raised plasma catecholamines in old and young patients with disproportionate systolic hypertension. *Clin Exp Hypertens* A4(7):1107–1120.
9. Domanski MJ, Davis BR, Pfeffer MA, et al. (1999) Isolated systolic hypertension: prognostic information provided by pulse pressure. *Hypertension* 34:375–380.
10. MacMahon S, Rodgers A (1993) The effects of blood pressure reduction in older patients: an overview of five randomized controlled trials in elderly hypertensives. *Clin Exp Hypertens* 15:967–978.
11. SHEP Cooperative Research Group (1991) Prevention of stroke by antihypertensive drug treatment in older persons with isolated systolic hypertension: final results of the Systolic Hypertension in the Elderly Program (SHEP). *JAMA* 65:3255–3264.
12. The Sixth Report of the Joint National Committee on Prevention, Detection, Evaluation, and Treatment of High Blood Pressure (1997) NIH publication no. 98-4080; November. Bethesda, MD: National Institutes of Health, National Heart, Lung, and Blood Institute, National High Blood Pressure Education Program.

3
Effects of Race on Blood Pressure

John M. Flack, MD, MPH

CONTENTS

PHYSIOLOGICAL PROFILE
GENERAL THERAPEUTIC PRINCIPLES
THERAPEUTIC TARGETS
PREFERRED DRUG THERAPIES
CONCLUSION
SUGGESTED READINGS

Hypertension is more prevalent and has an earlier onset in African Americans compared with the general population. The prevalence of the Sixth Joint National Committee on the Prevention, Detection, Evaluation and Treatment of High Blood Pressure (JNC VI) stage 3 hypertension is approx 8% among African Americans vs <1% in Caucasian hypertensive patients. Pressure-related target organ damage (TOD) (i.e., left ventricular hypertrophy) is more prevalent at any given blood pressure (BP) level in African Americans compared with Caucasians. Accordingly, African Americans have very high levels of absolute risk of pressure-related clinical complications such as stroke, renal insufficiency/end-stage renal disease, congestive heart failure (CHF), and myocardial infarction. Nevertheless, African Americans have been shown to experience similar, or even better, clinical cardiovascular disease outcomes as Caucasians when access to hypertension care was similar. In addition, the practitioner infrequently treats hypertension in African-American individuals with concurrent diabetes mellitus and/ or renal insufficiency.

From: *Hypertension Medicine*
Edited by: M. A. Weber © Humana Press Inc., Totowa, NJ

PHYSIOLOGICAL PROFILE

It has long been assumed that in African Americans, plasma volume is expanded; however, the actual data on this are conflicting. Yet, there is little doubt regarding the fact that African Americans, particularly women, prominently manifest salt sensitivity. Salt sensitivity is an important intermediate BP phenotype for a multiplicity of reasons. First, salt sensitivity has been linked to obesity in both Caucasians and African Americans. Although my focus is on hypertensive individuals, normotensive individuals also manifest salt sensitivity but to a lesser degree than among hypertensive individuals. I recently showed that the link of salt sensitivity with body size in African Americans was virtually all attributable to fat notlean body mass. Moreover, I and others have shown that the abnormal diurnal BP variation—an attenuation or absence of the nocturnal BP fall—has been linked to obesity and, in turn, to salt sensitivity. Salt sensitivity also increases BP medication requirements, although to a lesser degree for diuretics and calcium antagonists than for other drug classes. This makes attainment of adequate trough BP reductions—a surrogate marker of 24-h BP control—perhaps more difficult in salt-sensitive patients. Salt-sensitivity has also been linked to a pattern of abnormal intrarenal hemodynamics (raised intraglomerular pressure, increased intrarenal vascular resistance and filtration fraction) that, if sustained over time, could lead to progressive renal injury.

African Americans are also noted for their tendency to manifest suppressed circulating renin levels as well as a lesser stimulation of circulating renin with provocative volume-depleting stimuli. Suppression of circulating renin levels can be a marker for several physiologic and hemodynamic states, including high levels of dietary sodium intake, high levels of tissue angiotensin II in the juxtaglomerular cells of the renal afferent arteriole, high BP levels, and plasma volume expansion. The totality of evidence, though largely circumstantial, points to a central role for the renin-aldosterone-kinin system in the pathogenesis of elevation and pressure-related TOD in African Americans.

Although it is beyond the scope of this chapter, several other pathophysiologic aberrations have been described in African Americans. However, it is important for the reader to understand that these racial differences represent quantitative, not qualitative, differences. In addition, within any racial or ethnic group, there is tremendous variation in the actual expression of any of the aforementioned physiologic traits.

Finally, whether racial/ethnic physiologic tendencies represent primary (genetic) or secondary phenomena, perhaps attributable to BP *per se,* remains speculative.

GENERAL THERAPEUTIC PRINCIPLES

The general therapeutic approach to hypertension does not vary significantly by race or ethnic group. Once the diagnosis of hypertension has been confirmed, the patient should undergo comprehensive history, physical, and laboratory examinations that focus on identifying the status of related target organs (brain, kidneys, and heart) that may have been damaged by hypertension and/or other coexisting cardiovascular conditions such as diabetes mellitus or hyperlipidemia. An assessment of patient well-being is extremely important.

Lifestyle modifications such as weight loss, salt and alcohol restriction, and increased physical activity are particularly useful, either alone or in combination with antihypertensive drug treatments, in lowering BP. Weight loss is particularly effective in lowering BP. Moreover, weight loss attenuates the pressure response to dietary sodium intake, which, in turn, lowers antihypertensive medication requirements to achieve a given BP level. Reducing sodium intake is also an important lifestyle change in hypertensive African Americans because the majority of hypertensive African Americans are salt sensitive. Thus, lowering sodium intake to approx 2 to 3 g (87–131 mmol/d) will augment the BP-lowering response of virtually all antihypertensive drug classes, particularly those with the renin-angiotensin-aldosterone-kinin system as their primary site of action. Appropriate levels of regular aerobic physical activity lower BP as well as contribute to the maintenance of normal body weight. African-American women, particularly those residing in the southeastern United States, are disproportionately overweight compared with Caucasian women. In addition, many African-American women report low levels of physical activity. Nevertheless, hypertensive African Americans of both sexes will benefit from prudent initiation of the aforementioned lifestyle modifications. However, if the patient is unable to effectively adopt these lifestyle modifications, the practitioner should avoid the trap of allowing the patient's lack of success to become a wedge to the patient-practitioner relationship. Finally, there must be ample consideration and respect of individual preference, which may be deeply rooted in cultural tradition and beliefs.

THERAPEUTIC TARGETS

Appropriate therapeutic targets can be set only after comprehensive evaluation of the patient. The minimum therapeutic goal for those with uncomplicated hypertension is <140/90 mmHg. However, a minimum BP of <130/85 mmHg should be the therapeutic goal in hypertensive patients with renal insufficiency, diabetes mellitus, and/or CHF. When proteinuria exceeds 1 g/24 h, the appropriate BP target is even lower at <125/75 mmHg. Gradual attainment of these BP levels over many weeks to months is preferable to more rapid BP normalization if overmedication and treatment-related side effects are to be avoided. African-American hypertensive patients will not infrequently be a candidate for initiation of drug therapy at BP levels <140/90 mmHg because of their high prevalence of coexisting diabetes, renal insufficiency, and/or CHF.

Likewise, a significant number of African Americans also will qualify for lower target BP levels well below 130/85 mmHg. Nevertheless, certain drugs may be preferred within a multidrug regimen. The avenues available to express such preference are highlighted in the Preferred Drug Therapies section. The practitioner should remember the low likelihood of achieving target BP in persons with JNC VI stage 3 hypertension with monotherapy.

Race or ethnicity is not an appropriate criterion on which to base the selection of antihypertensive drug therapy for individual patients. A widespread clinical perception has been that β-blockers and angiotensin-converting enzyme (ACE) inhibitors are ineffective in African-American hypertensive patients. Concern has been raised that the currently marketed angiotensin II receptor antagonists are also ineffective hypotensive agents in African Americans. However, careful consideration of the published data, particularly regarding the ACE inhibitors and β-blockers, is that at low doses these agents are less effective in lowering BP in African Americans relative to Caucasians. Moreover, among African Americans, when used as monotherapy these agents also appear to be less effective than diuretics and calcium antagonists for lowering BP. On the other hand, the data are relatively persuasive that uptitration of ACE inhibitors into the upper part of their dosing range results in a substantial narrowing or obliteration of racial BP response differentials, and also improves the BP-lowering response of these agents relative to that obtained with calcium antagonists and diuretics.

Dietary sodium intake attenuates the magnitude of BP lowering with virtually all antihypertensive drug classes. The attenuation of the BP-lowering effect can be overcome, at least in part, by several strategies: (1) reduce the sodium intake, (2) uptitrate the drug dose, or (3) add a diuretic. Perhaps one major reason that diuretics and calcium antagonists have been widely perceived as the most effective antihypertensive monotherapy for the African-American hypertensive patient is because their BP lowering efficiency is less attenuated than other drug classes in the setting of usual (physiologically high) amounts of dietary sodium. It is reasonable to give an adequately dosed antihypertensive agent about 6 wk to fully manifest its BP-lowering effect at a given dose. When a therapeutic trial of sufficient duration has been given to a drug and BP remains uncontrolled, the practitioner must decide whether to substitute or add another drug from a different therapeutic class. When BP levels are in the high JNC VI stage 2 range (170–179/105–109 mmHg), strong consideration should be given to adding a second antihypertensive agent as opposed to substituting another drug.

PREFERRED DRUG THERAPIES

African Americans and Native American Indians will not infrequently have coexisting cardiovascular-renal conditions for which selected drug therapies should be preferred. For example, both diabetic and nondiabetic renal insufficiency represents conditions for which ACE inhibitors have proven benefit. Thus, the practitioner can show preference for an ACE inhibitor by initiating therapy with an ACE, pushing the dose into the upper therapeutic range, and adding a second agent from a different class when monotherapy with the ACE inhibitor fails to achieve the BP goal. Even when monotherapy with the ACE inhibitor has been ineffective in reaching the BP goal, the added agent will manifest a steeper dose-response curve when prescribed concurrently with the ACE than when taken at the same dose as monotherapy. It has been repeatedly shown that African Americans with CHF have ACE inhibitors prescribed less often than their Caucasian counterparts. A similar scenario can be construed for a β-blocker or long-acting calcium antagonist to be a preferred drug class in hypertensive African Americans with symptomatic coronary ischemia. α_1 Antagonists are particularly useful, either alone or in combination, in diabetic persons because these agents improve insulin sensitivity, and they also have a favorable effect on all lipoprotein fractions. A key concept regarding a preferred drug dose is that it should not be abandoned solely because of inadequate BP lowering.

CONCLUSION

The ultimate goal of antihypertensive drug therapy in African Americans is to improve patient well-being as well as to prevent pressure-related complications such as stroke, cognitive dysfunction, heart failure, renal insufficiency, and myocardial infarction. Patient characteristics that may attenuate the BP response to various antihypertensive drugs—renal function, obesity, sodium intake—are disproportionately prevalent in African Americans. However, when treating an individual patient, race is an inadequate criterion on which to base drug selection. African Americans will require combination drug therapy more often than their Caucasian counterparts to achieve their target BP. Nevertheless, the benefits of successful BP treatment to goal or lower levels will confer tremendous benefit, to both patient well-being and overall cardiovascular health in this high-risk population.

SUGGESTED READINGS

Flack JM, Neaton JD, Daniels B, Esunge P (1993) Ethnicity and renal disease: lessons from multiple risk factor intervention trial and the Treatment of Mild Hypertension Study. *Am J Kidney Dis* 21(4) (Suppl. 1):31–40.

Flack JM (1988) Therapy of hypertension in primer on kidney diseases. In: Greenberg, A, ed. Cheung AK, et al., assoc. ed). *Primer on Kidney Diseases,* 2nd ed., San Diego: Academic, pp 506–516.

Flack JM, Staffileno B (1998) Hypertension in Blacks. In: Johnson R, ed. *Comprehensive Clinical Nephrology,* London: Mosby International.

Ooi WL, Budner NS, Cohen H, Madhavan S, Alderman MH (1989) Impact of race on treatment response and cardiovascular disease among hypertensives. *Hypertension* 14(3):227–234.

Weir MR, Hall PS, Behrens MT, Flack JM (1997) Salt and blood pressure responses to calcium antagonism in hypertensive patients. *Hypertension* 30(3) (Pt. 1):422–427.

Joint National Committee on Prevention, Detection, Evaluation, and Treatment of High Blood Pressure (1997) The Sixth Report of the Joint National Committee on Prevention, Detection, Evaluation, and Treatment of High Blood Pressure. *Arch Intern Med* 157:2413–2446.

4
Genetics in Hypertension

Joel M. Neutel, MD
and David H.G. Smith, MD

Hypertension as a disease process was borne out of epidemiolog studies demonstrating that people with elevated blood pressure (BP) had a greater risk of developing strokes and heart attacks than matched people with normal BP. The hope was that treating hypertension would reduce the risk of cardiovascular disease to the rates seen in normotensive subjects. However, epidemiologic studies performed in the past 10–20 yr have demonstrated that the treatment of hypertension has resulted in very impressive reductions in the incidence of strokes among hypertensive patients, but very disappointing decreases in the incidence of coronary artery disease (CAD) *(1,2)*. Poor BP control rates among hypertensive patients are undoubtedly contributing to the disappointing reduction in CAD in hypertensive subjects *(3)*, and this is certainly an

From: *Hypertension Medicine*
Edited by: M. A. Weber © Humana Press Inc., Totowa, NJ

area that requires urgent attention. However, even in well-controlled hypertensive patients, the rate of CAD remains higher than in normotensive subjects with similar BPs *(4)*. The main reason for this discrepancy is probably related to hypertension not being simply a disease of high numbers but, rather, a complex inherited syndrome of cardiovascular risk factors, all of which contribute to heart disease in hypertensive patients. Furthermore, because high BP may be a late manifestation of this disease process, it is possible that patients with the hypertension syndrome may develop cardiovascular disease before they develop high BP. Thus, it is becoming obvious that simply treating BP is not enough. The treatment plan should include aggressive management of the syndrome as a whole rather than isolated treatment of the various risk factors.

This chapter demonstrates that hypertension is an inherited syndrome of cardiovascular risk factors, all of which appear to be genetically linked, clinically manifest independent of one another, and contribute to the development of cardiovascular disease in these patients. This realization has many important implications toward our approach to the treatment of patients with this syndrome. The management plan and the selection of antihypertensive agents need to focus both on reducing BP to goal levels and on achieving this with "syndrome friendly" drugs.

LIPIDS IN THE HYPERTENSION SYNDROME

Hypertension and lipid abnormalities often coexist. Each is an independent risk factor for cardiovascular events. Moreover, the likelihood of coronary events appears to be exaggerated when the two problems occur together *(5)*. The explanation for this phenomenon is not clear. However, studies in models of genetic hypertensive rats indicate that the vascular smooth muscle of these animals binds with a greater affinity to low-density lipoprotein than do the cells from normotensive controlled animals *(6)*.

The presence of high BP and hyperlipidemia is so common in hypertensive patients that many have argued that the high BP itself may play a role in altering lipid metabolism, resulting in lipid abnormalities. Recent data, however, have demonstrated that high BP and hyperlipidimia are genetically inherited and probably genetically linked, but are separate variables that may frequently present independently of one another. In a study comparing age-, sex-, and body mass index (BMI)-matched normotensive patients with and without a family history of hypertension, the patients with a family history of hypertension (hypertensive-prone patients) had significantly greater total cholesterol levels than those without a family history of hypertension *(7)*. This would suggest that the abnormalities of lipids precede the abnormalities of BP in patients likely to develop high BP over the next few years. Thus, we see two important cardiovascular risk factors in these hypertensive prone patients, both of which appear to be inherited, occur independently of one another, and contribute to the development of heart disease. This may have important therapeutic implications, because studies using the occurrence of coronary events to judge the success of treatment of hypertensive patients have shown that the treatment of hypertension alone, or hypercholesterolemia alone, produces only modest results. Only when both problems were controlled simultaneously was there a marked reduction in CAD *(8)*.

LEFT VENTRICULAR HYPERTROPHY

Left ventricular hypertrophy (LVH) is commonly regarded as a "normal" finding in hypertensive patients with little consequence. There is, however, a very strong relationship between left ventricular muscle mass and the incidence of cardiovascular events. A recent report from the Framingham Heart Study has confirmed that echocardiographically measured LVH, independent of other associated risk factors, is a powerful predictor of cardiovascular events or death *(9)*. Hypertensive patients with LVH have a fivefold increased risk of myocardial infarction (MI) and a threefold increased risk of sudden death compared with similar hypertensive patients who do not have LVH *(9)*.

Echocardiography M-mode techniques have made it possible to measure the thickness of the left ventricular walls and chamber size, thus enabling accurate calculations of left ventricular muscle mass *(10)*. Because of the sensitivity of the echocardiographic measurements, the prevalence of LVH in hypertension is now known to be far greater than previously supposed. In a survey of an unselected clinic population of hypertensive patients, ECG and chest radiographic estimates of the prevalence of LVH were in the range of 5–10%. Echocardiography in the same patients indicated that almost 50% had increased left ventricular muscle mass *(11)*.

Although sustained high BP can produce hypertrophy of the left ventricle, there is good evidence that LVH can develop early on in the course of hypertension and may actually precede the onset of high BP.

In a study of young individuals (age <30 yr) with mild hypertension, it was found that approximately half of these patients had values for septal and posterior wall thickness that were greater than the highest values found in an age-control group *(12)*. Interestingly, subsequent BP measurements indicated that many of these young hypertensive patients had normal or borderline BP values; the echocardiographic wall thickness in this subgroup, however, was not different from the increased measurements in the patients whose BP was in the hypertensive range.

In a separate study, in which echocardiographic findings in normotensive children of normotensive patients were compared with those of age-, sex-, and BMI-matched normotensive children of hypertensive parents, the offspring with hypertensive families had significantly greater left ventricular wall thickness and muscle mass *(13)*. Thus, in hypertensive-prone patients, abnormalities of left ventricular muscle mass may occur prior to the development of high BP. LVH is therefore another risk factor that is commonly associated with high BP, but presents independent of high BP and frequently before its onset.

It is generally believed that regression of LVH as a result of antihypertensive treatment will be associated with a reduction in cardiovascular outcomes. However, this has not been shown in outcome studies, and current *(14)* studies are under way to assess the impact of LVH regression on cardiovascular mortality and mobility. Nonetheless, the selection of a drug that will reduce BP and cause regression of left ventricular hypertrophy in hypertensive patients appears to be logical, although the final results of the outcome studies are still pending.

VENTRICULAR AND ARTERIAL COMPLIANCE

Hypertension is characterized by structural changes in the arterial circulation. Hypertrophy and hyperplasia of arterial and ventricular walls in association with increased laying down of connective tissue elements are common findings in hypertensive patients *(14)*. These changes stiffen the walls, resulting in reduced arterial compliance and reduced ventricular compliance (diastolic dysfunction). Comparisons of normotensive and hypertensive subjects have established that changes in cardiovascular compliance frequently precede the increase in BP in hypertensive subjects. Moreover, studies have suggested that abnormalities of compliance can precede the abnormalities of BP and may not worsen the increasing BP *(15)*. In a recent study comparing arterial function in normotensive subjects from hypertensive parents with that of normotensive subjects from normotensive parents, it was demonstrated that the patients with a family history of hypertension (hypertensive-prone patients) had abnormalities of arterial function despite the fact that they were still normotensive *(16)*. Similarly, in a study using an invasive technique to measure arterial compliance, normotensive subjects from hypertensive parents demonstrated a significant reduction in arterial compliance (arterial stiffening) compared with normotensive subjects from normotensive parents *(17)*. These findings suggest that the abnormalities of arterial structure and function frequently associated with hypertension may precede the onset of high BP and, in fact, may play a role in the pathogenesis of increasing BP.

A similar patient model was used to assess ventricular compliance in hypertensive-prone subjects. Transmitral flow characteristics, measured by Doppler echocardiography, have been used as an index of left ventricular filling during diastole; an increased ratio of late to early left ventricular filling reflects reduced compliance of the left ventricular wall. In advance stages, this may result in congestive heart failure in hypertensive patients *(18)*. It appears likely that the changes in ventricular compliance in hypertensive patients also precede the onset of high BP. Among a group of normotensive male college students, matched for age, blood pressure, and left ventricular mass, those with a family history of hypertension had delayed diastolic filling compared with those who did not have a family history of hypertension *(18)*.

Thus, the changes in compliance, frequently associated with hypertension, appear to precede the onset of BP and occur independently of BP. Furthermore, it has been demonstrated that reduced compliance causes an increase in BP and therefore may play a role in the pathogenesis of increased BP.

ABNORMAL GLUCOSE AND INSULIN METABOLISM

In recent years there has been growing interest in the presence of insulin resistance (syndrome X) in hypertensive patients. Multiple clinical studies have now demonstrated that there is an increased relative risk of cardiovascular events in patients who have insulin resistance *(19)*. Physicians have long been aware that diabetes mellitus and hypertension often coexist. There is growing evidence that many hypertensive patients can be characterized as having borderline glucose intolerance and insulin resistance. These patients usually have normal fasting blood glucose concentrations and are not regarded as having clinical diabetes. A large-scale population survey *(20)* has indicated that approx 50% of untreated hypertensive patients have glucose intolerance as measured by plasma glucose levels 2 h after glucose load. This prevalence is far higher than in normotensive control subjects. The explanation for this finding appears to be resistance to the action of insulin. In a recent study of well-matched groups of normal volunteers and hypertensive patients given a standard oral glucose tolerance test, glucose levels were found to be slightly higher in the hypertensive group than in the normotensive control subjects *(21)*. More impressive, this study showed that plasma insulin concentrations were significantly higher in the hypertensive patients than in their normotensive counterparts during much of the 3-h study. The study also demonstrated that the problem is exaggerated by thiazide treatment, especially when β-blockers are added. Thus, patients with insulin resistance may have almost normal blood glucose levels but still spend significant proportions of the day hyperinsulinemic.

These findings are potentially important in explaining the high instances of atherosclerotic disease in hypertensive patients. Insulin is a powerful growth factor that directly stimulates smooth muscle cell proliferation. In addition, it plays an important role in promoting the action of other growth factors on vascular tissue. Moreover, insulin appears to enhance the formation of atherosclerotic plaques by facilitating the transport of atherogenic lipid particles into the media of the vessel wall. In a recent comparison of patients with increased and normal plasma insulin levels, those with higher insulin levels had increased concentrations of triglycerides and total cholesterol and decreased levels of high-density lipoprotein (HDL) *(23)*. Increased insulin levels also appear to be associated with higher BP. Several actions of insulin may result in increased BP. It stimulates the sympathetic nervous system probably through a glucose-mediated effect on the hypothalamus. It also causes readsorption of sodium by the kidney *(24,25)*. These observations provide a possible explanation for the association of noninsulin-dependent diabetes mellitus (NIDDM) and hypertension *(26)*. Other important effects of hyperinsulinemia may include an increase in the pressor action of angiotensin II *(27)* and angiotensin II–stimulated production of aldosterone *(28)*. In one study, chronic administration of insulin to rats increased BP, which remained increased for several days after the insulin was discontinued *(29)*.

It appears that insulin resistance and elevated insulin levels may precede the onset of high BP. In a study comparing age-, sex-, and BMI-matched normotensive patients with and without a family history of hypertension, insulin levels were significantly higher in patients with a family history of hypertension than in those without a family history of hypertension *(7)*. Furthermore, the insulin:glucose ratio, which correlates well with insulin resistance measured by the euglycemic clamp technique *(30)*, demonstrated that patients with a family history of hypertension were less sensitive to their own insulin than those without a family history of hypertension, despite the presence of normal BP *(7)*. Similar findings were reported in a study of young African-American men; fasting plasma insulin concentrations were significantly greater in patients with borderline hypertension than in normal control subjects, and the young hypertensive subjects exhibited a diminished capacity to clear glucose from their plasma *(31)*. A similar picture of impaired glucose tolerance and compensatory hyperinsulinemia has been observed in normal offspring of patients with type II diabetes *(32)*, suggesting a possible link between the mechanisms that mediate an increase in BP and diabetes.

There is good evidence that insulin resistance and hyperinsulinemia are important cardiovascular risk factors. Early evidence linking diabetes and atherosclerosis came from the International Atherosclerosis Project *(33)*. Later, in prospective population studies, increased insulin concentrations were implicated in the development of CAD *(34,35)*. These studies have also shown that hyperinsulinemia is associated with increased triglycerides and decreased concentrations of HDL *(34)* cholesterol. Other studies have shown that changes in lipoprotein composition that are characteristic of NIDDM are extremely atherogenic *(36)*. In the Paris Prospective Study, plasma insulin concentrations were a patient-independent predictor of CAD. The Helsinki Policemen Study *(39)*, a prospective study of 982 men, showed that high plasma insulin was predictive of CAD, death, or nonfatal MI over a 9.5-yr follow-up. In the prospective Cardiovascular Munster study *(40)*, hypertension, NIDDM and hyperinsulinemia were shown to be independent risk factors for CAD.

Thus, abnormalities of glucose and insulin metabolism are yet another genetically determined cardiovascular risk factor that may occur in patients prone to the development of hypertension. These abnormalities appear to be genetically determined and linked to hypertension. However, they appear to clinically manifest independent of BP. Furthermore, they may play a role in the development of atherosclerotic disease and reduce arterial compliance, which ultimately may also be important in the pathogenesis of high BP.

OBESITY

Recent large studies have demonstrated that hypertensive patients had a greater BMI than well-matched normotensive male and female subjects in every age group (41). Obesity is associated with metabolic complications that are considered to be risk factors for cardiovascular disease, including insulin resistance, hyperinsulinemia, glucose intolerance-NIDDM, hypertension, and changes in the concentrations of plasma lipids and lipoproteins (42–44). Only recently has truncal obesity, characterized by a large waist:hip ratio (apple shape obesity), been shown to predict the risk of CAD (45). The mechanisms that link obesity and hypertension-lipid abnormalities are not clear. In view of the efficacy of weight loss and exercise in reducing BP, it has been speculated that insulin provides the link between obesity and increases sympathetic nervous system activity (46). The hyperglycemic clamp technique has been used to compare obese hypertensive patients with obese normotensive patients and lean control subjects to determine whether additional hyperinsulinemia and insulin resistance is associated with obesity when hypertension was also present (47). Both of these groups were similar and showed greater insulin concentrations and insulin resistance than their lean counterparts, but obesity and hypertension were not additive in these effects (46). When obese and nonobese patients with NIDDM with and without hypertension were compared, it was shown that there was a greater insulin resistance and that hypertension was present in lean individuals with NIDDM, but not in their obese counterparts (48).

ENDOCRINE CHANGES

The sympathetic nervous system and the renin angiotensin system are believed to play an important role in the pathogenesis of high BP. Many of the modern antihypertensive drugs function by interrupting these systems in order to reduce BP. It has been demonstrated, in recent studies, that plasma neuroendocrine levels and plasma renin activity were significantly elevated in normotensive subjects with hypertensive parents compared with matched normotensive subjects from normotensive parents *(7)*. It is interesting that these increases in neuroendocrine levels occur prior to the development of elevated BP and that hypertensive-prone patients with significantly elevated neuroendocrine and angiotensin II levels can be absolutely normotensive. These findings suggest that the hypertensive effects of these hormonal systems are not entirely owing to their vasoconstrictor properties, but may also be owing to their influences on the structure and function of cardiovascular smooth muscle.

RENAL CHANGES

Because of recent interest in milder forms of hypertension, early changes in renal function have been observed. It has been demonstrated that there are differences in renal functional reserve in children of normotensive compared with children of hypertensive parents. Thus, despite apparently normal renal function, children of hypertensive parents appear to be less able than children of normotensive parents to increase their creatinine clearance in response to protein load and also are more likely to exhibit microalbuminurea. These data were confirmed in a later study that demonstrated significantly more microalbuminurea in normotensive adults with a family history of hypertension than matched normotensive adults without a family history of hypertension *(20)*.

These data suggest that early changes in renal function may precede the development of high BP and may occur independently of high BP. Moreover, the reduction in renal function may play a role in causing high BP.

NORMOTENSIVE SUBJECTS WITH HYPERTENSION SYNDROME VS HYPERTENSIVE SUBJECTS

There are convincing data to suggest that many of the components of the hypertension syndrome precede the onset of high BP. Furthermore, normotensive subjects who are prone to developing hypertension (by virtue of a strong family history of hypertension) have significantly more cardiovascular risk factors than matched normotensive subjects without a family history of hypertension, and are thus more likely to develop cardiovascular disease. The question arises: How do normotensive subjects with a family of hypertension (who are seldom treated) compare with true hypertensive subjects (who are usually treated) in terms of cardiovascular risk factors?

A recent study *(49)* comparing the cardiovascular risk factor in normotensive patients with a family history of hypertension with hypertensive patients (matched for age and BMI) with and without a family history of hypertension, no differences were found in the plasma levels of insulin, norepinephrine, renin activity, and cholesterol. There were also no differences in insulin sensitivity, microalbuminuria, or systolic BP response to exercise. All three groups, however, were significantly worse in each of these parameters than the control group (normotensive subjects without a family history of hypertension).

Thus, in terms of cardiovascular risk, "normotensive hypertensive" subjects (who are not treated) have a similar cardiovascular risk factor profile and therefore are at similar risk of cardiovascular disease as hypertensive subjects (who are treated to protect them from developing cardiovascular disease). The only difference is that the normotensive subjects have not yet developed high BP, which seems to be a late manifestation of this disease. Because, universally, BP measurement is used to isolate patients with the hypertension syndrome in order to initiate treatment to protect them from developing heart disease, it is possible that physicians are treating these patients too late in the disease process. If physicians were to isolate and treat these patients earlier, before they develop high BP, there might be a bigger impact on the course of this disease, thereby possibly protecting the patients from developing high BP, and from developing heart disease.

It is conceivable, although by no means proven, that the hypertension syndrome may be reversible prior to the onset of high BP and that the development of high BP is a marker of irreversible vascular changes after which physicians can only control the disease. Evidence for this statement is the fact that early in the disease process, aerobic exercise may frequently reverse many of the cardiovascular risk factors associated with hypertension and may prolong or prevent the onset of high BP. This is not the case in hypertension, which is not weight induced. In addition, studies of controlled hypertensive patients have demonstrated that cardiovascular disease in these patients is more common than in age-matched, sex-matched, normotensive subjects, suggesting that there is more to hypertension than high BP *(49)*.

CONCLUSION

There are increasing data to suggest that in many patients, high BP may be a late manifestation of a complex inherited syndrome of cardiovascular risk factors. Moreover, it is possible that patients with the hypertension syndrome will develop cardiovascular disease prior to the development of high BP. It appears that high BP may represent a late phase of the disease process, indicating advanced or even irreversible vascular damage, and that in order to significantly affect these patients, treatment would have to be started prior to the onset of the increase in BP.

The problem is that BP is the tool used to isolate patients with the disease syndrome. We may be missing the boat. We need to investigate tools that will help isolated patients early in the course of the disease. One possibility would be the use of noninvasive measures of arterial compliance, which appears, in most patients, to be abnormal years before the onset of the increase of BP.

Another dilemma is the approach to treatment of these patients. Exercise and diet are clearly beneficial and may often be the only modality required. But, it would appear that in some patients, early drug intervention with drugs such as angiotensin-receptive blockers and angiotensin-converting enzyme inhibitors may be quite helpful in reversing the disease and perhaps preventing the onset of high BP.

REFERENCES

1. Samuelsson OG, Wilhelmson LW, Svardsudd KF, Pennert KM, Wedel H, Berglund GL (1987) Mortality and morbidity in relation to systolic blood pressure in two populations with different management of hypertension: the study of men born in 1913 and the multifactorial primary prevention trial. *J Hypertens* 5:57–66.
2. Grimm RH Jr, Flack JM, Byington R, Bond G, Brugger S (1990) A comparison of antihypertensive drug effects on the progression of extracranial carotid atherosclerosis: The Multicenter Isradipine Diuretic Atherosclerosis Study (MIDAS). *Drugs* 40:38–43.
3. Burt VC, Cutler JA, Higgins M (1995) Trends in the prevalence, awareness, treatment and control of hypertension in the adult US population: data from the Health Examinations Surveys, 1960 to 1991. *Hypertension* 26(1):60–69.
4. Havlik H, La Croix A, Kleinman J, Ingram D, Harris T, Cornoni-Huntley J (1989) Antihypertensive drug therapy and survival by treatment status in a national survey. *Hypertension* 13(Suppl. 1):1-28–1-32.
5. The Pooling Project Research Group (1978) Relationship of blood pressure, serum

cholesterol, smoking habit, relative weight and ECG abnormalities to incidence of major coronary events: final report of the Pooling Project. *J Chron Dis* 31:201–206.

6. Scannapieco G, Pauletta P, Pagnan A (1988) Lipoprotein binding to cultured aortic smooth muscle cells from normotensive and hypertensive rats. *J Hypertens* 6(Suppl. 4):S269–S271.

7. Neutel JM, Smith DHG, Graettinger WF, Winer RL, Weber MA (1992) Heredity and hypertension: impact on metabolic characteristics. *Am Heart J* 124:443–440.

8. Sammelsson O, Wilmhelmsen L, Andeson OK, Pinnert K, Berglund G (1987) Cardiovascular morbidity in relation to change in blood pressure and serum cholesterol levels in treated hypertension. *JAMA* 285:1768–1776.

9. Levy D, Garrison RJ, Savage DD, Kennel WB, Castelli WP (1990) Prognostic implications of echocardiographically determined left ventricular mass in Framingham Heart Study. *N Engl J Med* 332:1561–1566.

10. Devereux RB, Reichek N (1977) Electrocardiographic determination left ventricular mass in man: anatomic validation of the method. *Circulation* 66:613–618.

11. Savage DD, Drayer JIM, Henry WL (1979) Echocardiographic assessment of cardiac anatomy and function in hypertensive subjects. *Circulation* 59:623–632.

12. Drayer JIM, Weber MA, Laragh JH (1981) Echocardiography in the evaluation of patient with mild to borderline hypertension. In Weber MA ed. *Treatment Strategies in Hypertension,* Miami: Symposia Specialist, pp. 21–32.

13. Celentano A, Galderisis M, Garafalo M (1988) Blood pressure and cardiac morphology in young children of hypertensive subjects. *J Hypertens* 6(Suppl. 4):S107–S109.

14. Giligan JP, Spector S (1994) Synthesis of collagen in cardiac and vascular hypertension. *Hypertension* 6(Suppl. 3):1144–1149.

15. Safar ME, Laurent S, Pannier BM, London GM (1987) Structural and functional modification of peripheral large arteries in hypertensive patients. *J Clin Hypertens* 3:360–367.

16. Taddei S, Virdis A, Mattei P, Arzilli F, Salvetti A (1992) Endothelium-dependent forearm vasodilation in reduced in normotensive subjects with family history of hypertension. *J Cardiovasc Pharmacol* 20(Suppl. 12):S193–S195.

17. Neutel JM, Smith DHG, Graettinger WF, Weber MA (1992) Dependency of arterial compliance on circulating neuroendocrine and metabolic factors. *Am J Cardiol* 69:1340–1344.

18. Graettinger WF, Neutel JM, Smith DHG, Weber MA (1991) Left ventricular diastolic filling alterations in normotensive young adults with a family history of systemic hypertension. *Am J Cardiol* 68:51–56.

19. Ruige JB, Assendelft WJ, Dekker JM, Kostense PJ, Heine RJ, Bouter LM (1998) Insulin and risk of cardiovascular disease: a meta-analysis. *Circulation* 97(10):996–1001.

20. Modan M, Halkin H, Almog S (1985) Hyperinsulinemia: a link between hypertension, obesity and glucose intolerance. *J Clin Invest* 75:809–817.

21. Neutel JM, Smith DHG, Graettinger WF (1993) Metabolic characteristics of hypertension: importance of family history. *Am Heart J* 126:924–929.

22. Banskota NK, Taub R, Zellner K (1989) Characterization of induction of protooncogene c-myc and cellular growth in human vascular smooth muscle cells in insulin and IGF-1. *Diabetes* 38:123–129.

23. Zavaroni I, Bonora E, Palgliara M (1989) Risk factors for coronary artery disease in healthy persons with hyperinsulinemia and normal glucose tolerance. *N Engl J Med* 320:702–706.

24. Williams RR, Hunt SC, Hassted SJ, Stephenson SH, Hopkins PN (1990) Multigenic human hypertension: evidence for subtypes and hope for haplotypes. *J Hypertens* 8(Suppl.):S39–S46.

25. Gupta AK, Clark RV, Kirchner KA (1992) Effect on insulin on renal sodium excretion. *Hypertension* 19(Suppl. 1):8–82.

26. Reaven GM, Hoffman BB (1987) A role for Insulin in the aetiology and course of hypertension. *Lancet* ii:435–437.

27. Tuck M, Corry D, Trujillo A (1990) Salt-sensitive blood pressure and exaggerated vascular reactivity in the hypertension of diabetes mellitus. *Am J Med* 88:210–216.

28. Rocchini AP, Moorehead C, DeRemer S, Goodfriend TL, Ball DL (1990) Hyperinsulinemia and the aldosterone and pressor responses to angiotensin II. *Hypertension* 15:861–866.

29. Meehan WP, Buchanan TA, Shargil NS (1990) Chronic insulin administration elevates blood pressure in rates. *Circulation* 82:11–86 (abstract).

30. Caro JF (1991) Clinical review 26: insulin resistance in obese and non-obese men. *J Clin Endocrinol Metab* 73:691–695.

31. Fralkener B, Hulman S, Tannenbaum J, Kushner H (1990) Insulin resistance and blood pressure in young black men. *Hypertension* 16:706–711.

32. Warram JH, Maritn BC, Krolewski AS, Soeldner JS, Kahn R (1990) Slow glucose removal rate and hyperinsulinemia precede the development of type II diabetes in the offspring of diabetic parents. *Ann Intern Med* 113:909–915.

33. Robertson WB, Strong JP (1968) Atherosclerosis in persons with hypertension and diabetes mellitus. *Lab Invest* 18:538–551.

34. Stout RW (1990) Insulin and atheroma: 20-yr perspective. *Diabetes Care* 13:631–654.

35. Stout RW (1985) Overview of the association between insulin and atherosclerosis. *Metabolism* 34(Suppl.):7–12.

36. Uusitupa MI, Niskanen LK, Sitonen O, Voulitainen E, Pyorala K (1990) 5 year incidence of atherosclerotic vascular disease in relation to general risk factors, insulin level and abnormalities in lipoprotein composition in non-insulin-dependent diabetic and non-diabetic subjects. *Circulation* 82:27–36.

37. Fontbone A, Tchobroutsky G, Eschwege E, Richards JL, Claude JR, Roselin GE (1987) Coronary heart disease mortality risk: plasma insulin level in a more sensitive maker than hypertension or abnormal glucose tolerance in overweight male. The Paris Prospective Study. *Int J Obes* 12:557–565.

38. Fontbone A, Eschwega E (1987) Diabetes, hyperglycemia, hyperinsulinemia and atherosclerosis: epidemiological data. *Diabetes Metab* 13:350–353.

39. Pyorala K, Savolainen E, Kaukola S, Jaapakoski J (1985) Plasma insulin as coronary heart disease risk factor: relationship to other risk factors and predictive value during 9½ year follow-up of the Helsinski Policemen Study population. *Acta Med Scand* 701(Suppl.   ):38–52.

40. Depres JP, Moorjani S, Lupien PF, Tremblay A, Madaeu A, Bouchard C (1990) Regional distribution of body fat, plasma lipoproteins, and cardiovascular disease. *Arteriosclerosis* 10:497–511.

41. Laurenzi M, Mancini M, Menotti A, Stamler J, Stamler R, Trevisan M, Zanchetti A (1990) Multiple risk factors in hypertension: results from the Gubbioi study. *J Hypertens* 8(1) (Suppl.   ):S7–S12.

42. Kaplan NM (1989) The deadly quartet: upper-body obesity, glucose intolerance, hypertriglyceridemia, and hypertension. *Arch Interm Med* 149:1514–1520.

43. Depres JP, Moorjani S, Lupien PJ, Tremblay A, Nadeau A, Bouchard C (1990)

Regional distribution of body fat, plasma, lipoproteins, and cardiovascular disease. *Arteriosclerosis* 10:497–511.

44. Raison J, Bonithon KC, Egloff M, Ducimetiere P, Guy-Grant B (1990) Hormonal influences on the relationship between body fatness, body fat distribution, lipid, lipoproteins, glucose and blood pressure in French working women. *Arteriosclerosis* 85:185–192.

45. Ducimetiere P, Richard J, Cambien F (1986) The pattern of subcutaneous fat distribution in middle-aged men and the risk of coronary heart disease: the Paris Prospective Study. *Int J Obes* 10:229–240.

46. Krieger DR, Landberg L (1988) Mechanisms in obesity related hypertension: role of insulin and catecholamines. *Am J Hypertens* 1:84–90.

47. Bonora E, Moghetti P, Zenere M, Tosi F, Travia D, Muggeo M (1990) B cell secretion and insulin sensitivity in hypertensive and normotensive obese subjects. *Int J Obes* 14:735–742.

48. Laakso M, Sarlund H, Mykkanen L (1989) Essential hypertension and insulin resistance in non-insulin dependant diabetes. *Eur J Clin Invest* 19:518–526.

49. Neutel JM, Smith DHG, Graettinger WF (1992) Heredity and hypertension: impact on metabolic characteristics. *Am Heart J* 124:435–440.

5 Sodium and Other Dietary Factors

Myron H. Weinberger, MD

Contents

The most recent report of the Sixth Joint National Committee on the Prevention, Detection, Evaluation and Treatment of High Blood Pressure (JNC VI) *(1)* has recommended a trial of lifestyle intervention as initial therapy in individuals with high-normal (130–139 mmHg systolic/85–89 diastolic) or stage I (140–159/90–99 mmHg) blood pressure (BP) levels without end-organ disease, concomitant cardiovascular disease, or diabetes mellitus. This chapter examines the evidence in support of dietary alterations and their effect on BP. The constituents that are considered include calories (body weight), salt (sodium chloride), potassium, calcium, and combinations of these minerals, other dietary components, and alcohol. Rather than attempting an encyclopedic review of the studies of all these dietary elements, this chapter succinctly summarizes what is currently known.

From: *Hypertension Medicine*
Edited by: M. A. Weber © Humana Press Inc., Totowa, NJ

BODY WEIGHT

Body weight has long been linked to BP levels. More recent findings indicate that the distribution of body fat may be a more important determinant of BP elevation and the risk for cardiovascular disease. An increase in visceral abdominal fat (the central or "apple" form) in contrast to the lower body adiposity pattern (the "pear" shape) is linked not only to BP elevation but also to insulin resistance, dyslipidemia, and an increased risk for cardiovascular events. These associations have been based largely on epidemiologic evidence. However, there are now several intervention trials in which it has been demonstrated that weight loss, often as little as 5 kg rather than a reduction to "ideal" body weight, is associated with a decrease in BP and an improvement in insulin sensitivity. Studies on both humans and experimental animals suggest that the sympathetic nervous system (SNS) is involved in the pathophysiology of the weight–blood pressure–insulin resistance relationship, but therapeutic interventions based on these findings are not yet available to confirm this connection.

Another mediator of the body weight–blood pressure relationship appears to be the kidney. In experimental animals, obesity has been associated with alterations in renal blood flow and glomerular filtration rate or intraglomerular pressure. In humans, urinary microalbumin excretion was increased among obese subjects, supporting an abnormality in renal function in humans as well. Moreover, microalbuminuria has been linked to an increased risk of cardiovascular events in hypertensive individuals.

SALT (SODIUM CHLORIDE)

The relationship between dietary salt consumption and elevated BP is well-known (2). The prevalence of hypertension and its consequences is linearly related to dietary salt intake in societies throughout the world. Hypertension and its sequelae are virtually absent in societies in which habitual salt intake is <50–100 mmol/d. However, there are other differences between these groups and those that habitually consume larger amounts of salt. The "low-salt" societies tend to be isolated, genetically homogeneous, physically fit, and consume increased amounts of potassium and calcium in the form of fresh fruits and vegetables. Increased salt intake is associated with societal "accultura-tion." This implies a crowded and sedentary lifestyle as well as many other behavioral factors that may affect BP and cardiovascular risk. In addition, the age-related increase in BP is observed only in societies in which salt intake is high. Many of the elderly individuals in low-salt cultures have BP levels that are no higher than those of young adults.

Despite this convincing evidence, controversy still exists concerning the importance of salt in human BP in general, in hypertension, and as a treatment modality. Without considering the various reasons for this controversy, suffice it to say that the magnitude of the effect of salt intake on BP is diluted by the fact that there is substantial heteroge-neity in the BP responses of humans to alterations in salt intake *(2)*. Numerous studies have demonstrated that salt-sensitive and salt-resis-tant individuals can be identified within both the hypertensive and normotensive populations *(3)*. Salt-sensitive subjects will demonstrate a decrease in BP with dietary sodium reduction, usually to the level of 100 mmol/d (2.4 g/d). The human need for sodium is about 10 mmol/d (230 mg/d). Thus, the threshold for BP responsiveness to a reduction in salt intake is many times higher than the physiologic requirements. It is often difficult to differentiate between salt-sensitive and salt-resistant subjects without sophisticated research techniques. However, a trial of modest dietary salt restriction or diuretic adminis-tration should identify those most likely to benefit from this dietary intervention. Moreover, there have been no adverse reports when a modest reduction in salt intake such as 80–100 mmol/d has been followed.

Certain population groups have been reported to be more likely to be salt sensitive than others *(2)*. Hypertensive individuals are more salt sensitive than those with normal BP. Among hypertensive subjects, salt sensitivity of BP is more frequent among African-Americans (75%) than Caucasians (50%) *(3)* and increases with increasing age *(4)*. The latter finding is also observed in the normotensive population, with the finding that significant salt sensitivity of BP is not seen until the age decade of 60 yr or more. Individuals with reduced renin responses to sodium and volume depletion, the so-called low-renin subjects, are more likely to be salt sensitive than those with brisk renin responses *(5)*.

In addition to a possible permissive effect of sluggish renin responses to salt sensitivity, a variety of substances have been reported to be involved in the pathophysiology of salt sensitivity of BP. An extensive scientific critique of the many studies that have been conducted in this area is beyond the scope of this chapter; however, note that the SNS, endothelin, insulin sensitivity, atrial natriuretic factor, alterations in renal hemodynamics, and leptin have all been implicated in the pathophysiology of salt sensitivity. It remains to be determined which of these many factors are primary events and which are simply compensatory responses or epiphenomena.

It has been shown that salt sensitivity requires the administration of sodium as the chloride salt and that other forms of sodium do not have the same pressor effect. However, this is a moot point because >95% of the sodium found in foods is in the chloride form. Moreover, most of the salt found in food is added in the preparation, processing, and preservation of food, and only 15% is added as the discretionary form (as table salt). Thus, it is important for the food preparer as well as the patient to become familiar with identifying the salt content of foods at the grocery store and restaurant as well as in cooking.

Another important recent finding related to salt and BP is the observation that long-term follow-up of salt-sensitive normotensive subjects over a period of 10 yr or more demonstrated an eightfold greater rate of BP increase compared with those who were initially salt resistant *(4)*. This finding supports the epidemiologic observations relating the age-associated rise in BP to increased salt intake.

POTASSIUM

As already mentioned, in societies in which there is a low prevalence of hypertension and its complications as well as little age-related increase in BP, people tend to consume increased amounts of potassium (and calcium, as discussed in the next section) and follow a reduced salt diet. Fewer studies have examined the relationship between potassium and BP than those involving sodium. However, the findings regarding potassium tend to be consistent. In general, the effect of potassium is smaller than that of sodium based on interventional trials *(6)*. Again, heterogeneity in responsiveness of BP to alterations in potassium intake or balance has been demonstrated. Among potassium-replete normotensive subjects, typically those consuming 60 mmol/d of potassium or more, little effect on BP can be demonstrated with additional potassium administration. However, in hypertensive populations, particularly those comprising substantial numbers of individuals in whom dietary potassium intake is traditionally deficient (the elderly, African Americans) or those in whom diuretic-induced potassium loss occurs, potassium supplementation has been shown to lower BP. It has also been observed that potassium is more likely to lower BP in hypertensive individuals consuming a high salt intake, further suggesting a link between sodium and potassium intake in their effects on BP.

The amount of potassium intake required for optimal reduction in BP in those who are sensitive to this mineral is not clear. Most studies indicate that dietary potassium deficiency begins at levels of intake <50 mmol/d and is clearly observed at intakes of 30 mmol/d or less. Dietary sources of potassium are largely fresh fruits and vegetables. In environments where these are scarce, e.g., because of cold climate or high cost, potassium deficiency is more likely. Among a group of normotensive nurses in whom dietary intakes of potassium, calcium, and magnesium were deficient, only potassium supplementation reduced BP *(7)*. Recent studies using diets involving multiple mineral manipulations, such as the Dietary Approaches to Stop Hypertension (DASH) trial *(8)*, are discussed in the Combination Diets section.

CALCIUM

Epidemiologic surveys have suggested a relationship between reduced dietary calcium intake and hypertension. Several studies have demonstrated a small and inconsistent effect of calcium supplementation to lower BP. Again, this appears to be largely owing to the heterogeneity in human responses to calcium supplementation. Subgroup analyses of some of the larger studies suggest that those in whom dietary calcium intake is often reduced (African-Americans, the elderly) are more likely to demonstrate a reduction in BP with calcium supplementation than other groups in whom intake is higher. Because both subgroups are traditionally salt sensitive, we conducted a study of calcium supplementation in a group of normal and hypertensive subjects who had been previously categorized with respect to salt sensitivity of BP *(9)*. We found no significant effect of calcium supplementation on BP for the entire group. However, when the subjects were separated on the basis of salt-sensitivity status, we found a significant decrease in BP when the salt-sensitive subjects received calcium supplements and a significant increase in BP when calcium was given to the salt-resistant subjects. These findings suggested a reciprocal relationship between the effects of calcium and sodium on BP that was confirmed by the results of the DASH trial (*see* Combination Diets section).

OTHER DIETARY CONSTITUENTS

There is, at present, no convincing evidence to link alterations in magnesium intake with BP, and thus the JNC VI report did not advocate an increase in this mineral for the purpose of lowering BP *(1)*. Caffeine may raise BP acutely in caffeine-naïve individuals but does not appear to be a factor in the chronic elevation of BP. Moreover, there is no evidence that withdrawal of caffeine in habitual consumers produces a decrease in BP. Although some studies have suggested a beneficial effect of large amounts of omega-3 fatty acids in reducing BP, intolerance of these doses makes this an impractical approach for most individuals.

COMBINATION DIETS

A variety of studies have examined the effect of combined dietary approaches on BP as nonpharmacologic treatment of hypertension or for the prevention of hypertension in those at increased risk (high-normal BP). These combined studies have been fraught with problems resulting from recidivism, inadequate achievement of dietary goals, or relatively short duration. In general, it can be stated that weight loss appears to be the most effective single intervention as long as the weight loss can be maintained. There does not appear to be an additive benefit when potassium supplementation is combined with modest dietary salt restriction beyond that seen with salt restriction alone. However, in the DASH trial, when a specific diet incorporating modest salt restriction with an increase in fresh fruits and vegetables and low-fat dairy products (presumably increasing potassium, calcium, and magnesium intake) was followed, a significant reduction in BP was observed over the 8-wk study period *(8)*. This benefit appeared to be greatest among African-Americans and those with higher initial BP levels *(10)*. Another study examining multiple dietary changes was a subgroup of the Nurses Health Study II *(7)*, which compared the effects of supplemental potassium, calcium, magnesium, or all three minerals to placebo in normotensive nurses in whom dietary deficiencies of these minerals were documented. As previously mentioned, potassium supplementation alone, but not combination supplementation, lowered BP.

ALCOHOL

Alcohol consumption has been shown to have a biphasic effect on BP. Small amounts of alcohol appear to lower BP, presumably secondary to a vasodilator effect, but as alcohol consumption increases, BP rises. The dose-response characteristics vary from individual to individual and may be based on factors such as body surface area, gender, and race. The racial differences may be explicable, in part, by virtue of genetic differences in alcohol metabolism. The mechanism for the alcohol-induced increase in BP appears to be related to activation of, or increased responsiveness to, the SNS. This is manifested by an increase in cardiac output when more than one ounce of alcohol is consumed. Thus, a prudent recommendation to hypertensive subjects is to limit their daily alcohol consumption to no more than 2 oz (60 mL) of 100-proof spirits (or 2.5 oz of 80-proof whiskey), 24 oz (720 mL) of beer, or 10 oz (300 mL) of wine. For those hypertensive individuals in whom habitual alcohol consumption exceeds these levels, a reduction in intake may lower BP or make it easier to control.

CONCLUSION

A variety of dietary and lifestyle factors can influence BP. The ideal recommendation for individuals who are hypertensive or are at increased risk for its development are to maintain a body weight as close to ideal as possible; to consume a diet modest in salt content and enriched with fresh fruits, vegetables, and low-fat dairy products, and to consume no more than the recommended optimal amounts of alcohol.

REFERENCES

1. The Joint National Committee on Prevention, Detection, Evaluation, and Treatment of High Blood Pressure: the Sixth Report (JNC VI) (1997) *Arch Intern Med* 157:2413–2446.
2. Weinberger MH (1996) Salt sensitivity of blood pressure in humans. *Hypertension* 27 (Pt. 2):481–490.
3. Weinberger MH, Miller JZ, Luft FC, et al. (1986) Definitions and characteristics of sodium sensitivity and blood pressure resistance. *Hypertension* 8(Suppl. 2):127–134.
4. Weinberger MH, Fineberg NS (1991) Sodium and volume sensitivity of blood pressure: age and blood pressure change over time. *Hypertension* 18:67–71.

5. Weinberger MH, Stegner JE, Fineberg NS (1993) A comparison of two tests for the assessment of blood pressure responses to sodium. *Am J Hypertens* 6:179–184.
6. Whelton PK, He J, Cutler JA, et al. (1997) Effects of oral potassium on blood pressure. *JAMA* 277:1624–1632.
7. Sacks FM, Willett WC, Smith A et al. (1998) Effect on blood pressure of potassium, calcium, and magnesium in women with habitual low intake. *Hypertension* 31:131–138.
8. Appel LJ, Moore TJ, Obarzanek E, et al. (1997) The effect of dietary patterns on blood pressure: results from the Dietary Approaches to Stop Hypertension (DASH) Trial. *N Engl J Med* 336:1117–1124.
9. Weinberger MH, Wagner UL, Fineberg NS (1993) The blood pressure effects of calcium supplementation in humans of known sodium responsiveness. *Am J Hypertens* 6:799–805.
10. Svetkey LP, Simons-Morton D, Vollmer WM, et al. (1999) Effects of dietary patterns on blood pressure: subgroup analysis of the Dietary Approaches to Stop Hypertension (DASH) randomized clinical trial. *Arch Intern Med* 159:285–293.

6 Role of Stress in Development of Hypertension

Thomas G. Pickering, MD

The etiology of hypertension remains unknown, but one fact is clearly established: no single cause is responsible. High blood pressure (BP) is the end result of a number of factors, both genetic and environmental, that may be quantitatively and qualitatively different in different individuals. Furthermore, BP is distributed continuously in the population, with no clear separation between normal and raised BP. Any definition of hypertension is thus quite arbitrary.

For many years, it has been suspected that an adverse reaction between an individual and his or her environment may play a role in the development of hypertension, although conclusive evidence is still lacking. Four general approaches have been used to identify the potential role of such factors. The first is to study the effects of environmental stressors in epidemiologic studies, the second is to look for

From: *Hypertension Medicine*
Edited by: M. A. Weber © Humana Press Inc., Totowa, NJ

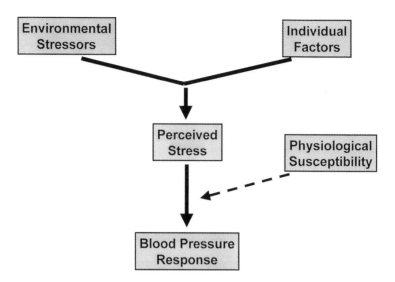

Fig. 6-1. Hypothetical interaction of factors that may contribute to behaviorally mediated hypertension.

personality differences between normotensive and hypertensive individuals, and the third is to examine the relevance of individual differences in susceptibility or reactivity to standardized stressors in a laboratory setting. Fourth, conducting animal experiments of stress-induced hypertension also is informative.

Figure 6-1 shows a convenient model for defining the roles of psychologic factors. There are three independent variables. First is the nature of the stressor, which is a characteristic of the environment. Second is the individual's perception of the stressor. This will depend on both the individual's personality and previous experience. What is stressful for one individual is not necessarily as stressful for another. The effects of the perceived stress on BP will in turn depend on the third factor, which is the individual's physiologic susceptibility. This may depend on genetic and environmental factors, e.g., a family history of hypertension, and the state of sodium balance. It seems reasonable to suppose that all three are important and that any effects on hypertension are likely to be interactive. This chapter discusses each of these three variables in turn, and also some of the possible physiologic mechanisms that might mediate their effects on BP.

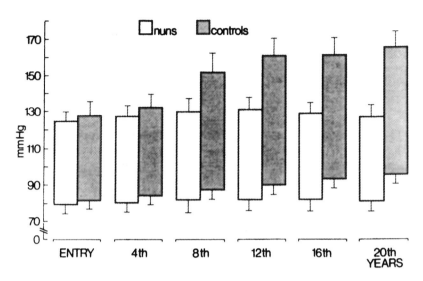

Fig. 6-2. BP in a group of Italian nuns living in a secluded order, compared with control subjects. Reproduced with permission from ref. *(123)*.

ENVIRONMENTAL SOURCES OF PSYCHOLOGIC STRESS

Although BP tends to rise with age, this is not an invariable phenomenon, and many societies have been described in which it remains low throughout life. The change with age appears to be determined culturally rather than genetically. A good example of this phenomenon is provided by a 30-yr observational study of Italian nuns living in a secluded order, reported by Timio *(1)*. The nuns were compared with a control group both at entry and after 30 yr. BPs were the same at entry, but by the end of the study were approx 30 mmHg higher in the control subjects than in the nuns (Fig. 6-2). The differences could not be explained by changes in body weight, by diet, or by childbearing. Timio *(1)* concluded that the differences were owing to the monastic and relatively stress-free environment in which the nuns were living.

The effects of social interactions on BP have also been studied in experimental animals. Figure 6-3, taken from a study by Hallbäck *(2)*, shows that in spontaneously hypertensive rats being reared in social isolation results in a lower BP than when rats are reared in colonies.

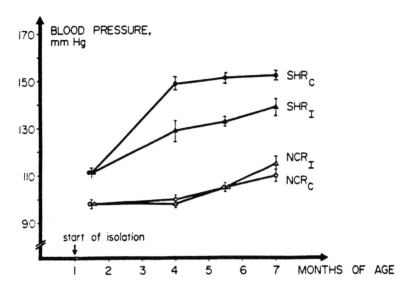

Fig. 6-3. In spontaneously hypertensive rats (SHR) social isolation (I) results in a lower BP than being reared in colonies (C). In normotensive control rats (NCR) this effect is not apparent. Reproduced with permission from ref. 2.

In normotensive control rats, however, this environmental difference is without effect.

A similar series of observations has been made in people who migrate from a stable traditional society to a Westernized one. Studies of the nomadic Samburo in Kenya *(3)* and of the bushmen of the Kalahari *(4)* have shown no increase in BP with age. Bushmen who abandon their traditional lifestyle, however, and become farm laborers, or even prisoners, have blood pressures 15 mmHg higher than the nomads *(5)*. And Samburo warriors who joined the Kenyan army also showed an increase in BP *(6)*. Numerous other studies could be quoted confirming the effects of acculturation from structured traditional societies to contemporary Western life, but the problem with nearly all of them is that it is difficult to know exactly what factors were responsible for the rise in BP. While stress may be one of them, there are also major dietary changes.

One of the most important of these studies is the Kenyan Luo migration study *(7)*, in which 355 subjects who migrated from rural villages to Nairobi were followed prospectively for 2 yr after they migrated, and were matched with a control group that stayed in the villages. Even as soon as 1 mo after migrating, the distribution curve

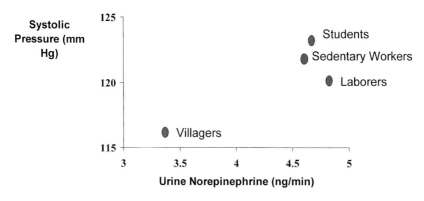

Fig. 6-4. Urine norepinephrine and BP in Samoans living a traditional village life or after acculturation to a Western lifestyle. Adapted from ref. *8.*

of BP had shifted to the right in the migrants. There were also significant increases in body weight, heart rate, and urinary sodium:potassium ratio. Over the 2-yr follow-up period, the differences in BP persisted, whereas those of body weight and heart rate did not. The authors suggested that the two factors responsible for the early increase in BP were sodium retention and increased sympathetic nervous system (SNS) activity occurring in response to the stress of migrating. As shown in Fig. 6-4, urine catecholamines tend to be higher in Westernized Samoans than in those living a traditional village life *(8)*.

Defense-Defeat Model

The defense reaction is a very fundamental response to challenges in the natural environment and consists of a generalized autonomic arousal, with an increase in BP and cardiac output, and increased blood flow to the skeletal muscles. Many years ago Brod et al. *(9)*, observed this reaction and found that these changes resemble those seen in young patients with borderline hypertension. It has been proposed by Neel *(10)* that "diseases of civilization" such as diabetes may occur as a result of natural selection, and that traits that confer red a survival advantage in primitive societies may be detrimental in modern society. Julius et al. *(11)* have extended this concept to include hypertension, and propose that a permanent hemodynamic pattern of the defense reaction would lead to hypertension and insulin resistance.

On the basis of an extensive series of studies of mice housed in colonies designed to promote social interaction and conflict, Henry et

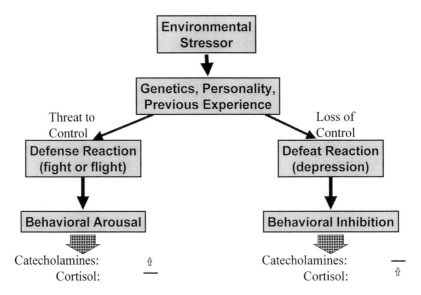

Fig. 6-5. The Defense-Defeat model of Henry *(12)*. The left-hand side shows the defense reaction, characterized by sympathetic activation, and the right-hand side the defeat reaction.

al. *(12)* proposed that two psychophysiologic patterns, which they referred to as the defense and defeat reactions (Fig. 6-5), might determine which individuals become hypertensive and which do not. Their mice were housed in population cages consisting of boxes connected by narrow tubing, wide enough to accommodate only one mouse at a time. This promotes the development of a social hierarchy, in which the dominant animals develop higher BPs than the subordinates. Subsequent work showed that the highest BPs (160 mmHg) were seen in subdominants attempting to achieve control; the BPs in stable unchallenged dominants was 145 mmHg, and in the subordinates 125 mmHg *(12,13)*. Similar results have been reported by Fokkema *(14)* in rats, in which the subdominant individuals again had the highest BPs *(14)*.

The subdominant animals are conceived as showing a chronic defense (fight or flight) reaction, characterized by activation of the SNS, whereas the subordinates exhibit the defeat reaction, in which there is activation of the pituitary-adrenal cortical axis.

Not surprisingly, comparable studies in humans are sparse. A situation analogous to the social interaction of mice in population cages was reported by D'Atri and Ostfeld *(15)*, who studied men confined to prison. The systolic blood pressure (SBP) of men who had lived for

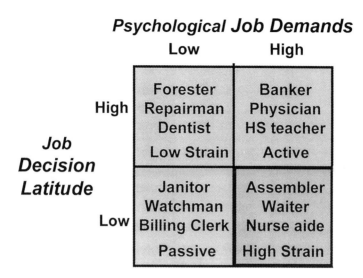

Fig. 6-6. The Demand-Control model of Karasek. The high-strain jobs are in the bottom right quadrant.

several months in a dormitory was 131 mmHg, whereas in men living in single-occupancy cells it was only 115 mmHg. Furthermore, transfer from a cell to a dormitory caused BP to increase, and vice versa *(16)*. These changes could not be attributed to diet, because all the prisoners ate the same food.

Demand-Control and Effort-Distress Models

The subdominant individuals in the social hierarchy of the Defense-Defeat model may be perceived as attempting to achieve control. Two models that originated in Sweden, and that closely resemble each other, have some similarity to the model of Henry et al. *(12)*. The first is the Job Strain model of Karasek and Theorell *(17)*, which was specifically designed to assess occupational stress. It has two orthogonal components: psychologic demands, and decision latitude, which is equivalent to control (Fig. 6-6). The most stressful (or "high-strain") jobs are those that are perceived to combine high demands and low decision latitude. This model has been used mainly for studying the effects of job strain on the development of coronary heart disease *(18,19)*, but, in my laboratory, we have shown that it may also be relevant in the development of hypertension. In the Cornell Worksite Study (originally

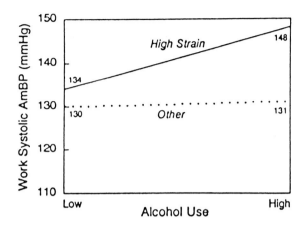

Fig. 6-7. Interaction between job strain and alcohol intake on BP. Reproduced with permission from ref. *21.*

a case-control study of men employed in a variety of jobs), we found that hypertensive individuals (the cases) were approximately three times as likely to be employed in high-strain jobs as the normotensive controls *(20)*. Exposure to job strain was also associated with an increased left ventricular mass, which would be consistent with the effects of a sustained elevation in BP. Subjects in high-strain jobs also had higher ambulatory BP *(21)*. Interestingly, this elevation in BP was seen not only during working hours but also while at home and during sleep. An important aspect of the results is that neither of the two components of job strain—demands and perceived control—were individually associated with any changes in BP; only the interaction of high demands and low control had an effect.

Two other interactive effects that were observed in our study are worth noting. The first was with alcohol intake. The highest BPs were observed in subjects who were in high-strain jobs and drank regularly (Fig. 6-7). However, alcohol intake had no discernible effect on BP in subjects with low-strain jobs. In the present context, alcohol intake may be regarded as another environmental pressor agent, whose intake is perhaps related to personality. The second interactive effect was with age. The effects of job strain on BP were much greater in older than in younger subjects. This finding could have at least two explanations: first, the effects are cumulative over many years, and, second, the physiological susceptibility of the older subjects might be greater. In a 3-yr follow-up of 195 men in the Cornell Worksite Study *(22),* we found that the cross-sectional relationships between job strain and BP were virtually identical 3 yr apart, although nearly half of the men had changed their job strain status. In addition, men who remained in high-strain jobs over the 3 yr had BPs at work and at home that were on average 11/7 mmHg higher than those in men in non-high-strain jobs at both times, and men who changed from a high-strain to a non-high-strain job showed a decrease of 5/3 mmHg. There was a small but insignificant increase in men who went from a non-high-strain to a high-strain job. These results strongly support the idea that the previously observed association between job strain and BP is causal.

These findings have received some support from other studies. Theorell et al. *(23)* studied 161 men with borderline hypertension with ambulatory monitoring and found that job strain (expressed by the ratio between psychologic demands and control) was significantly related to diastolic pressure during work and at night. Van Egeren *(24)* studied 11 subjects with high-strain jobs and 26 with low-strain jobs, and found higher BPs in both groups during work and while at home in the former. There was a less clearcut tendency for sleep BPs to be higher as well. A third study, by Light et al. *(25),* performed in 129 healthy young men and women found that job strain was associated with higher work BPs in men, but not in women.

A closely related model is the effort-distress model of Frankenhaueser *(26).* This also has two orthogonal components (*see* Fig. 6-5), which are termed *effort* and *distress*. Effort corresponds to demands in the job strain model, and distress to control. Effort is conceived as arousing the SNS, and distress the adrenocortical system. A typical example of this type of approach is provided by a study conducted by Lundberg and Frankenhaueser *(27)* in which normal subjects performed two tasks. The first was a monotonous vigilance task that was perceived to induce effort and distress, and the second was a more enjoyable self-paced reaction-time talk, which required effort but without distress. During the vigilance task, urinary excretion of both epinephrine and cortisol increased, whereas during the reaction-time task only epinephrine increased. This model has not yet been related to sustained hypertension, but it is relevant because epinephrine and cortisol are both potential pressor hormones.

Models of Socioecologic Stress

The studies of the effects of acculturation, which I have briefly reviewed, suggest that there is something about modern society that tends to elevate BP. Waldron et al. *(28)* pooled data from 84 different societies and concluded that higher BPs were associated with increasing emphasis on a market economy, increased economy competition, and decreased family ties. These associations appeared to be independent of salt intake, and in men, of obesity.

In another series of studies, Dressler and colleagues *(29–31)* have developed the concept of "lifestyle incongruity," which is defined as the extent to which a high status style of life exceeds an individual's occupational class. Its evaluation is relatively objective and is based on a match between occupation and income, on the one hand, and possession of material goods, on the other. Lifestyle incongruity has been found to be related to BP not only in developing countries *(29–31)* but also in African Americans in the United States *(32)*.

A somewhat similar approach has been used by James et al. *(33)*, who developed the concept of John Henryism to investigate the effects of socioecologic stress in African Americans. An individual who scores high on the John Henryism scale is one who believes that he can control environmental stressors through a combination of hard work and determination. In their first study, James et al. *(33)* found that men who scored below the sample median on education but above the median on John Henryism had higher BPs than men who scored above the median on both measures. In a subsequent study *(34)*, they found that men who had achieved a relatively high level of job success and scored high on John Henryism had higher diastolic pressures than men with similar levels of job success and low John Henryism. Another psychosocial factor that contributed to higher BPs in the more successful men was the perception that being African American had hindered their chances of success.

The effects of socioecologic stress on BP in African Americans *(32)* have also been documented in a study by Harburg et al. *(35)*. They performed a population survey of BP in different neighborhoods of Detroit, which were defined as either high stress or low stress according to the socioeconomic status of the inhabitants (defined by variables such as income, home ownership, and education) and instability variables (e.g., crime rate and marital instability). The highest BPs were seen in African-American males under the age of 40 living in high-stress neighborhoods; African-American and Caucasian males living in low-stress neighborhoods had similar BPs. More recent research conducted in U.S. cities has provided further evidence for a "neighborhood" effect on BP (people living in poorer neighborhoods have higher

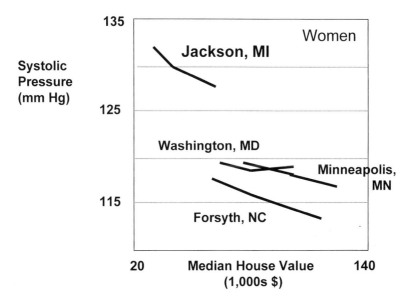

Fig. 6-8. The relationships between SBP and residential neighborhood (expressed as median house value) in women living in four US cities. The women in Jackson were predominantly African American, whereas those in the other three cities were Caucasian. Adapted from ref. *36*.

BP; *see* Fig. 6-8) *(36)*, which is related to psychosocial factors independently of the traditional environmental influences *(35,37)*.

Role of Genetic Factors and Race

As mentioned, hypertension evolves through an interaction of individual and environmental factors. Such individual factors are likely to be at least in part genetic. Thus, the mice in Henry et al.'s studies *(12)* were of a certain strain, and experiments in other strains have not been found to replicate the hypertension *(38,39)*. A good example of the role of genetic factors is provided by a study conducted by Henry et al. *(39)* in different strains of rats, using a design similar to the studies conducted previously in mice, in which social interaction raised BP. When subjected to the same protocol, there was no effect on BP in Wistar-Kyoto hyperactive rats, a modest increase in Sprague-Dawley rats, and a much more marked increase in Long-Evans rats.

Another animal model of stress-induced hypertension is the border-line hypertensive rat, which is a cross between the spontaneously hyper-tensive rat and the normotensive Wistar-Kyoto rat. When reared in a benign environment, the borderline hypertensive rat remains normoten-sive, but if subjected to continued environmental stress or a high-salt diet, it becomes hypertensive *(40)*.

In the United States, African Americans bear a greater burden of cardiovascular disease than Caucasians, and the prevalence of hyperten-sion is approximately double. This difference, however, is much greater in the United States than in other countries. Several studies have docu-mented that hypertension was traditionally relatively rare in Africa, with the exception of the big cities *(41)*. It is also clearly established in longitudinal studies conducted mostly in Africa (described above) that moving from village to city life is associated with an increase in BP, which suggests that environmental factors are predominantly responsible. A major unresolved issue is whether the higher prevalence of hypertension seen in African Americans in the United States com-pared with Caucasians is genetic or environmental. So far, attempts to identify genes or physiologic processes that distinguish "African-American hypertension" from "Caucasian hypertension" have proved disappointing *(41)*. Several studies have found that African Americans with darker skin have higher BPs than those with light skin, which could be explained by either genetic or cultural factors. Although there have been reports of racial differences in physiologic regulatory processes such as sodium sensitivity, the renin-angiotensin system, and kallikrein, there is no evidence that these differences, which are usually subtle, are causally related to the differing prevalence of hypertension *(41)*.

Considerable attention is currently being paid to identifying racial differences in genes that contribute to the development of hypertension, or that increase the susceptibility to environmental factors. An example is the angiotensinogen gene, in which a mutant allele has been reported to be related to BP in Caucasians *(42)*, and which has been found to occur much more frequently in African Americans in the United States and Nigeria *(43)*. It cannot, however, be assumed that this explains the higher prevalence of hypertension in African Americans, because within African Americans there is no correlation between the presence of the mutant allele and BP *(44)*. It is possible that there are gene-environment interactions that predispose African Americans to the pressor effects of environmental stimuli, but these are difficult to demonstrate in human studies, because they require evaluation of the expression of a genotype in different environments. The problem is compounded by the fact that

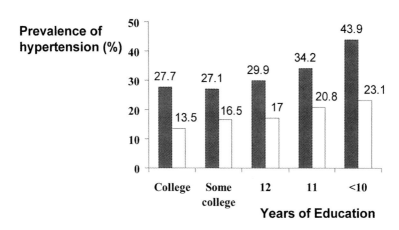

Fig. 6-9. Prevalence of hypertension in U.S. African American (■) and Caucasian (□) subjects according to years of education. Data from ref. *45.*

hypertension is almost certainly polygenic, so that the presence or absence of a particular allele is unlikely to account for more than a small effect on BP.

Presently, the higher prevalence of hypertension in African Americans in the United States can best be explained by environmental factors. The prevalence of hypertension is inversely proportional to educational status, particularly in African Americans *(45)* (Fig. 6-9). A proportion of the racial differential can be explained by obesity (particularly in African-American women) and mineral intake, but potentially stronger and also less well-defined factors are psychosocial stress and racism. The low prevalence of hypertension in rural Africa has already been referred to, and there are populations in which an African-American–Caucasian BP difference is absent or very small. One example is Cuba *(46)*, and another is factory workers in England *(47)*. In both populations it was concluded that the similarities of social class between the ethnic groups might account for the similarity in BPs. In the United States, there is such a strong association between race and socioeconomic status that it is quite difficult to separate the two.

INDIVIDUAL PSYCHOLOGIC FACTORS AND PERCEPTION OF STRESS

Two types of factors relevant to individual differences in the way in which potential stressors are perceived are the individual's personality, which is relatively immutable, and the individual's previous experience or learning, which obviously is not. Because there is no evidence that hypertension is a learned behavior pattern (although this remains an interesting possibility), my discussion is restricted to personality variables.

Personality Variables and Hypertension

The idea that there is a "hypertensive personality" has been mooted for many years, but is still unsettled. The concept originated with Alexander (48), who proposed that the hypertensive individual experiences repressed hostility, or "anger-in," which is channeled into the autonomic nervous system, resulting in increased BP. This theory has been reviewed by Shapiro (49). A potential problem with such studies is that characteristics such as anger and anxiety, which are frequently associated with hypertension, may be a consequence of making the diagnosis (a "labeling" phenomenon) rather than being etiologic factors, and there is always a problem of knowing what constitutes an appropriate control group. A more reliable method may be to study a randomly selected population. One such study was conducted by Harburg et al. (35), who found that in men, anger-in was correlated with BP. Two other personality variables that have been reported to be characteristic of hypertensive individuals are submissiveness (50) and alexithymia, which has been defined as an inappropriate affect, difficulty in expressing emotions, and an absence of fantasies. There is limited evidence for both (reviewed in ref. 51).

Type A Behavior Pattern, Anger, and Hostility

Several related personality characteristics have been investigated with regard to hypertension, which all relate to hostility and aggression. One of the earlier studies reporting this phenomenon was conducted by Wolf and Wolff (52), who evaluated personality measures using both interviews and questionnaires in 103 hypertensive patients, who were compared with 150 patients with allergies and 61 normotensive hospitalized patients. They concluded that the hypertensive patients had restrained aggression and excess inner tension. A more recent example of such a finding comes from a study by Perini et al. (53), who compared young subjects with borderline hypertension with age-matched normotensive controls with and without a family history of hypertension. The hypertensive patients showed less externalized aggression, more internalized aggression, and more submissiveness. They also demonstrated evidence of increased SNS activity, such as faster heart rates and higher plasma catecholamines. Although many other studies have reported varying degrees of association between inhibited aggression and BP (reviewed in ref. *51*), others have reported negative or inconsistent results.

The Type A behavior pattern, which is generally regarded as being at least in part a personality variable, has been most closely related to coronary heart disease. Most studies have not found any close relationship with hypertension *(54)*, perhaps because most of them used only one or two BP measurements. An example was the Western Collaborative Group Study, in which 3524 men were followed for 8 yr *(55)*. In their study, Irvine et al. *(54)* compared the prevalence of type A in 109 untreated hypertensive subjects and 109 demographically matched control subjects, whose BP was measured five times over 5 mo. Type A behavior was assessed by the structured interview and was significantly more prevalent in the hypertensive subjects (78%) than in the normotensive subjects (60%). Hostility, which is now considered to be one of the most important components of coronary-prone behavior *(56)*, was also higher in the hypertensive subjects.

Everson et al. *(57)* found that anger (whether expressed or repressed) is associated with an increased risk of developing hypertension over a 4-yr follow-up period. Hostility has also been shown to have an interactive effect with occupational stress on BP, at least over the short term. In a study of paramedics who wore an ambulatory BP monitor during a workday, Jamner et al. *(58)* found that subjects who scored high on hostility and defensiveness demonstrated higher diastolic pressures while in the hospital, but not while waiting for a call at the ambulance station.

Anxiety and Panic Disorder

Associations between anxiety and depression with hypertension and cardiovascular morbidity have been observed in cross-sectional studies *(59–62)*. Panic disorders also occur more commonly in hypertensive than in normotensive individuals, although whether the panic disorder precedes or follows the hypertension is unknown *(62,63)*. One prospective study has found that individuals who report high levels of symptoms of anxiety or depression are at increased risk of hypertension 9 yr later *(64)*.

INDIVIDUAL DIFFERENCES IN SUSCEPTIBILITY TO PSYCHOLOGIC FACTORS

The effects that a given level of perceived stress will have on the cardiovascular system will depend to some extent on the physiologic susceptibility of the individual. In other words, for a given intensity of a stressor, some individuals will be more reactive than others. In practice, it may be difficult to separate the physiologic and psychologic components of reactivity, but conceptually this distinction is important. Of all the components of the potential interactions between stress and BP, reactivity has received much more attention than any other, and perhaps more than it deserves.

Reactivity Hypothesis

In its simplest form, the reactivity hypothesis states that individuals who show increased cardiovascular reactivity to psychologically stressful stimuli are at increased risk of developing cardiovascular disease. The latter is often taken to include hypertension and coronary heart disease as if they were a single entity, which of course they are not. Two forms of the hypothesis as it relates to hypertension have been proposed: in one, the "Recurrent Activation Model," the response to laboratory tests, is assumed to be correlated with intermittent pressor responses to stress occurring in everyday life, whereas in the other, the "Prevailing State Model," the laboratory response predicts the average level of BP *(65)*. It has also been suggested that stressors initially produce transient elevations in BP by neurohormonal mechanisms, and that these elevations may in turn induce structural changes in the arterial wall, which eventually results in a sustained increase in vascular resistance and hence BP *(66)*. This mechanism is usually thought to be elicited by stimuli that are psychologically stressful, but there is no clear reason why it should not also apply to physically stressful stimuli such as exercise.

It must be admitted, however, that direct evidence in support of this mechanism is limited. It has recently been demonstrated, e.g., that neurogenically produced pressor episodes do not on their own lead to any sustained increase in the basal BP level, although they can produce left ventricular hypertrophy *(67)*. And exercise training, which certainly produces intermittent neurogenically mediated pressor episodes, results in a reduction in the resting BP level *(68)*.

Some of the criteria that this hypothesis must satisfy have been reviewed elsewhere *(69)*. First, the degree of reactivity for an individual subject should be stable over time; second, it should, to some extent, be generalizable from one type of challenge to another; third, it should be generalizable from the laboratory to the stresses of everyday life; and fourth, reactivity should be an independent predictor of disease.

The test-retest reliability of BP changes measured during reactivity testing is not very good, with correlation coefficients ranging from about 0.4 to 0.7 *(65,70–73)*. Surprisingly, few studies have systematically examined the extent to which an individual subject's response to one task will predict his or her response to another. Parati et al. *(74)* found that the responses to two predominantly mental tasks (mental arithmetic and mirror drawing) were quite well correlated with each other ($r =$ 0.78, $p<0.01$), and also the response to two predominantly physical tasks (isometric exercise and the cold pressor test), but correlations between the responses to the mental and physical tasks were not significant. Fredrikson et al. *(75)* examined the correlation between the change scores for four tasks: an attentional demands task, mental arithmetic, the cold pressor test, and isometric exercise. The only significant correlation for systolic pressure was between mental arithmetic and isometric exercise in normotensive subjects; for hypertensive subjects none of the correlations was significant. By contrast, Turner et al. *(76)* found significant correlations between four tasks (two involving speech and two mental arithmetic) ranging from 0.62 to 0.80 for systolic pressure, and considerably lower for diastolic. These results suggest that there is limited evidence for generalizability of reactivity across dissimilar tasks, and that characterizing an individual as being generally "hyper-reactive" has little validity at the present time.

Physiologic and Demographic Factors Affecting Reactivity

Several studies have compared BP reactivity in normotensive and hypertensive subjects. We reviewed a selection of these that gave adequate details of the actual BP levels and statsistical comparison *(69)*. The two most extensively studied tests have been mental arithmetic and the cold pressor test. We concluded that there is a tendency for hypertensive subjects to show increased reactivity to behavioral, but not physical tasks. A more formal meta-analysis was undertaken by Fredrikson and Matthews *(77)*. They concluded that patients with essential hypertension (with BPs of at least 165/95 mmHg) showed an

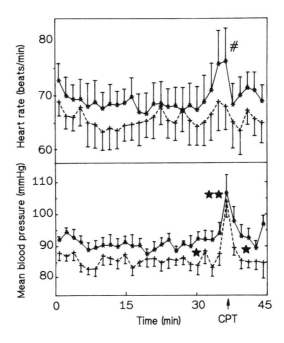

Fig. 6-10. Mean BP and heart rate in an informed (solid lines) and uninformed group (dotted lines) at rest and during a cold pressor test (CPT). # and * indicate significant group differences (*$p < 0.05$; **$p < 0.01$). Reproduced with permission from ref. 79.

exaggerated SBP response to passive stressors (including the cold pressor test), in comparison to normotensive controls, although this was seen in only 31 of 63 studies. Overall, borderline hypertensive subjects showed a significantly greater response to active stressors (in 8 of 25 individual studies).

The only population-based study, conducted in 169 men and 120 women by Julius et al. *(78)* in Tecumseh, Michigan, did not find any correlation between reactivity to mental arithmetic or isometric exercise and the resting level of BP. They pointed out that one reason for the discrepancy between their findings and those of other studies comparing normotensive and hypertensive subjects was that their subjects were not necessarily aware of which diagnostic group they were in, whereas in most other studies they were. The importance of this is that it has been shown by Rostrup and Ekeberg *(79)* that labeling subjects as hypertensive increases their BP reactivity (Fig. 6-10).

Several studies have examined the influence of family history of hypertension on reactivity, and many have dealt with children. The meta-analysis by Fredrikson and Matthews *(77)* concluded that 13 of 30 studies demonstrated an increased BP or heart rate reactivity in association with a positive family history, and that overall this effect was significant in comparison with subjects without a family history. The difference was more reliable for active than passive tasks. However, one study reported that the BP response to dynamic exercise was exaggerated in subjects with a family history of hypertension in comparison to those without one *(80)*. A more recent study of normotensive young adults found that subjects with a positive family history (either one or both parents hypertensive) had higher baseline BPs (measured both in the laboratory and during ambulatory monitoring) but did not show an exaggerated BP response to four different stressors *(81)*. The Tecumseh study did not find any association between BP reactivity and family history *(78)*.

Psychologic Factors Influencing Differences in Reactivity

As already reviewed, attempts to relate a specific personality type with hypertension have been, on the whole, disappointing. The picture is a little better with BP reactivity: in a meta-analysis of 71 studies comparing cardiovascular reactivity in type A and type B individuals, Harbin *(82)* concluded that type A men showed a consistently greater reactivity of systolic (but not diastolic) pressure and heart rate to cognitive challenges. In parallel with these findings, it has also been reported that men and women scoring high on tests of hostility have a larger BP reactivity when attempting a frustrating task *(83)*.

With mental challenge tasks requiring an active response by the subject, it is to be expected that the subject's attitude to the task will affect the response. This has been confirmed in a study by Smith et al. *(84)*, who found that the increase in BP occurring during talking is much greater if the person who is talking is trying to persuade another person to change his or her opinion about something, compared to just talking alone.

Does Reactivity Measured in the Laboratory Predict BP Changes During Everyday Life?

The rationale generally proposed for the use of laboratory tests of cardiovascular reactivity is that an individual's response to such a test may predict how he or she will respond to stressful situations in real life. Until quite recently, it has not been possible to test this assumption, but with the introduction of ambulatory monitoring techniques it can now be attempted.

Four studies have compared the response to laboratory stressors with BP variability measured with the intra-arterial technique of ambulatory monitoring *(85–88)*. Several studies have used noninvasive ambulatory monitoring techniques *(70,73)*. Because BP is recorded intermittently rather than continuously by this technique, the characterization of BP variability and reactivity is inevitably less precise than with intra-arterial monitoring. All these studies found very low or absent correlations between BP reactivity (measured as change scores) and ambulatory BP.

Viewed as a whole, these studies suggest that if there is an association between reactivity measured in the laboratory and the BP variability or reactivity of daily life, it is rather weak, or is obscured by the problems of measurement error. Furthermore, it appears to be quite nonspecific; that is, it can be demonstrated equally well (or poorly) with laboratory challenges both with and without a strong behavioral component. The simplest explanation of the few positive findings is that there are significant interindividual differences in BP variability that may be detected both by laboratory testing and by ambulatory monitoring. As they stand, the results of these studies provide little evidence that the type of reactivity testing commonly used in the laboratory is an ecologically valid representation of the stresses of everyday life. Yet, the assumption of such validity is the basis for much of the work being done in this field. It seems clear that a great deal of research must be done in this area before conclusions can be drawn.

In the Tecumseh population study *(78)* of 169 men and 120 women, two indices of reactivity (mental arithmetic and isometric exercise) were related to two measures of target organ damage (left ventricular mass and minimal forearm vascular resistance). Subjects classified as hyperreactors to mental arithmetic did not show any greater signs of vascular damage than the others.

Prognostic Significance of BP Reactivity

BP is not the only factor that can be used to predict hypertension. A family history of hypertension is also of major importance. In Thomas's *(89)* prospective precursors study of medical students at Johns Hopkins University, it was found that subjects who had two hypertensive parents and a high initial clinical systolic pressure (above 125 mmHg) were 12.6 times as likely to become hypertensive over a 30-yr follow-up period as subjects without these risk factors. The study also found that reactivity to the cold pressor test failed to predict future hypertension, but a subsequent analysis, published in 1989, and using more sophisticated statistical techniques *(90)*, found that after adjusting for age, obesity, baseline BP, and smoking, an exaggerated response to the cold pressor test did predict the development of hypertension after an interval of 20 yr. Without these adjustments there was still no association, however. Other prospective studies have reported mixed results, mostly negative *(91–94)*.

Two studies have reported that the reactivity to mental arithmetic, which has more of a psychologic component than the cold pressor test, does predict future BP. The first, by Falkner et al. *(95)*, followed 80 adolescents with borderline hypertension for up to 5 yr. The development of hypertension was predicted both by a positive family history and by an exaggerated BP response to mental arithmetic. The relative importance of the two was not evaluated. The second study, by Borghi et al. *(96)*, reported that subjects with a positive family history and borderline hypertension showed an increased reactivity to both behavioral and physical challenges, and that they were more likely to become hypertensive over a 5-yr period. Overall, the evidence that BP reactivity is an independent predictor of future BP status is unconvincing.

PHYSIOLOGIC MECHANISMS THAT MIGHT MEDIATE STRESS-INDUCED HYPERTENSION

Since the evidence that chronic stress contributes to the development of hypertension is not yet widely accepted, it is not surprising that relatively little is known about the underlying physiological mechanisms. It can be assumed that the brain is the prime mover, but there are in principle two types of mechanism that could be involved. First, there might be a direct effect, for example via stress leading to increased activity of the sympathetic nervous system. Second, there might be an indirect effect such as a stress-induced increase in sodium intake.

Sympathetic Nervous System

For any postulated mechanism linking the brain and BP, the autonomic nervous system is the primary candidate. There is increasing evidence for a subtle overactivity of the SNS in the early stages of essential hypertension *(97,98)*, which raises the question, What is the origin of such overactivity? Although it may well be genetic, it is equally plausible that environmental stressors play a role. It is relatively easy to show that stress can cause a transient elevation in BP. However, this is of doubtful relevance to sustained hypertension, which appears to be primarily a disorder of the tonic regulation of BP rather than of its short-term variability. It is therefore appropriate to examine the time course of the effects of stress on BP, and the mechanisms by which the cardiovascular effects of a stressor may outlast the stimulus.

The SNS is normally regarded as being primarily responsible for the short-term regulation of BP, and other mechanisms such as the role of the kidney *(99)* or structural changes in the resistance vessels *(66,100)* regulate the tonic level. This poses a problem for those who believe that stress may influence the development of hypertension. How is it that transient increases of sympathetic activity can lead to a sustained increase in BP? There are in fact a number of possible mechanisms.

A series of pharmacologic studies, predominantly conducted by Majewski et al. *(101,102)*, have identified a potential mechanism by which adrenaline (epinephrine) might mediate stress-linked hypertension. It has been shown by both in vitro and in vivo studies that infusion of epinephrine in low doses (equivalent to the levels seen during naturally occurring stress) can enhance norepinephrine release from sympathetic nerve terminals *(102)*. This effect is thought to be mediated by prejunctional β_2 receptors, because it can be blocked by β-blocking agents. Furthermore, circulating epinephrine may be taken up by the sympathetic nerve terminals, stored with norepinephrine as a cotransmitter, and released with it during sympathetic nerve stimulation. There are two crucial components to this mechanism that make it relevant to stress-induced hypertension. First, the release, reuptake, and presynaptic facilitation of norepinephrine release acts as a positive feedback loop. Second, whereas the half-life of epinephrine in the plasma is only a few minutes, for epinephrine stored in the sympathetic nerves it may be many hours, providing the potential for producing sustained effects.

Human studies have also implicated this mechanism. An acute infusion of epinephrine produces a tachycardia, with an increased systolic and slightly decreased diastolic pressure. When the infusion is terminated, the plasma epinephrine level rapidly returns to normal, although the tachycardia and increased systolic pressure persist for an hour or two, and diastolic pressure rises to above baseline levels *(103)*. The most impressive demonstration of the delayed pressor effect of epinephrine was provided in a study conducted by Blankenstijn et al. *(104),* who infused epinephrine, norepinephrine, or dextrose for 6 h in normal volunteers, and monitored the effects on BP over the next 26 h using intra-arterial monitoring. The infusion was given between 10:00 AM and 4:00 PM, and the subjects were in bed from midnight to 8:00 AM. Arterial pressure was at first reduced by the epinephrine, but by the end of the infusion was above the baseline value, and remained elevated throughout the night. Infusion of norepinephrine produced an initial elevation in pressure, but no sustained effects. The pressor effect of epinephrine was most marked during periods of increased sympathetic activity, e.g., when the subjects were active, and not when they were at rest. The increased BP following epinephrine infusion was not accompanied by any changes in heart rate. However, a more direct test of the epinephrine hypothesis was recently reported by Goldstein et al. *(105),* who found that local infusion of epinephrine does not enhance norepinephrine release. This casts doubt on the proposed mechanism of this phenomenon.

Another mechanism is via the renal sympathetic nerves, which promote sodium retention and renin release as well as increase renal vascular resistance. DiBona et al. *(106)* have shown that air-jet stress leads to an increased activity in the renal sympathetic nerves, and that enhanced sympathetic responsiveness to air-jet stress cosegregates with arterial pressure in a back-cross experiment between the borderline hypertensive and the Wistar-Kyoto rat strains *(107).* The SNS may also influence the permeability of vascular smooth muscle cells to sodium *(108),* and there may also be trophic effects an cardiac and vascular muscle *(109).*

Renin-Angiotensin System

Several studies have implicated the renin-angiotensin system in the development of stress-induced hypertension, an effect that could be mediated by the influence of sympathetic nerves on renin release. Thus, in the borderline hypertensive rat, 10 d of air-jet stress can induce sustained hypertension, but this is prevented by pretreatment with captopril *(40).* Plasma catecholamines were unaffected by either the exposure to stress or treatment with captopril, suggesting that the SNS was not the prime mover in this model of hypertension. Plasma renin activity was increased in Henry's mice subjected to chronic social stress, and captopril also lowered the BP *(110)*.

Endogenous Opioid System

There has recently been a lot of interest in the possibility that endogenous opioids may modulate the effects of stress on BP, stemming from human studies using opioid antagonists such as naloxone and naltrexone. It has been shown that pretreatment with these agents can increase the BP, catecholamine, and glucocorticoid response to psychologic stress *(111,112)*. Young adults who are presumed to be at low risk for future hypertension (e.g., those who have a low casual pressure or who are physically fit) show a more developed opioid inhibition of the stress response or reactivity than those at higher risk. And a study using ambulatory monitoring to evaluate the effects of naturally occurring stress found that opioid blockade had no effect on the resting pressure, but did enhance the BP response during periods of stress *(112)*.

Structural Changes in the Heart and Resistance Vessels

It is well recognized that in the majority of patients with sustained hypertension, peripheral resistance is increased. That this is not wholly attributable to neurohumoral influences has been argued most forcefully by Folkow *(66)*, on the basis of both anatomical and functional studies. Thus, even during maximal vasodilation such as occurs following a period of ischemia, hypertensive subjects still show an increased resistance to blood flow *(66)*. These changes are largely owing to medial hypertrophy, and can be regarded as an adaptive process in the presence of increased pressure and for flow. The extent to which stress can produce such changes is unclear, but there is evidence that the growth of vascular smooth muscle can be influenced by a number of stress-related factors, including angiotensin, catecholamines, and corticosteroids *(100)*.

Sodium Retention and the Kidney

The case for the dominant role of the kidneys in the long-term regulation of BP has been proposed by Guyton *(99)* on the basis of the phenomenon of pressure natriuresis: an increase in arterial pressure (by any mechanism) causes increased sodium and water excretion, which will tend to lower the blood volume and hence also the pressure.

Sustained hypertension occurs only when the set point of the renal-volume mechanism for pressure control is reset to a higher level of pressure. This could occur either because of sodium and volume retention or because of a change occurring in the kidney (e.g., an increase in prerenal resistance).

There is increasing evidence from animal experiments that environmental stress can cause sodium retention mediated via renal sympathetic nerve activity *(113,114)*. The same phenomenon has also been described in humans *(115)*. In addition, mental stress results in a greater increase in BP in salt-sensitive than in salt-resistant subjects *(116)*, which would be consistent with the observation of Anderson et al. *(114)* that experimental hypertension is more readily produced when environmental stress is combined with a high salt intake.

In the borderline hypertensive rat, chronic exposure to conflict stress for 2 h a day can lead to sustained hypertension *(117)*. In the early stages of this process, however, exposure to the conflict situation produces only a slight increase in BP. Analysis of the hemodynamic pattern shows that there is a profound renal and mesenteric vasoconstriction that is offset by skeletal muscle vasodilation *(118)*. An analogous observation by Hollenberg et al. *(119)* showed that the effects of a behavioral challenge on renal blood flow lasted much longer than the effects on BP.

Role of Glucocorticoids

An important physiologic component of Frankenhaeuser's *(26)* Effort-Distress model is the increase of cortisol that occurs in the "high effort-high distress" situation. Although most of the attention has been given to the SNS as the prime mediator of stress-induced increases in BP, there is also evidence to suggest that glucocorticoids may be involved. The effects of glucocorticoids on BP are complex and not well understood, although there is agreement that they tend to have a pressor effect, as reviewed recently by Whitworth *(120)*. They may also increase the reactivity to adrenergic stimulation, particularly to epinephrine *(121)*, although this effect is less certain in humans *(120)*. Whitworth et al. *(122)* gave four different synthetic steroids to normal subjects for 5 d, at doses that had similar glucocorticoid activity, but that had little or no mineralocorticoid effect. All four raised BP without any accompanying sodium retention. The effects on the diurnal profile of BP were not evaluated; it might be expected that the increase in BP would be particularly pronounced at night.

CONCLUSION

Attempts to find a single cause of hypertension have proven universally frustrating. This applies no less to psychologic than to physiologic
causes. It thus seems plausible that hypertension may be the result of
the interaction of a variety of factors, whose contribution may vary in
different individuals. It is well established that BP is socially and
culturally determined, but the precise factors responsible for group
and individual differences remain elusive. Although dietary habits are
undoubtedly important, they cannot explain the observed differences,
and there is a growing body of evidence to suggest that psychosocial
stressors also play a role. Several different factors and models to explain
their effects have been proposed, and a common feature to all is an
element of discord between the individual and his or her social setting.
In the job strain, or demand-control model, there is the conflict between
demands and control. Thus, most of those models rely on an interaction
of two or more factors to produce hypertension, rather than by any
one factor acting in its own. Because human behavior is infinitely
complex, these models are not mutually exclusive. For example, we
should not necessarily expect a model that predicts hypertension in
African Americans living in Detroit to work in Italian nuns living in
a convent.

The role of individual factors must also be acknowledged to be
important. Personality variables have been the subject of much attention.
Repressed anger and submissiveness are the two that are most frequently
invoked, but the findings are quite mixed. In part, this may be a measurement issue, because of the difficulties in quantifying something as
nebulous as personality, but it may also mean that we should be focusing
on subsets of patients (e.g., those with high renin levels) in whom
personality variables contribute to BP, perhaps in conjunction with
environmental stressors.

The most extensively studied individual factor is BP reactivity, but
despite an enormous amount of research on the subject, the relevance
of increased cardiovascular reactivity to the development and consequences of hypertension remains unclear. There is no consensus as to
which test should be used to define reactivity, and the generalization
of an individual's responses from one test to another cannot be assumed.
Hypertensive subjects tend to show greater reactivity than normotensive
subjects, particularly to behavioral challenges, but this may be a consequence rather than a cause of the hypertension. The reactivity hypothesis
requires that reactivity predict the development of hypertension.

Attempts to demonstrate this have met with varying success, and in some of the reportedly positive studies, it has not been established that reactivity is independent of other predictors. These considerations lead us to conclude that on the basis of present evidence, increased BP reactivity to behavioral stimuli is unlikely to play a primary role in the development of hypertension. The evidence that chronic exposure to environmental stressors can accelerate the development of hypertension, on the other hand, is quite encouraging. Whether or not such stressors produce a more pronounced effect in individuals who have a particular personality type, or who are hyperactive, remains unclear, but may prove to be a productive area for future research.

REFERENCES

1. Timio M (1997) Blood pressure trend and psychosocial factors: the case of the nuns in a secluded order. *Acta Physiol Scand Suppl* 640:137.
2. Hallback M (1975) Consequence of social isolation on blood pressure, cardiovascular reactivity and design in spontaneously hypertensive rats. *Acta Physiol Scand* 93:455.
3. Shaper AG (1962) Cardiovascular studies in the Samburo tribe of Northern Kenya. *Am Heart J* 63:437.
4. Kaminer B, Lutz W (1968) Blood pressures in Kalahari bushmen. *Circulation* 22:289.
5. Truswell AS, Kennelly BM, Hansen JD, et al. (1972) Blood pressures of Kung bushmen in Northern Botswana. *Am Heart J* 84:5.
6. Shaper AG, Leonard PJ, Jones KW, et al. (1969) Environmental effects on the body build, blood pressure and blood chemistry of nomadic warriors serving in the army in Kenya. *East Afr Med J* 46:282.
7. Poulter NR, Khaw KT, Hopwood BE, et al. (1990) The Kenyan Luo migration study: observations on the initiation of a rise in blood pressure. *BMJ* 300:967.
8. James GD, Jenner DA, Harrison GA, et al. (1985) Differences in catecholamine excretion rates, blood pressure and lifestyle among young Western Samoan men. *Hum Biol* 57:635.
9. Brod J, Fencl V, Hejl Z, et al. (1959) Circulatory changes underlying blood pressure elevation during acute emotional changes in normotensive and hypertensive subjects. *Clin Sci* 18:269.
10. Neel JV (1962) Diabetes mellitus: a "thrifty" genotype rendered detrimental by "progress"? *J Hum Genetics* 14:353.
11. Julius S, Gudbrandsson T, Jamerson K, et al. (1992) The interconnection between sympathetics, microcirculation, and insulin resistance in hypertension. *Blood Press* 1:9.
12. Henry JP, Stephens PM, Ely DL (1986) Psychosocial hypertension and the defence and defeat reactions. *J Hypertens* 4:687.
13. Ely DL (1981) Hypertension, social rank, and aortic arteriosclerosis in CBA/J mice. *Physiol Behav* 26:655.

14. Fokkema DS (1985) *Social Behavior and Blood Pressure (a study of rats). Dissertation for Doctorate in Natural Sciences.* Netherlands: Groningen University.

15. D'Atri DA, Ostfeld AM (1975) Crowding: its effects on the elevation of blood pressure in a prison setting. *Prev Med* 4:550.

16. D'Atri DA, Fitzgerald EF, Kasl SV, et al. (1981) Crowding in prison: the relationship between changes in housing mode and blood pressure. *Psychosom Med* 43:95.

17. Karasek R, Baker D, Marxer F, et al. Job decision latitude, job demands, and cardiovascular disease: a prospective study of Swedish men. *Am J Public Health* 71:694.

18. Alfredsson L, Karasek R, Theorell T (1982) Myocardial infarction risk and psychosocial work environment: an analysis of the male Swedish working force. *Soc Sci Med* 16:463.

19. Karasek RA, Theorell T, Schwartz JE, et al. (1988) Job characteristics in relation to the prevalence of myocardial infarction in the US Health Examination Survey (HES) and the Health and Nutrition Examination Survey (HANES). *Am J Public Health* 78:910.

20. Schnall PL, Devereux RB, Pickering TG, et al. (1992) The relationship between 'job strain,' workplace diastolic blood pressure, and left ventricular mass index: a correction. *JAMA* 267:1209 (letter; comment).

21. Schnall PL, Schwartz JE, Landsbergis PA, et al. (1992) Relation between job strain, alcohol, and ambulatory blood pressure. *Hypertension* 19:488.

22. Schnall PL, Schwartz JE, Landsbergis PA, et al. (1998) A longitudinal study of job strain and ambulatory blood pressure: results from a three-year follow-up. *Psychosom Med* 60:697.

23. Theorell T, de Faire U, Johnson J, et al. (1991) Job strain and ambulatory blood pressure profiles. *Scand J Work Environ Health* 17:380.

24. Van Egeren LF (1992) The relationship between job strain and blood pressure at work, at home, and during sleep. *Psychosom Med* 54:337.

25. Light KC, Turner JR, Hinderliter AL (1992) Job strain and ambulatory work blood pressure in healthy young men and women. *Hypertension* 20:214.

26. Frankenhaueser M (1983) The sympathetic-adrenal and pituitary-adrenal response to challenge: comparison between the sexes. In Dembroski TM, Schmidt T, Blumchen G, eds. *Biobehavioral Bases of Coronary Heart Disease.* Basel: Karger, p. 91.

27. Lundberg U, Frankenhaueser M (1984) Pituitary-adrenal and sympathetic-adrenal correlates of distress and effort. *J Psychosom Res* 24:125.

28. Waldron I, Nowotarski M, Freimer M, et al. (1982) Cross-cultural variation in blood pressure: a quantitative analysis of the relationships of blood pressure to cultural characteristics, salt consumption and body weight. *Soc Sci Med* 16:419.

29. Dressler WW (1982) *Hypertension and Culture Change: Acculturation and Disease in the West Indies.* South Salem, MA: Redgrave Publishing.

30. Dressler WW, Mata A, Chavez A, et al. (1987) Arterial blood pressure and individual modernization in a Mexican community. *Soc Sci Med* 24:679.

31. Dressler WW (1987) Arterial blood pressure and modernization in Brazil. *Am Anthropol* 89:389.

32. Dressler WW (1990) Lifestyle, stress, and blood pressure in a southern black community. *Psychosom Med* 52:182.

33. James SA, Hartnett SA, Kalsbeek WD (1983) John Henryism and blood pressure differences among black men. *J Behav Med* 6:259.
34. James SA, La Croix AZ, Kleinbaum DG, et al. (1984) John Henryism and blood pressure differences among black men. II. The role of occupational stressors. *J Behav Med* 7:259.
35. Harburg E, Erfurt JC, Hauenstein LS, et al. (1973) Socio-ecological stress, suppressed hostility, skin color, and Black-White male blood pressure: Detroit. *Psychosom Med* 35:276.
36. Diez-Roux AV, Nieto FJ, Muntaner C, et al. (1997) Neighborhood environments and coronary heart disease: a multilevel analysis. *Am J Epidemiol* 146:48.
37. Harburg E, Blakelock EHJ, Roeper PR (1979) Resentful and reflective coping with arbitrary authority and blood pressure: Detroit. *Psychosom Med* 41:189.
38. Harrap SB, Louis WJ, Doyle AE (1984) Failure of psychosocial stress to induce chronic hypertension in the rat. *J Hypertens* 2:653.
39. Henry JP, Liu YY, Nadra WE, et al. (1993) Psychosocial stress can induce chronic hypertension in normotensive strains of rats. *Hypertension* 21:714.
40. Coste SC, Qi Y, Brooks VL, et al. (1995) Captopril and stress-induced hypertension in the borderline hypertensive rat. *J Hypertens* 13:1391.
41. Cooper R, Rotimi C (1997) Hypertension in blacks. *Am J Hypertens* 10:804.
42. Jeunemaitre X, Soubrier F, Kotelevtsev YV, et al. (1992) Molecular basis of human hypertension: role of angiotensinogen. *Cell* 71:169.
43. Rotimi C, Cooper RS, Ward RH, et al. (1993) The role of the angiotensinogen gene in human hypertension: absence of an association among African Americans. *Genet Epidemiol* 10:339 (abstract).
44. Lifton RP, Warnock D, Acton RT, et al. (1993) High prevalence of hypertension-associated angiotensinogen variant T235 in African Americans. *Clin Res* 41:260A (abstract).
45. Hypertension detection and follow-up program cooperative group (1987) Educational level and 5-year all-cause mortality in the Hypertension Detection and Follow-up Program. *Hypertension* 9:641.
46. Ordunez-Garcia PO, Espinosa-Brito AD, Cooper RS, et al. (1998) Hypertension in Cuba: evidence of a narrow black-white difference. *J Hum Hypertens* 12:111.
47. Cruickshank JK, Jackson SH, Beevers DG, et al. (1985) Similarity of blood pressure in blacks, whites and Asians in England: the Birmingham Factory Study. *J Hypertens* 3:365.
48. Alexander F (1939) Emotional factors in essential hypertension. *Psychosom Med* 1:173.
49. Shapiro AP (1988) Psychological factors in hypertension: an overview. *Am Heart J* 116:632.
50. Harburg E, Julius S, McGinn NF, et al. (1964) Personality traits and behavioral patterns associated with systolic blood pressure levels in college males. *J Chronic Dis* 17:405.
51. Cottier C, Perini C, Rauchfleisch U (1987) Personality traits and hypertension: an overview. In: Julius S, Bassett DR, eds. *Handbook of Hypertension (vol. 9): Behavioral Factors in Hypertension,* Amsterdam: Elsevier, p. 123.
52. Wolf S, Wolff HG (1951) A summary of experimental evidence relating life stress to the pathogenesis of essential hypertension in man. In Bell ET, ed. *Hypertension,* Minneapolis: University of Minnesota Press.
53. Perini C, Muller FB, Rauchfleisch U, et al. (1990) Psychosomatic factors in

borderline hypertensive subjects and offspring of hypertensive parents. *Hypertension* 16:627.

54. Irvine J, Garner DM, Craig HM, et al. (1991) Prevalence of Type A behavior in untreated hypertensive individuals. *Hypertension* 18:72.

55. Rosenman RH, Brand RJ, Jenkins D, et al. (1975) Coronary heart disease in Western Collaborative Group Study: final follow-up experience of 8 1/2 years. *JAMA* 233:872.

56. Williams RBJ (1987) Refining the type A hypothesis: emergence of the hostility complex. *Am J Cardiol* 60:27J.

57. Everson SA, Goldberg DE, Kaplan GA, et al. (1998) Anger expression and incident hypertension. *Psychosom Med* 60:730.

58. Jamner LD, Shapiro D, Goldstein IB, et al. (1991) Ambulatory blood pressure and heart rate in paramedics: effects of cynical hostility and defensiveness. *Psychom Med* 53:393.

59. Coryell W, Noyes RJ, House JD (1986) Mortality among outpatients with anxiety disorders. *Am J Psychiatry* 143:508.

60. Simonsick EM, Wallace RB, Blazer DG, et al. (1995) Depressive symptomatology and hypertension-associated morbidity and mortality in older adults. *Psychosom Med* 57:427 (comments).

61. Paterniti S, Alperovitch A, Ducimetiere P, et al. (1999) Anxiety but not depression is associated with elevated blood pressure in a community group of French elderly. *Psychosom Med* 61:77.

62. Davies SJ, Ghahramani P, Jackson PR, et al. (1999) Association of panic disorder and panic attacks with hypertension. *Am J Med* 107:310.

63. Davies SJ, Ghahramani P, Jackson PR, et al. (1997) Panic disorder, anxiety and depression in resistant hypertension—a case-control study. *J Hypertens* 15:1077.

64. Jonas BS, Franks P, Ingram DD (1997) Are symptoms of anxiety and depression risk factors for hypertension? Longitudinal evidence from the National Health and Nutrition Examination Survey I Epidemiologic Follow-up Study. *Arch Fam Med* 6:43.

65. Manuck SB, Schaefer DC (1978) Stability of individual differences in cardiovascular reactivity. *Physiol Behav* 21:675.

66. Folkow B (1978) The fourth Volhard lecture: cardiovascular structural adaptation; its role in the initiation and maintenance of primary hypertension. *Clin Sci Mol Med* 4(Suppl.):3S–22S.

67. Julius S, Li Y, Brant D, et al. (1989) Neurogenic pressor fail to cause hypertension, but do induce cardiac hypertrophy. *Hypertension* 13:422.

68. Jennings GL, Nelson L, Esler MD, et al. (1984) Effects of changes in physical activity on blood pressure and sympathetic tone. *J Hypertens* (Suppl. 3):S139–S149.

69. Pickering TG, Gerin W (1990) Reactivity and the role of behavioral factors in hypertension: a critical review. *Ann Behav Med* 12:3.

70. McKinney ME, Miner MH, Ruddel H, et al. (1985) The standardized mental stress test protocol: test-retest reliability and comparison with ambulatory blood pressure monitoring. *Psychophysiology* 22:453.

71. Parati G, Pomidossi G, Ramirez A, et al. (1983) Reproducibility of laboratory tests evaluating neural cardiovascular regulation in man. *J Hypertens* (Suppl. 2):S88–S90.

72. Langewitz W, Ruddel H, Noack H, et al. (1989) The reliability of psychophysiological examinations under field conditions: results of repetitive mental stress testing in middle-aged men. *Eur Heart J* 10:657.
73. Van Egeren LF, Sparrow AW (1989) Laboratory stress testing to assess reallife cardiovascular reactivity. *Psychosom Med* 51:1 (comments).
74. Parati G, Omboni S, Staessen J, et al. (1988) Limitations of the difference between clinic and daytime blood pressure as a surrogate measure of the 'whitecoat' effect. Syst-Eur investigators. *J Hypertens* 16:23.
75. Fredrikson M, Dimberg U, Frisk-Holmberg M, et al. (1985) Arterial blood pressure and general sympathetic activation in essential hypertension during stimulation. *Acta Med Scand* 217:309.
76. Turner JR, Girdler SS, Sherwood A, et al. (1990) Cardiovascular responses to behavioral stressors: laboratory-field generalization and inter-task consistency. *J Psychosom Res* 34:581.
77. Fredrikson M, Matthews KA (1990) Cardiovascular responses to behavioral stress and hypertension: a meta-analytic review. *Ann Behav Med* 12:30.
78. Julius S, Jones K, Schork N, et al. (1991) Independence of pressure reactivity from pressure levels in Tecumseh, Michigan. *Hypertension* 17:(3)12.
79. Rostrup M, Ekeberg O (1992) Awareness of high blood pressure influences on psychological and sympathetic responses. *J Psychosom Res* 36:117.
80. Molineux D, Steptoe A (1988) Exaggerated blood pressure responses to submaximal exercise in normotensive adolescents with a family history of hypertension. *J Hypertens* 6:361.
81. Ravogli A, Trazzi S, Villani A, et al. (1990) Early 24-hour blood pressure elevation in normotensive subjects with parental hypertension. *Hypertension* 16:491 (comments).
82. Harbin TJ (1989) The relationship between the type A behavior pattern and physiological responsivity: a quantitative review. *Psychophysiology* 26:110.
83. Weidner G, Friend R, Ficarrotto TJ, et al. (1989) Hostility and cardiovascular reactivity to stress in women and men. *Psychosom Med* 51:36.
84. Smith TW, Allred KD, Morrison CA, et al. (1989) Cardiovascular reactivity and interpersonal influence: active coping in a social context. *J Pers Soc Psychol* 56:209.
85. Melville DI, Raftery EB (1981) Blood pressure changes during acute mental stress in hypertensive subjects using the Oxford intra-arterial system. *J Psychosom Res* 25:487.
86. Parati G, Pomidossi G, Albini F, et al. (1987) Relationship of 24-hour blood pressure mean and variability to severity of target-organ damage in hypertension. *J Hypertens* 5:93.
87. Floras JS, Hassan MO, Jones JV, et al. (1987) Pressor responses to laboratory stresses and daytime blood pressure variability. *J Hypertens* 5:715.
88. Watson RD, Stallard TJ, Flinn RM, et al. (1980) Factors determining direct arterial pressure and its variability in hypertensive man. *Hypertension* 2:333.
89. Thomas DB, Duszynski KR (1982) Blood pressure levels in young adulthood as predictors of hypertension and the fate of the cold pressor test. *Johns Hopkins Med J* 151:93.
90. Menkes MS, Matthews KA, Krantz DS, et al. (1989) Cardiovascular reactivity to the cold pressor test as a predictor of hypertension. *Hypertension* 14:524.

91. Harlan WR, Osborne RK, Graybiel A (1964) Prognostic value of the cold pressor test and the bassal blood pressure: based on an 18-year follow-up study. *Am J Cardiol* 13:683.
92. Wood DL, Sheps SG, Elveback LR, et al. (1984) Cold pressor test as a predictor of hypertension. *Hypertension* 6:301.
93. Eich RH, Jacobsen EC (1967) Vascular reactivity in medical students followed for 10 yr. *J Chronic Dis* 20:583.
94. Carroll D, Davey SG, Sheffield D, et al. (1996) Blood pressure reactions to the cold pressor test and the prediction of future blood pressure status: data from the Caerphilly study. *J Hum Hypertens* 10:777.
95. Falkner B, Onesti G, Hamstra B (1981) Stress response characteristics of adolescents with high genetic risk for essential hypertension: a five year follow-up. *Clin Exp Hypertens* 3:583.
96. Borghi C, Costa FV, Boschi S, et al. (1986) Predictors of stable hypertension in young borderline subjects: a five-year follow-up study. *J Cardiovasc Pharmacol* 8(Suppl. 5):S138.
97. Goldstein DS (1983) Plasma catecholamines and essential hypertension: an analytical review. *Hypertension* 5:86.
98. Julius S, Nesbitt S (1996) Sympathetic overactivity in hypertension: a moving target. *Am J Hypertens* 9:113S.
99. Guyton AC (1989) Dominant role of the kidneys and accessory role of whole-body autoregulation in the pathogenesis of hypertension. *Am J Hypertens* 2:575.
100. Lever AF (1986) Slow pressor mechanisms in hypertension: a role for hypertrophy of resistance vessels? *J Hypertens* 4:515.
101. Majewski H, Tung LH, Rand MJ (1981) Hypertension through adrenaline activation of prejunctional beta-adrenoceptors. *Clin Exp Pharmacol Physiol* 8:463.
102. Majewski H, Hedler L, Starke K (1982) The noradrenaline rate in the anaesthetized rabbit: facilitation by adrenaline. *Naunyn Schmiedebergs Arch Pharmacol* 321:20.
103. Brown MJ, Dollery CT (1984) Adrenaline and hypertension. *Clin Exp Hypertens* 6:539.
104. Blankestijn PJ, Man i, V, Tulen J, et al. (1988) Support for adrenaline-hypertension hypothesis: 18 hour pressor effect after 6 hours adrenaline infusion. *Lancet* 2:1386 (comments.
105. Goldstein DS, Golczynska A, Stuhlmuller J, et al. (1999) A test of the "epinephrine hypothesis" in humans. *Hypertension* 33:36.
106. Di Bona GF, Jones SY (1995) Analysis of renal sympathetic nerve responses to stress. *Hypertension* 25:531.
107. Di Bona GF, Jones SY, Sawin LL (1996) Renal sympathetic neural mechanisms as intermediate phenotype in spontaneously hypertensive rats. *Hypertension* 27:626.
108. Hermsmeyer K (1976) Cellular basis for increased sensitivity of vascular smooth muscle in spontaneously hypertensive rats. *Circ Res* 38:53.
109. Bevan RD (1984) Trophic effects of peripheral adrenergic nerves on vascular structure. *Hypertension* 6(3):III19–III26.
110. Vander AJ, Henry JP, Stephens PM, et al. (1978) Plasma renin activity in psychosocial hypertension of CBA mice. *Circ Res* 42:496.
111. McCubbin JA, Surwit RS, Williams RBJ (1988) Opioid dysfunction and risk for hypertension: naloxone and blood pressure responses during different types of stress. *Psychosom Med* 50:8.
112. McCubbin JA, Bruehl S, Wilson JF, et al. (1998) Endogenous opioids inhibit

ambulatory blood pressure during naturally occurring stress. *Psychosom Med* 60:227.

113. Koepke JP, Jones S, Di Bona GF (1988) Stress increases renal nerve activity and decreases sodium excretion in Dahl rats. *Hypertension* 11:334.

114. Anderson DE, Dietz JR, Murphy P (1987) Behavioural hypertension in sodium-loaded dogs is accompanied by sustained sodium retention. *J Hypertens* 5:99.

115. Light KC, Koepke JP, Obrist PA, et al. (1983) Psychological stress induces sodium and fluid retention in men at high risk for hypertension. *Science* 220:429.

116. Deter HC, Buchholz K, Schorr U, et al. (1997) Psychophysiological reactivity of salt-sensitive normotensive subjects. *J Hypertens* 15:839.

117. Lawler JE, Barker GF, Hubbard JW, et al. (1980) The effects of conflict on tonic levels of blood pressure in the genetically borderline hypertensive rat. *Psychophysiology* 17:363.

118. Knardahl S, Sanders BJ, Johnson AK (1989) Haemodynamic responses to conflict stress in borderline hypertensive rats. *J Hypertens* 7:585.

119. Hollenberg NK, Williams GH, Adams DF (1991) Essential hypertension: abnormal renal vascular and endocrine responses to a mild psychological stimulus. *Hypertension* 3:11.

120. Whitworth JA (1987) Mechanisms of glucocorticoid-induced hypertension. *Kidney Int* 31:1213 (clinical conference).

121. Kalsner S (1969) Mechanism of hydrocortisone potentiation of responses to epinephrine and norepinephrine in rabbit aorta. *Circ Res* 24:383.

122. Whitworth JA, Gordon D, Andrews J, et al. (1989) The hypertensive effect of synthetic glucocorticoids in man: role of sodium and volume. *J Hypertens* 7:537.

7

Neuroendocrine Factors

*Role of Sympathetic Nervous and
Renin Angiotensin Systems*

Stevo Julius, MD, ScD

CONTENTS

Both the renin-angiotensin system (RAS) and the sympathetic nervous system (SNS) are frequently overactive in patients with hypertension. Whereas the activation of the RAS can be relatively easily assessed by relating plasma renin to urinary sodium levels, there are no reliable routine measurements to assess the sympathetic activity. Consequently, the elevation of renin in hypertension is a matter of record *(1)*, whereas the more indirect evidence for sympathetic overactivity merits a short review.

Each measurement of sympathetic overactivity has its limitations. Plasma catecholamine levels are too variable whereas the measurement of urinary catecholamines is rather insensitive. In spite of these limitations, it has been shown that norepinephrine and epinephrine are elevated in a substantial proportion of patients with hypertension. More complex measurements have also confirmed an elevation of sympathetic

From: *Hypertension Medicine*
Edited by: M. A. Weber © Humana Press Inc., Totowa, NJ

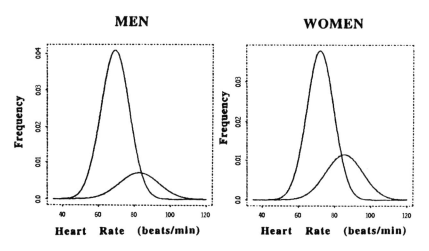

Fig. 7-1. Distribution of heart rates in the population of Tecumseh, MI (reprinted from ref. *4*).

tone in hypertension *(2)*, but, of necessity, these observations are limited to a small number of patients. The simplest and therefore best documented evidence for sympathetic overactivity stems from measurements of heart rate in hypertension. The evidence that tachycardia is important in hypertension *(3)* can be summarized as follows. In large population studies, heart rate is invariably positively correlated with blood pressure (BP). Fast heart rate in normotensive subjects is a predictor of future hypertension, and in most studies and at all ages hypertensive subjects have faster heart rate than normotensive subjects, and the distribution of the heart rate in these populations is bimodal (Fig. 7-1). The bimodal distribution *(4)* and the fact that the group with tachycardia also has higher BP suggest that the "hyperkinetic neurogenic" hypertension may be a separate, pathophysiologically distinctive entity. Data indicate that about 30% of patients with hypertension have tachycardia *(5)*.

The tachycardia in hypertensive patients can be abolished by a pharmacologic denervation of cardiac sympathetic and parasympathetic receptors, which, in turn, suggests that the tachycardia is neurogenic *(6)*.

CHANGING PHENOTYPE OF SYMPATHETIC OVERACTIVITY IN HYPERTENSION

An increased sympathetic tone in patients with the hyperkinetic state who have mild hypertension, tachycardia, and increased cardiac output has been demonstrated by measurements of catecholamine turnover, and by direct microneurography of sympathetic activity in peroneal nerves. The evolution from mild hyperkinetic to treatment requiring established hypertension has been confirmed in an important longitudinal cohort study *(7)*. However, as hypertension advances tachycardia is less pronounced *(3)*, and cross-sectional studies have suggested that with passage of time plasma norepinephrine levels and turnover cease to be elevated.

The absence of telltale signs of sympathetic overactivity in advanced hypertension has been used to challenge the significance of the SNS in hypertension. If sympathetic overactivity is indeed important in early phases of hypertension, why is it so hard to find signs of enhanced sympathetic tone among the "garden variety" patients with more advanced forms of hypertension?

The answer to this question lies in the changing responsiveness of cardiovascular organs to sympathetic stimulation. Prolonged sympathetic stimulation elicits a downregulation of the β-adrenergic responsiveness. A decreased chronotropic and inotropic responsiveness to infusions of isoproterenol has been demonstrated in hypertension *(8,9)*. As the exemplary and unique study by Lund-Johanasson et al. demonstrates *(7)*, the gradual decrease in heart rate in hypertension is associated with a similarly gradual decrease in the stroke volume and cardiac output. BP in these patients slowly increased, and after 20 yr their underlying hemodynamic pattern changed from a state of high cardiac output and tachycardia to a typical high-resistance type of established hypertension.

The increase in vascular resistance in later phases of hypertension can be best explained by vascular hypertrophy. As arterioles become hypertrophic, the thicker muscular (medial) layer protrudes into the lumen of the blood vessel. This is of little hemodynamic significance as long as the vessels are dilated. However, during vasoconstriction, the wall of such hypertrophic vessels abnormally and excessively encroaches on the lumen and thereby elicits a steep increase in vascular resistance. Infusion of norepinephrine or angiotensin into the brachial artery causes a substantially higher increase in forearm vascular resistance in hypertensive than in normotensive subjects *(10)*.

The excessive responsiveness of arterioles to vasoconstriction also provides an explanation for the gradual decrease in plasma norepinephrine values in the course of hypertension. In hypertension the brain seems to seek and maintain a constant elevation of the baseline BP levels. As peripheral vascular responsiveness to sympathetic stimulation increases, less sympathetic outflow is needed to maintain the same BP elevation. Under these circumstances, the plasma norepinephrine values in hypertensive patients are nominally similar to the ones in normotensive patients. However, in spite of the diminished tone, the central nervous system continues to maintain the BP at hypertensive levels. Details supporting this hypothesis are given elsewhere *(11)*.

INTERACTION OF SNS AND RAS

As is the case with many systems that regulate important functions in the body, the SNS and RAS interact and mutually reinforce each other's actions. Sympathetic stimulation via renal β-adrenergic receptors elicits the release of renin from the kidneys. Renin, in turn, releases angiotensin from its substrate. Angiotensin increases the sympathetic discharge from the brain and, peripherally, potentiates the sympathetic cardiovascular responses. In view of this, it is not surprising that patients with elevated plasma renin activity also have increased norepinephrine values *(2)*.

In addition to a direct mutual potentiation, the RAS and SNS potentiate each other's physiologic actions. A good example is fluid and sodium balance in which both systems induce retention but through very different mechanisms: angiotensin via aldosterone, sympathetics through a direct renal action. Similar potentiation of physiologic outcomes through different mechanisms occurs regarding the trophic effect of both systems on smooth muscle hypertrophy and regarding the enhancement of coagulation. As discussed next, in the pathophysiologic setting of hypertension, these physiologic interactions promote cardiovascular complications.

SYMPATHETIC OVERACTIVITY AND CORONARY RISK IN HYPERTENSION

The authoritative meta-analysis of large antihypertensive trials by Collins et al. *(12)* shows that antihypertensive therapy is fully capable of reducing strokes but that the effect on reduction of coronary events is less than anticipated. The failure to reduce coronary outcomes is particularly clear in younger patients.

To a student of physiology, such an outcome is not at all surprising because elevation of BP is only one of multiple pathophysiologic abnormalities in hypertension. Many of these abnormalities are in their own right and independently of BP are conducive to excessive coronary events. The interaction between the overactivity of the RAS and the SNS is one of the most important pressure-independent coronary risk factors in hypertension.

Trophic Effects

Both the RAS and the SNS favor cardiac and vascular hypertrophy. Whereas hypertrophy in the short term enhances the functional performance of cardiovascular organs, long-standing and advanced hypertrophy carries negative prognostic implications. A hypertrophic heart becomes stiffer, which impedes the diastolic filling and function. In due course the hypertrophic myocardium outgrows its blood supply, which eventually causes ischemic heart disease. It is therefore not surprising that left ventricular hypertrophy is an independent potent predictor of cardiovascular mortality *(13)*.

As indicated earlier, hypertrophic arterioles become hyperresponsive and this leads to acceleration of hypertension. Because of the thicker wall, the hypertrophic vessels are also less capable of vasodilation. The insufficient vasodilation is further aggravated by pressure-related endothelial dysfunction. These processes lead to a substantial decrease in coronary reserve in hypertension.

Tachycardia

It is generally assumed that tachycardia is a benign sign, which is typical for nervous people whose BP is only temporarily elevated. However, epidemiologic data do not provide support for such an interpretation. A fast heart rate is a strong and independent predictor of cardiovascular mortality and morbidity. The importance of heart rate could be predicted from physiology; the work of the heart is a product of both heart rate and BP. Furthermore, the excessive and frequent pulsatile flow has a deleterious effect on coronary blood vessels and tachycardia is conducive to arrhythmias. Support for these statements can be found in a recent review (*see* ref. *3*).

Procoagulant Properties

Hypertension is frequently associated with elevated hematocrit values. High hematocrit, possibly because it increases the viscosity of blood, is a predictor of coronary mortality *(14)*. The red blood cell volume in hypertension is normal and the high hematocrit is owing to a decrease in plasma volume *(15)*. The decreased plasma volume in hypertension can be best explained by an increase in the capillary pressure, which causes a translocation of a small amount of plasma from the intravascular to the interstitial space. It is likely that one of the factors that increases the capillary pressure in hypertension is an excessive postcapillary α-adrenergic venoconstriction. In healthy humans, an infusion of sympathomimetic amines or an unopposed α-adrenergic tone causes a quick decrease in plasma volume. Furthermore, an association of indices of higher sympathetic tone with higher hematocrit values has been found in the Tecumseh *(5)* epidemiologic study.

In addition to elevated hematocrit, an increased sympathetic tone (reflected in higher epinephrine values) has also been associated with signs of platelet overactivity in hypertension. Infusion of angiotensin II increases plasma fibrinogen inhibitor levels, which impedes fibrinolysis. Unfortunately, measurements of platelet overactivity and plasma fibrinolysis are not simple and their value as predictors of coronary risk has not been tested in epidemiologic studies. It stands to reason, however, that akin to high hematocrit, these procoagulant abnormalities may be conducive to excessive coronary thrombosis.

Insulin Resistance and Metabolic Syndrome

An elevated fasting plasma insulin is a sign of insulin resistance, a condition in which the insulin-mediated glucose uptake decreases. In such resistant individuals, higher insulin levels are needed to maintain normal blood glucose levels. Insulin resistance is intimately associated with dyslipidemia. An elevated plasma insulin level, independent of dyslipidemia, is a strong coronary risk factor *(16)*.

High plasma insulin levels have been frequently found in hypertension *(17)*. It has been proposed and experimentally verified *(18)* that that α-adrenergic vasoconstriction may cause insulin resistance. In short, most of the insulin-mediated glucose uptake occurs in skeletal muscle cells. α-Adrenergic vasoconstriction decreases the nutritional blood flow to skeletal muscles and thereby impedes the glucose uptake by metabolically active myocytes. Because less glucose is cleared, the pancreatic secretion of insulin increases in order to enhance the glucose clearance. The end result is a steady state of high insulin and near normal glucose. Support for this concept has been described in detail elsewhere *(17)* and is based on the following observations. First, a decreased skeletal muscle capillary density has been found in insulin-resistant states of hypertension, obesity, and type II diabetes. Second, antihypertensive drugs that cause vasoconstriction worsen insulin resistance and those that cause vasodilation improve insulin sensitivity. Third, exercise training improves insulin sensitivity and increases skeletal muscle capillary density.

IMPLICATIONS FOR PRACTICE

The understanding that hypertension is associated with multiple coronary risk factors and that both the RAS and SNS overactivity contribute to pressure-independent cardiovascular morbidity in hypertension ought to affect clinical practice. It is logical that antihypertensive drugs, which centrally decrease the sympathetic outflow or peripherally interfere with angiotensin's action, may be particularly useful in patients with multiple cardiovascular risk factors. However, currently a clinician's enthusiasm for sympatholytic agents is restrained by the awareness that drugs such as reserpine, aldomet, and clonidine can cause considerable side effects. The new imidazoline agonists appear to be equally effective as clonidine while causing fewer side effects, but they are not available in the United States. Problems with the clinical diagnosis of neurogenic hypertension are another impediment to the use of sympatholytic agents. How is a physician to know which patient has a neurogenic form of hypertension? The answer is reasonably simple. In the absence of other causes (hyperthyroidism, anemia, pulmonary disease), a resting sitting heart rate of 75 beats/min or higher is a good indicator of sympathetic overactivity in hypertension.

Whereas on conceptual grounds the use of drugs that antagonize the renin angiotensin system appears to offer additional benefits, physicians will not change their prescribing habits until there is some demonstration that these theoretical properties can be translated into practical advantage. Several comparative trials of old vs new antihypertensive drugs are under way. Should these trials prove the superiority of new agents, physicians will use them more frequently.

Currently, decreasing BP by any of the available drugs remains the primary clinical objective. It is, however, reasonable to tailor the treatment to an individual patient's clinical condition. Personally, in a patient who has signs of sympathetic overactivity, I prefer to start with an angiotensin-converting enzyme inhibitor, an angiotensin receptor blocking agent, or possibly with an α-adrenergic blocking agent. β-Blockers decrease BP but aggravate both the dyslipidemia and insulin resistance and should not be the primary drug for patients with a metabolic syndrome.

REFERENCES

1. Laragh JH, Baer L, Brunner HR, Buhler FR, Sealey JE, Vaughan ED, Jr. (1972) Renin, angiotensin and aldosterone system in pathogenesis and management of hypertensive vascular disease. *Am J Med* 52:633–652.
2. Esler M, Julius S, Zweifler A, Randall O, Harburg E, Gardiner H, DeQuattro V (1977) Mild high-renin essential hypertension: neurogenic human hypertension? *N Engl J Med* 296:405–411.
3. Palatini P, Julius S (1997) Heart rate and the cardiovascular risk. *J Hypertens* 15:1–15.
4. Palatini P, Casiglia E, Pauletto P, Staessen J, Kaciroti N, Julius S (1997) Relationship of tachycardia with high blood pressure and metabolic abnormalities: a study with mixture analysis in three populations. *Hypertension* 30:1267–1273.
5. Julius S, Jamerson K, Mejia A, Krause L, Schork N, Jones K (1990) The association of borderline hypertension with target organ changes and higher coronary risk. Tecumseh Blood Pressure Study. *JAMA* 264:354–358.
6. Julius S, Pascual AV, London R (1971) Role of parasympathetic inhibition in the hyperkinetic type of borderline hypertension. *Circulation* 44:413–418.
7. Lund-Johansen P, Omvik P (1990) Hemodynamic patterns of untreated hypertensive disease. In: Laragh JH, Brenner BM, eds. *Hypertension: Pathophysiology, Diagnosis, and Management,* New York: Raven, pp. 305–327.
8. Julius S, Randall OS, Esler MD, Kashima T, Ellis CN, Bennett J (1975) Altered cardiac responsiveness and regulation in the normal cardiac output type of borderline hypertension. *Circ Res* 36–37 (Suppl. I):I-199–I-207.
9. Trimarco B, Volpe M, Ricciardelli B, Picotti GB, Galva MA, Petracca R, Condorelli M (1983) Studies of the mechanisms underlying impairment of beta-adrenoceptor-mediated effects in human hypertension. *Hypertension* 5:584–590.
10. Egan B, Panis R, Hinderliter A, Schork N, Julius S (1987) Mechanism of increased alpha-adrenergic vasoconstriction in human essential hypertension. *J Clin Invest* 80:812–817.
11. Julius S (1988) Editorial review: the blood pressure seeking properties of the central nervous system. *J Hypertens* 6:177–185.
12. Collins R, Peto R, MacMahon S, Hebert P, Fiebach NH, Eberlein KA, Godwin J, Qizilbash N, Taylor JO, Hennekens CH (1990) Blood pressure, stroke, and coronary heart disease. Part 2, short-term reduction in blood pressure: overview of randomized drug trials in their epidemiological context. *Lancet* 1990; 335:827–838.
13. Levy D, Garrison RJ, Savage DD, Kannel WB, Castelli WP (1990) Prognostic

implications of echocardiographically determined left ventricular mass in the Framingham heart study. *N Engl J Med* 322:1561–1566.

14. Smith SD, Julius S, Jamerson K, Amerena J, Schork N (1994) Hematocrit levels and physiologic factors in relationship to cardiovascular risk in Tecumseh, Michigan. *Hypertension* 12:455–462.

15. Julius S, Pascual A, Reilly K, London R (1971) Abnormalities of plasma volume in borderline hypertension. *Arch Intern Med* 127:116–119.

16. Pyorala K, Savolainen E, Kaukola S, Haapakoski J (1985) Plasma insulin as a coronary heart disease risk factor: relationship to other risk factors and predictive value during 9 1/2 year follow-up of the Helsinki Policemen Study population. *Acta Med Scand Suppl* 701:38–52.

17. Anderson EA, Sinkey CA, Lawton WJ, Mark AL (1989) Elevated sympathetic nerve activity in borderline hypertensive humans: evidence from direct intraneural recordings. *Hypertension* 14:177–183.

18. Jamerson KA, Julius S, Gudbrandsson T, Andersson O, Brant DO (1993) Reflex sympathetic activation induces acute insulin resistance in the human forearm. *Hypertension* 21(5):618–623.

8 Left Ventricular Hypertrophy and Diastolic Dysfunction

George A. Mansoor, MD
and William B. White, MD

Contents

Our understanding of systemic hypertension and its vascular complications has been expanding steadily in the past two decades. This progress has refined methods for the measurement of hypertensive disease complications and allowed an inquiry into the clinical factors that may accelerate them. The heart is a prime target for hypertensive damage, suffering accelerated coronary atherosclerosis, left ventricular hypertrophy (LVH), arrhythmias, and congestive heart failure (CHF) *(1)*.

From: *Hypertension Medicine*
Edited by: M. A. Weber © Humana Press Inc., Totowa, NJ

LVH is initially a compensatory mechanism for the increased systemic vascular resistance that occurs in hypertension, but this hypertrophy eventually becomes deleterious and can result in inadequate myocardial perfusion and cardiac dysfunction. LVH has emerged as an
independent cardiovascular risk factor with prognostic precision that
may be better than blood pressure (BP) itself. Primary care physicians
must therefore be aware of the importance of LVH as a cardiovascular
risk factor, understand the methods of detecting LVH and diastolic
dysfunction, and be aware of current methods of treating LVH.

EPIDEMIOLOGY OF HYPERTENSIVE CARDIAC HYPERTROPHY

BP is the major determinant of left ventricular mass index (left
ventricular mass corrected for body surface area) with better correlation
with 24-h ambulatory BP measurement than office BP *(2)*. This is
probably because of the greater reproducibility of ambulatory BP compared with office BP and the fact that it more closely represents overall
BP levels. Similar to other hypertensive complications, systolic (both
basal and exercise BP) rather than diastolic BP is more consistently
related to left ventricular mass index. The prevalence of LVH among
hypertensive subjects varies from 3 to 50%, depending on whether
electrocardiography (ECG) or echocardiography is used for diagnosis
and whether treated or untreated patients are studied *(3)*. This variability
not only reflects differences in the populations studied, the severity of
hypertension, but the methods and normal values used to define LVH.
It is apparent that LVH is a common finding in hypertensive subjects.
    Although the overall hemodynamic load is certainly the prime ele-
ment in the development of LVH, several other clinical factors affect
the clinical expression of left ventricular mass. Epidemiologic studies
such as The Framingham Study *(4)* have shown that the prevalence of
LVH increases slowly with age with a sharp rise in subjects over 60
yr. However, this increase in LVH with age may be dependent on other
factors such as the prevalence of hypertension or obesity. It has also
been revealed that women have less LVH than similarly aged men
until about the sixth decade, after which the rates are higher in women.
The effects of body mass index (BMI) on cardiac mass are noteworthy
because for any given level of BP the prevalence of LVH increases
sharply as BMI increases. Thus, it is appropriate to express left ventricular mass indexed for body surface area, body weight, or height. Many

Table 8-1
Clinical and Pathophysiologic Factors Linked to Increase in
Left Ventricular Mass

Clinical Factors	Pathophysiologic Factors
BP	Glucose intolerance
Age	Sympathetic nervous system activity
BMI	Renin-angiotensin system activity
Alcohol intake	Insulin and growth hormone
Sodium intake	
Race and family history	
Valvular heart disease	
Uremia	

other clinical and pathophysiologic factors have been suggested to play a role in the development of LVH (Table 8-1). One contentious issue is whether race is itself an independent factor in the higher prevalence of LVH in African Americans. This remains an unresolved but debated area *(5)*.

PATHOPHYSIOLOGY OF LVH

Current thinking about the pathogenesis of LVH is that of an adaptive process initially. It is thought to be initiated by sustained or episodic increases in BP that impart added work on the heart with increases in wall stress (Laplace's law) and myocardial oxygen consumption (Fig. 8-1). This then leads, through several cellular mechanisms, to hypertrophy of myocytes as well as other supporting tissue. Note that cardiac myocytes cannot undergo hyperplasia because adult myocytes are terminally differentiated and cannot replicate. Because there is inadequate capillary increase to keep up with the cardiac hypertrophy, the relative capillary density is reduced with a possibility for inadequate coronary flow to meet the demands of the bigger myocardium. The increase in cardiac mass is associated with an increase in left ventricular end-diastolic pressure, which may eventually lead to reductions in filling for the ventricle. Furthermore, the hypertensive heart becomes more dependent on left atrial emptying to maintain cardiac output. In extreme forms of diastolic dysfunction with abnormalities of left atrial function, clinical CHF may develop.

$T = PR/2$

where T = wall tension, P = pressure, R = radius of chamber. Increases in pressure must cause increases in tension. But

$S = T \div h$

S = wall stress, t = wall tension, h = average wall thickness.

Therefore

$P = (S \cdot h \cdot 2) \div R$

Therefore any *increase* in wall stress must be accompanied by *increases* in h/R, which is the relative wall thickness. The typical change in the heart is an increase in both septal and posterior wall thickness giving concentric left ventricular hypertrophy.

Fig. 8-1. Explanation of ventricular hypertrophy based on Laplace's law.

ADVERSE CONSEQUENCES OF LVH

Several large epidemiologic and prospective studies have shown that ECG or echocardiographic LVH is a serious finding and increases the risk for coronary artery disease (CAD), CHF, stroke, cardiac arrhythmias, and sudden death *(4–7)*. Subjects with LVH suffer about two to four times the cardiac complications of hypertension as their hypertensive counterparts with no LVH. Furthermore, these findings have been reported in a variety of patient populations: subjects with and without hypertension and with and without CAD. In one report from The Framingham Study, the cardiovascular mortality in a group of subjects with ECG-determined LVH with ST-T wave changes was about seven times higher than that of an age-matched group with normal ECG. Other work has shown that patients with LVH who experience a myocardial infarction (MI) have a higher death rate than similar subjects without LVH with an acute MI. Further data published from The Framingham Study *(6)* on a group of 3220 subjects over age 40 and who were clinically free of cardiovascular disease show that echocardiographic determination of left ventricular mass was associated positively with the incidence of cardiovascular disease and death from cardiovascular disease (Fig. 8-2). Similar results have been obtained on a group of elderly patients from the same database. Therefore, LVH is a cardiovascular risk factor similar in importance to diabetes, hypertension, and hypercholesterolemia. In fact, the Sixth Joint National Committee on the Prevention, Detection, Evaluation and Treatment of High Blood Pressure (JNC VI) has included LVH as one of the factors in stratifying patients into the high-risk category *(8)*.

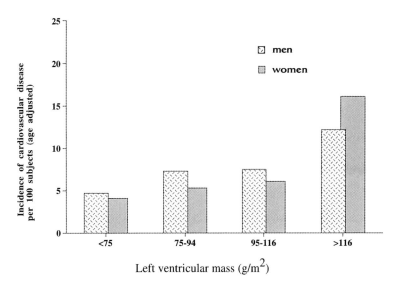

Fig. 8-2. The age-adjusted incidence of cardiovascular disease over 4 yr with left ventricular mass index. Reproduced from ref. *6* with permission.

From a practical point of view, the finding of LVH on ECG with ST-T wave abnormalities should be as ominous to the primary care physician as the finding of old q-waves indicative of a previous MI. Similarly, an echocardiographic report of LVH based on an increase in relative wall thickness and normal chamber size should also alert the clinician that the subject is at increased risk.

LEFT VENTRICULAR MASS, HYPERTENSION, AND DIASTOLIC DYSFUNCTION

Diastolic dysfunction *(9)* may be seen in patients with enlargement of the heart (either LVH or hypertrophic cardiomyopathy), with infiltrative disease, or with CAD. The type of diastolic dysfunction of interest here is that found in many hypertensive patients with and without ECG-LVH. As the extent of LVH increases, so does the incidence of diastolic dysfunction. With time, the impaired relaxation of the ventricle during left ventricular filling is severe enough to produce symptoms during exertion or during atrial fibrillation. The fact that many patients with LVH will become symptomatic during atrial fibrillation is explained by the increased contribution of atrial contraction to left ventricular filling in these subjects. Loss of the atrial contribution to left ventricular filling during atrial fibrillation precipitates symptoms owing to increased pulmonary wedge pressure. Note that diastolic dysfunction may also be accompanied by systolic dysfunction and a reduced left ventricular ejection fraction. However, systolic function is typically preserved in most hypertensive subjects without CAD and diastolic perturbations predominate.

DETECTION OF LVH AND DIASTOLIC DYSFUNCTION

LVH *(10)* can be detected noninvasively using 12-lead ECG (Fig. 8-3) as well as echocardiography. ECG is still recommended in the routine evaluation of hypertensive subjects whereas echocardiography should be reserved for selected patients *(8)*. Electrocardiographic detection of LVH has lower sensitivity than echocardiography but has strong risk prediction when ST-T wave abnormalities are also present. It has been suggested that these ST-T wave changes may be indicative of myocardial ischemia—hence the high risk for coronary events in this group of patients.

Echocardiographic detection of LVH can be done using both M-mode and 2-D echocardiography; it is well established and gives information about anatomical hypertrophy. A limited M-mode study can provide the wall thickness and left ventricular diastolic dimensions to calculate left ventricular mass. The data obtained from echocardiography also allow the separation of the types of LVH into concentric, eccentric, and concentric remodeling. Currently, however, whether such an analysis provides major additional prognostic significance beyond left ventricular mass is not clear. More detailed examination with Doppler technology can provide objective measures of left ventricular filling. Many of the noninvasive indices used are not specific for hypertensive diastolic dysfunction and may be seen in diastolic dysfunction secondary to CAD and various metabolic or infiltrative diseases.

The most common index used to infer diastolic dysfunction is an alteration in the E:A wave velocity ratio of left ventricular filling. The E wave represents the early active filling phase in diastole and the A wave represents atrial filling. The normal ratio varies with age but is usually >1.0, and in general a ratio <0.5 is clearly abnormal. Other Doppler changes seen in situations of impaired relaxation include prolonged deceleration time and an increased isovolumetric relaxation time. In the hypertrophied ventricle, a low E wave is seen with a tall

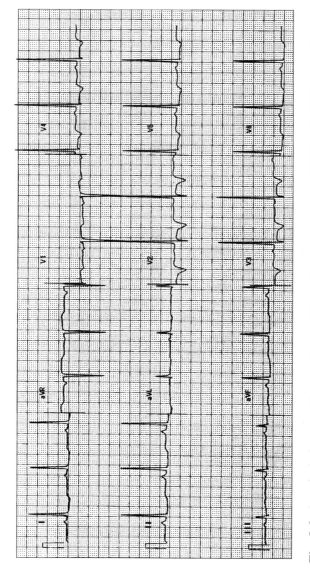

Fig. 8-3. A typical electrocardiogram from a 65-yr-old woman showing LVH with ST-T wave changes. She had poorly controlled hypertension for many years.

A wave indicative of reduced early filling and late filling promoted by enhanced left atrial contraction. The primary care physician may be told that there has been a reduction in the E:A ratio. These patterns are also affected by age, and preload and considerable care is necessary in interpretation.

These Doppler-based abnormalities of flow are common. Even in relatively young untreated subjects with mild hypertension and without LVH, ECG shows that about 20–25% have abnormal left ventricular filling. The abnormalities of diastolic function may antedate overt LVH.

REGRESSION OF LVH AND OUTCOME

It makes intuitive sense that therapy to reverse LVH should reduce cardiovascular risk in these patients. Diastolic dysfunction improves appreciably when LVH is reversed by antihypertensive therapy, and such improvement may be seen in a few months (11). Furthermore, reversal of LVH should translate into a reduction in cardiovascular risk. Several studies now indicate that this may indeed be true (12). In the most recent of these studies (13), 430 patients with essential hypertension were followed for an average of 2.8 yr. All patients were studied with ECG and ambulatory BP monitoring and cardiovascular events ascertained over time. The group of patients in whom there was an increase of left ventricular mass during follow-up had a higher rate of cardiovascular events than the group in whom there was a decrease in left ventricular mass. Furthermore, in the subgroup with LVH at commencement of the study, there was a higher event rate among those whose left ventricular mass increased during therapy compared with those in whom left ventricular mass decreased with follow-up. It therefore appears that a reduction in left ventricular mass predicts a lower risk than in those patients whose left ventricular mass increases over time. A large multicenter trial, Losartan Intervention for Endpoints, with hard cardiovascular end points is nearing completion and is comparing the angiotensin II receptor blocker losartan to atenolol in patients with established ECG-LVH.

A controversial issue remains whether certain antihypertensive agents are superior in reducing left ventricular mass and therefore reducing risk. Current data do not support one class of antihypertensive agent over others except that vasodilators that induce reflex tachycardia are to be avoided as monotherapy. Our practice is to reduce elevated

BP by whatever methods possible, including lifestyle modifications. If there is an unusually large left ventricular mass for a patient with stage 1 to 2 hypertension, then some consideration should be given to performing ambulatory BP monitoring to document sleep BP, which may exaggerate LVH if elevated. Additional recommendations should include reduction of salt and alcohol intake and attainment of ideal body weight if possible. The antihypertensive drugs of choice for these subjects should be guided by compelling indications and concomitant diseases as outlined in the JNC VI report.

ROLE OF LVH AND DIASTOLIC DYSFUNCTION IN HEART FAILURE

The presence of diastolic dysfunction as a contributing factor to CHF is significant *(14)*. The clinical features of both systolic and diastolic forms of heart failure are similar, making routine noninvasive evaluation of ventricular function during the episode mandatory in these patients *(14)*. Echocardiography not only detects diastolic dysfunction but also excludes coexisting valvular, pericardial, and restrictive disease. In many patients with preserved systolic function but clinical evidence for heart failure, ischemia may be playing a role and should be actively excluded. In as many as one third of subjects with clinical heart failure, diastolic dysfunction is the cause or major contributor to their disease process *(15)*. Although subjects with diastolic heart failure have lower mortality rates than their counterparts with systolic failure, the morbidity and mortality is still substantial. Also of interest is the finding that the incidence of CHF with isolated diastolic dysfunction as the cause increases impressively with age *(16)*.

The best therapies for subjects with hypertensive diastolic heart failure are not known. Empiric suggestions derived from clinical experience include careful diuretic use to eliminate congestive symptoms, maintenance of sinus rhythm, and use of antihypertensive agents that slow heart rate and increase filling time. The use of digoxin should be limited to patients with atrial fibrillation. The goal BP in these subjects remains unclear although office BP of 135/85 mmHg may be a reasonable goal. Serial echocardiographic measures of left ventricular mass, though of limited reproducibility, may be useful to confirm regression of LVH.

CONCLUSION

Unfortunately, too many hypertensive patients develop LVH. The presence of LVH among hypertensive patients should be treated with concern because it is not a mere cardiac manifestation of hypertension but portends a worsened clinical outcome. Ideally, prevention of LVH should be the goal by maintaining good BP control, ideal body weight, and reduced salt intake. LVH is accompanied initially by minor echocardiographic abnormalities of diastolic function, but as time progresses these worsen and can induce heart failure. There is promising evidence that antihypertensive therapy to reduce left ventricular mass is beneficial. Suggested therapy for isolated diastolic heart failure associated with LVH includes maintenance of sinus rhythm and control of heart rate, relief of pulmonary congestion, and good BP control in the long term. Hypertensive heart disease, once identified, remains a major challenge to treat.

REFERENCES

1. Frohlich ED, Apstein C, Chobanian AV, Devereux RB, Dustan HP, Dzau V, Fauad-Tarazi F, Horan MJ, Marcus M, Massie B, Pfeffer MA, Re RN, Rocella EJ, Savage D, Shub C (1992) The heart in hypertension. *N Engl J Med* 327:998–1008.
2. White WB (1994) Hypertensive target organ involvement and 24-hour ambulatory blood pressure measurement. In: Waeber B, Brunner H, eds. *Ambulatory Blood Pressure Monitoring,* New York: Raven.
3. Devereux RB (1990) Hypertensive cardiac hypertrophy. In: *Hypertension, Pathophysiology, Diagnosis and Management.* Laragh JH, Brenner BM, eds, New York: Raven.
4. Levy D, Anderson KM, Savage DD, Kannel WB, Christiansen JC, Castelli WP (1988) Echocardiographically detected left ventricular hypertrophy, prevalence and risk factors. The Framingham Study. *Ann Intern Med* 108:7–13.
5. Devereux RB, Okin PM, Roman MJ (1998) Pre-clinical cardiovascular disease and surrogate end-points in hypertension: does race influence target organ damage independent of blood pressure? *Ethnicity Dis* 8:134–148.
6. Levy D, Garrison RJ, Savage DD, Kannel WB, Castelli WP (1990) Prognostic implications of echocardiographically determined left ventricular mass in the Framingham Heart study. *N Engl J Med* 322:1561–1566.
7. Bikkina M, Levy D, Evans JC, Larson MG, Benjamin EJ, Wolf PA, Castelli WP (1994) Left ventricular mass and risk of stroke in an elderly cohort. The Framingham Heart Study. *JAMA* 272:33–36.
8. Joint National Committee on Prevention, Detection, Evaluation and Treatment of High Blood Pressure: The Sixth Report (1997) *Arch Intern Med* 157:2413–2446.
9. Cohen GI, Pietrolungo JF, Thomas JD, Klein AL (1996) A practical guide to

assessment of ventricular diastolic function using doppler echocardiography. *J Am Coll Cardiol* 27:1753–1760.

10. Devereux RB, Pini R, Aurigemma GP, Roman MJ (1997) Measurement of left ventricular mass: methodology and expertise. *J Hypertens* 15:801–809.

11. White WB, Schulman P, Karimeddini MK, Smith VE (1989) Regression of left ventricular mass is accompanied by improvement in rapid left ventricular filling following antihypertensive therapy with metoprolol. *Am Heart J* 117:145–150.

12. Lip GY, Lydakis C, Zarifis J, Messerli FH (1998) Regression of LVH or improved prognosis (or both): what is the question? *J Hum Hypertens* 12:423–425.

13. Verdecchia P, Schillaci G, Borgioni C, Ciucci A, Gattobigio R, Zampi I, Reboldi G, Porcellati C (1998) Prognostic significance of serial changes in left ventricular mass in essential hypertension. *Circulation* 97:48–54.

14. Vasan RS, Benjamin EJ, Levy D (1995) Prevalence, clinical features and prognosis of diastolic heart failure: an epidemiological perspective. *J Am Coll Cardiol* 26:1565–1574.

15. European Study Group on Diastolic Heart Failure (1998) How to diagnose diastolic heart failure. *Eur Heart J* 19:990–1003.

16. Tresch DD (1997) The clinical diagnosis of heart failure in older patients. *J Am Geriatr Soc* 45:1128–1133.

9 Role of Endothelium in Hypertension

Ellis R. Levin, MD

CONTENTS

VASOACTIVE HORMONES
DIABETES AND HYPERTENSION
CONCLUSION
REFERENCES

The endothelial lining of blood vessels is the one-cell-thick innermost layer and comprises endothelial cells. The endothelium plays an important role in the dynamic regulation of blood pressure (BP) (Fig. 9-1). Through hormones, cytokines, and other vasoactive factors, the endothelium communicates to and regulates the function of vascular smooth muscle tone. This is critical to the dynamic equilibrium of basal BP, and our understanding of how the body rapidly adjusts to changes in position or blood volume. Abnormalities of the endothelium are reflected in altered basal control of BP, and clearly contribute to the development of hypertension. In this chapter, I explore the important endothelial participants in BP control and suggest ways to modify these factors to yield normotension.

VASOACTIVE HORMONES

Endothelin

The regulation of basal BP must be understood as a dynamic state, in which factors that stimulate vasodilation are balanced by vaso-constricting factors. The endothelium makes both factors, and local

From: *Hypertension Medicine*
Edited by: M. A. Weber © Humana Press Inc., Totowa, NJ

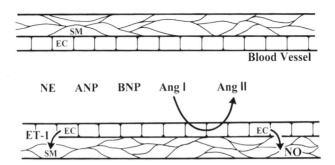

Fig. 9-1. Dynamic regulation of vasomotor tone and arterial pressure by cardiovascular hormones. Vasodilators, such as (nitric oxide) (NO), and atrial natriuretic peptide (ANP) or brain natriuretic peptide (BNP) are opposed in their action by catecholamines (norepinephrine) or vasoconstrictor peptides angiotensin II (Ang II) or endothelin-1 (ET-1). This endocrine/paracrine system acts locally on vascular endothelial cells (EC) and smooth muscle cells (SM).

regulation within the blood vessel is the most important contributor to normotension. One important peptide hormone that is made in the endothelial cell is the peptide ET-1. This peptide is the most potent vasoconstrictor in the body. It is 100 times as potent as the previous endogenous champion, the catecholamine norepinephrine, which is manufactured in nerve endings that communicate to the adventitial (outer) layer of blood vessels. ET-1 is a paracrine hormone, which means that 75% of it is secreted toward the adjacent vascular smooth muscle cell, where it binds and induces contraction and elevates BP. Since ET-1 was discovered in 1989 *(1)*, intense research in animals and humans has led us to understand the importance of this hormone in human health and disease. As with any hormone, this peptide binds a protein receptor and triggers a variety of biochemical events in the vascular smooth muscle cell, which results in vasoconstriction. Haynes and Webb *(2)* reported that infusing an ET-1 receptor antagonist into normal human volunteers resulted in a 68% decrease in basal BP and vasomotor tone. This suggests that ET-1 is indispensable for the normal regulation of BP.

Further studies in humans support this idea. In human patients with mild to moderate hypertension, administration of an ET receptor antagonist reduced the diastolic blood pressure by 6 mmHg, which was identical to the reduction in response to enalapril (angiotensin-converting enzyme [ACE] inhibitor) in this same study *(3)*. The fact that inhibition of the angiotensin system or the ET system afforded the same degree of BP reduction is not surprising. In heart failure, Ang II is felt to play a major role in the increased vascular resistance, cardiac hypertrophy followed by dilation, and altered hemodynamics in this decompensated state. In several animal models, inhibition of the ET system markedly resetored normal cardiac and vascular parameters and prevented the effects of administered or endogenous Ang II. Thus, ET production is stimulated by angiotensin and mediates the actions of angiotensin on both the heart and blood vessels. It is predicted that the development of ET antagonists will be used in conjunction with or in place of angiotensin antagonists in the future (*see* below).

ET-1 has also been shown to play an important role in other forms of hypertension. ET-1 levels are greatly elevated in the pulmonary blood vessels of patients with pulmonary hypertension, and both animal and human studies have shown impressive decreased pulmonary capillary pressures in response to endothelin antagonists *(4)*. It is expected that the ET receptor antagonists will play an important role in the prevention and treatment of pulmonary hypertension, and thereby prevent the sequelae of right-sided heart failure. In transplant patients, administration of cyclosporine is necessary to prevent rejection of the organ. Cyclosporine has precipitated renovascular hypertension through effects on the afferent renal blood vessels. ET-1 is liberated in response to cyclosporine in these vessels, and ET receptor antagonists markedly decrease the intrarenal BPs that contribute to the failure of the transplanted kidney, or the overall state of BP in other organ transplant recipients *(5,6)*.

At least four pharmaceutical companies are actively developing ET receptor antagonists. There are also positive effects of these antagonists in preventing ischemia-induced arrhythmias. Therefore, it is not farfetched to propose that in the setting of a myocardial infarction, IV delivery of ET receptor antagonists may prevent further damage to the myocardium by preventing overconstriction of injured blood vessels and stabilize the heart to arrhythmias. Furthermore, modifying the ET system may be part of a treatment plan to prevent the cardiovascular and cerebrovascular sequelae of poorly controlled hypertension.

Angiotensin II

It is in the endothelium that the precursor hormone angiotensin I is converted to Ang II by a converting enzyme. Angiotensin is a vasoconstrictor. The role of the angiotensin system in essential hypertension is supported in that the genetics of this human disease point out that an abnormality of this system strongly correlates to the development of this disorder *(7)*. More specific information is not yet available. ACE inhibitors are the most widely prescribed pharmacologic agent for control of hypertension in the United States. Gene inactivation studies in mice clearly show the importance of this hormone in the maintenance of normal BP. This factor has been discussed herein and clearly makes an important contribution to the hemodynamic state of humans.

Other Vasoconstrictors

Heightened sympathetic overactivity is mediated at the level of the kidney and results in the retention of salt and water, leading to volume expansion and increased BP. In addition, some hypertensive individuals have high levels of circulating plasma catecholamines or increased sensitivity of target organs, such as the vascular smooth muscle cell, to normal levels of these vasoactive amines. In the first situation, decreased salt intake and contraction of the intravascular space with diuretics forms the mainstay of therapy. The use of α-adrenergic blockade to lower BP is an effective strategy in many hypertensive patients. The rare patient who has a pheochromocytoma can be identified by measuring urinary catecholamines in a properly collected 24-h urine specimen. If the specimen is suggestive of pheochromocytoma, then measuring plasma catecholamines after the patient is recumbent and has an indwelling iv catheter for 30 min is indicated. Catecholamines >1,000 pg/mL support this diagnosis *(8)*. Appropriate radiologic scanning (renal scan or MIBG scan) will then confirm the presence of the tumor. Consultation with an endocrinologist and an experienced surgeon is then recommended.

Various other vasoconstricting agents have been identified, such as thromboxane, prostaglandin F, and endothelial-derived constricting factor. To date, there is no convincing evidence that abnormalities of these factors or their receptors play a role in the pathogenesis of human hypertension, and therefore no specific therapeutic interventions are appropriate.

Natriuretic Peptides

The family of natriuretic peptides has profound effects as natriuretic and diuretic hormones *(9)*. These actions result from multiple effects at target organs, including the kidney, vasculature, adrenal gland, and heart. ANP and BNP are synthesized in the heart, but only ANP appears to be relevant in the normal physiologic state. Based on animal gene inactivation studies, ANP is the most important endogenous defender against salt-induced hypertension, promoting a brisk natriuresis in response to salt challenge in humans *(9,10)*. ANP is also a potent vasodilator, acting mainly by opposing the vasoconstricting effects at the vascular smooth muscle cell, of ET-1, Ang II, and catecholamines. ANP inhibits aldosterone production and action, further limiting the propensity to retain salt and water in volume-overloaded states such as congestive heart failure (CHF) or some forms of hypertension. Through many actions, ANP reduces plasma volume and lowers peripheral vascular resistance in hypertensive patients. This suggests that administration of ANP may play a role in the treatment of hypertension in the future. Another member of the family, C-type natriuretic peptide, plays a local role in regulation of vascular tone and blood vessel remodeling, because it is made in the endothelial cell and does not appreciably circulate in plasma.

Another important role of the natriuretic peptides is to compensate for the sequelae of a failing heart. At a time when the clinical manifestations of heart failure are not evident, BNP secretion from the ventricle into plasma is greatly increased, and it is now gaining prominence as an early marker of this disease. Plasma ANP and BNP levels strongly parallel the severity of CHF, increasing 40-fold in the most severe forms of CHF *(12)*. This represents the body's desperate attempt to compensate for the failure of the heart to adequately perfuse vital organs, which leads to heightened renin-angiotensin-aldosterone production. Because ANP (and more potently BNP) reduces preload and afterload in CHF, plasma volume expansion is limited and a rise in BP is dampened. Intraveous administration of ANP has been a mainstay of the treatment of CHF in Japan for several years and results in salt and water excretion and decreased vascular resistance. Administration of BNP for treatment of these conditions is in clinical trial in the United States.

Nitric Oxide

One of the most important factors produced in the endothelium is the soluble gas NO. NO results from the breakdown of arginine to citrulline in various cells including endothelial cells. There are various forms of the enzyme that lead to the production of NO, and all forms are regulated by either calcium or a variety of peptides, growth factors, and cytokines. NO is the most potent endogenous vasodilator yet described *(13)*. It is the counter to many vasoconstrictors, and thereby limits the development of high BP. NO also inhibits the proliferation of vascular smooth muscle cells, thus preventing an initial step in the development of atherosclerosis.

It has been observed that the ability of atherosclerotic endothelium to produce NO is impaired. This leads to unopposed actions of vasoconstrictors such as ET-1, thereby increasing BP and systemic vascular resistance. Through either mechanism, this places an increased load on the heart and contributes to the development of cardiac hypertrophy.

Impaired NO production also plays an important role in another vascular disease—impotence. The failure to vasodilate penile arteries and veins is not different from that in other blood vessels, reflecting a more widespread problem in the patient with atherosclerosis. NO stimulates cyclic guanosine 5′-monophosphate (cGMP) generation as a second messenger of action, and this fact was used in the development of Viagra, which also generates cGMP, and therefore bypasses the need to generate NO in the penis. In arteries that exhibit moderate impairment of NO production, it has been suggested that providing substrate in the form of arginine tablets could lead to increased NO production, and therefore maintain the vasculature for a longer time *(14)*.

DIABETES AND HYPERTENSION

Over the last few years, it has been postulated that hyperinsulinemia and insulin resistance play a role in the development of hypertension in humans who are not diabetic. After many studies of this issue, there is little evidence to convincingly support this idea. However, there does appear to be an association between the development of diabetes mellitus and the subsequent development of hypertension. In diabetes, the normal vasodilator function of insulin has been found to be impaired *(15)*. This is owing to the inability of insulin to augment endothelium-related vasodilation, as part of the spectrum of insulin resistance *(16)*. This defect appears early on in the setting of diabetes, before macrovascular disease develops, and has been observed in the normal, first-degree relatives of diabetics. There are some data supporting the idea that insulin does not stimulate normal NO production, or that NO does not act normally in the diabetic vasculature. Furthermore, the target organs that bear the brunt of hyperglycemia and related metabolic disturbances in diabetes are also profoundly affected by hypertension. These include the retina, kidney, and large blood vessels. The kidney, in particular, suffers from the combined insult of diabetes and hypertension, and management of hypertension needs to be much more aggressive than in the nondiabetic patient. Because intrarenal hypertension or at least increased renin-angiotensin dynamics occurs in the diabetic kidney, ACE inhibitors should constitute the first line of therapy for the hypertensive diabetic. Indeed, development of proteinuria and progression to renal failure in normotensive diabetics, both type I and type II, can be markedly decreased by instituting ACE inhibitor treatment *(17)*.

CONCLUSION

The function of the endothelium includes the production of and response to a variety of vasoactive peptides and factors that regulate vascular tone. Working in conjunction with the medial layer of the blood vessel that contains vascular smooth muscle cells, the endothelium has the capacity to regulate moment-to-moment changes in BP. When the normal function is disrupted, e.g., by diabetes or arteriosclerosis, the noncompliant vessel results in increased hypertension in various vascular beds. Also, increased systemic vascular resistance occurs and leads to increased work on the heart, leading to hypertrophy and dilation.

REFERENCES

1. Yanagisawa M, Kurihara H, Kimura S, et al. (1988) A novel potent vasoconstrictor peptide produced by vascular endothelial cells. *Nature* 332:411–415.
2. Haynes WG, Webb DJ (1994) Contribution of endogenous generation of endothelin-1 to basal vascular tone. *Lancet* 344:852–854.
3. Krum H, Viskoper RJ, Lacourciere Y, Budde M, Charlon V (1998) The effect of an endothelin-receptor antagonist, bosentan, on blood pressure in patients with essential hypertension. Bosentan Hypertension Investigators. *N Engl J Med,* 338(12):784–790.
4. Giaid A, Yanagisawa M, Langleben D, Michel RP, Levy R, Shennib H, Kimura S, Masaki T, Duguid WP, Stewart DJ (1993) Expression of endothelin-1 in the lungs of patients with primary pulmonary hypertension. *New Engl J Med* 328:1732–1739.
5. Lanese DM, Conger JD (1993) Effects of endothelin receptor antagonist on cyclosporine-induced vasoconstriction in isolated rat renal arterioles. *J Clin Invest* 93:2144–2149.
6. Fogo A, Hellings SE, Inagami T, Kon V (1992) Endothelin receptor antagonism is protective in in vivo acute cyclosporine toxicity. *Kidney Int* 42:770–774.
7. Corvol P, Soubrier F, Jeunemaitre X (1997) Molecular genetics of the renin-angiotensin-aldosterone system in human hypertension. *Pathologie Biologie* 45(3):229–239.

8. Bravo EL, Gifford RW Jr (1993) Pheochromocytoma. *Endocrinol Metab Clin North Am* 22(2):329–341.

9. John SWM, Veress AT, Honrath U, et al. (1996) Blood pressure and fluid-electrolyte balance in mice with reduced or absent atrial natriuretic peptide. *Am J Physiol* 271:R109–R114.

10. Kishimoto I, Dubois SK, Garbers DL (1996) The heart communicates with the kidney exclusively through the guanylyl cyclase-A receptor: acute handling of sodium and water in response to volume expansion. *Proc Natl Acad Sci USA* 93:6215–6219.

11. Hunt PJ, Espiner EA, Nichols MG, Richards AM, Yandle TG (1996) Differing biological effects of equimolar atrial and brain natriuretic peptide infusions in normal man. *J Clin Endocrinol Metab* 81:3871–3876.

12. Burnett JC Jr, Kao PC, Hu DC, et al. (1986) Atrial natriuretic peptide elevation in congestive heart failure in the human. *Science* 231:1145–1147.

13. Ignarro LJ (1993) Nitric oxide-mediated vasorelaxation. *Thromb Haemost* 70(1):148–151.

14. Maccario M, Oleandri SE, Procopio M, Grottoli S, Avogadri E, Camanni F, Ghigo E (1997) Comparison among the effects of arginine, a nitric oxide precursor, isosorbide dinitrate and molsidomine, two nitric oxide donors, on hormonal secretions and blood pressure in man. *J Endocrinol Invest* 20(8):488–492.

15. Baron AD (1996) Insulin and the vasculature—old actors, new roles. *J Invest Med* 44(8):406–412.

16. Pieper GM (1998) Review of alterations in endothelial nitric oxide production in diabetes: protective role of arginine on endothelial dysfunction. *Hypertension* 31(5):1047–1060.

17. Penno G, Chaturvedi N, Talmud PJ, Cotroneo P, Manto A, Nannipieri M, Luong LA, Fuller JH (1998) Effect of angiotensin-converting enzyme (ACE) gene polymorphism on progression of renal disease and the influence of ACE inhibition in IDDM patients: findings from the EUCLID Randomized Controlled Trial. EURODIAB Controlled Trial of Lisinopril in IDDM. *Diabetes* 47(9):1507–1511.

II DIAGNOSIS AND SPECIAL TESTS

10 Systolic, Diastolic, Mean, or Pulse Pressure

Which Is the Best Predictor of Hypertensive Cardiovascular Risk?

Stanley S. Franklin, MD

CONTENTS

The relative importance of diastolic blood pressure (DBP), systolic blood pressure (SBP), mean arterial pressure (MAP), and pulse pressure (PP) as hypertensive cardiovascular risk factors has been controversial. The cardiovascular risks of hypertension result primarily from mechanical stresses to the left ventricle and to the vascular endothelium and media of blood vessels supplying the heart, brain, and kidneys. With

From: *Hypertension Medicine*
Edited by: M. A. Weber © Humana Press Inc., Totowa, NJ

the application of the sphygmomanometer to clinical medicine at the beginning of the twentieth century, DBP was thought to be initially the best measure of this risk. In the 1990s, however, authorities advocated that both SBP and DBP, whichever is higher, be used in classifying hypertensive cardiovascular risk. There are problems with the present guidelines, in that SBP and DBP represent only two inflection points on the propagated arterial pulse wave that is measured by cuff readings at the peripheral brachial artery.

CONCEPT OF PULSATILE AND STEADY-STATE HEMODYNAMICS

The arterial pulse wave is better described as consisting of a pulsatile component (PP) during systole and a steady component (MAP) during diastole. PP, the difference between peak SBP and end DBP, represents the pressure increment over and above the existing DBP that results from ventricular contraction and ejection of arterial blood into the aorta. At any given ventricular ejection, cardiac output and heart rate, large-artery stiffness, and early wave reflection determine PP. PP, therefore, is the surrogate measurement of pulsatile opposition to blood flow during systole. By contrast, MAP is influenced by cardiac output and peripheral vascular resistance (PVR) in the absence of pulsations, and is calculated from the following standard equation: MAP = ($\frac{2}{3}$) DBP + ($\frac{1}{3}$) SBP (in mmHg). MAP is thought to be the surrogate measure of static resistance to blood flow provided by the arterioles and small arteries during diastole.

Both elevations in static resistance and pulsatile arterial stiffness contribute to left ventricular vascular load and, hence, to hypertensive cardiovascular risk. The principal question to be answered in this chapter is: Which BP component is the best predictor of hypertensive cardiovascular risk?

HOW DO HEMODYNAMIC MECHANISMS IMPACT BP COMPONENTS?

Both increased resistance and increased stiffness elevate SBP. By contrast, DBP rises with increased PVR but falls with increased stiffness; the relative contribution of each determines the ultimate DBP. Two clinical patterns of BP elevation can be recognized with systolic

BP ≥ 140 mmHg. If PVR increases greatly and there is a mild increase in arterial stiffness, DBP rises to a least 90 mmHg, in a condition classified as combined systolic/diastolic hypertension. If arterial stiffness increases greatly and there is a mild increase in resistance, DBP remains <90 mmHg, in a condition classified as isolated systolic hypertension.

Aging affects BP hemodynamics. There is a linear rise in SBP with aging from adolescence onward that is paralleled by increases in DBP and MAP until about age 50 (Fig. 10.1). The almost parallel rise in SBP, DBP, and MAP up to age 50 can best be explained by an increase in PVR. After age 50–60, DBP declines, PP rises steeply, and MAP levels off while SBP continues to show a linear increase throughout the geriatric years. The BP pattern from age 50 onward is best explained by a predominance of large-artery stiffness. With age-related stiffening of the aorta, there is a decreased elasticity and a greater peripheral runoff of stroke volume during systole. With less blood remaining in the aorta at the beginning of diastole, and with diminished elastic recoil, DBP decreases and the diastolic decay curve becomes steeper. Moreover, the fall in DBP secondary to the increase in large-artery stiffness explains why the MAP equation grossly underestimates PVR after age 50.

IMPORTANCE OF PULSE WAVE PROPAGATION AND REFLECTION

The heart, brain, and kidneys are not exposed to peripheral artery pressure but instead to the pressure in the aorta and its immediate branches. Brachial cuff pressure provides only a limited view of the arterial tree, whereas elevated aortic pressure is crucial in the development of cardiovascular complications. Although vascular resistance is almost identical in both peripheral and central arteries, significant discrepancies between central and brachial artery PP may exist as a result of pulse wave propagation and reflection.

In young subjects with elastic arteries, there is a progressive increase in the amplitude of PP from the central to the peripheral arteries as a result of reflected waves reinforcing incident waves (Fig. 10.2). Because of this amplification phenomenon, central artery BPs in young normotensive subjects with highly elastic aortas are lower than those recorded at the brachial artery. Furthermore, there is a beneficial boost in coronary perfusion as the reflected wave impacts on the heart during diastole.

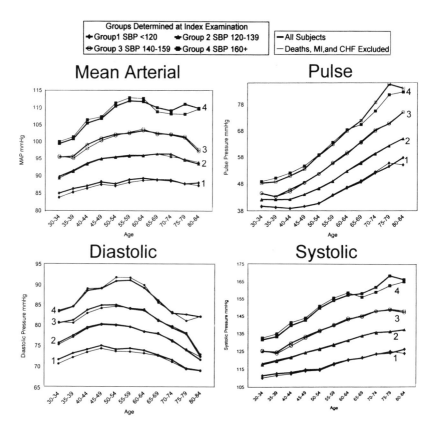

Fig. 10-1. Arterial pressure components by age. Group-averaged data for all subjects and with deaths, MI, and CHF are excluded. Averaged BP levels are from all available data from each subject within 5-yr age intervals (30–34 through 80–84) by SBP groupings 1–4. Thick line represents entire study cohort (2036 subjects); thin line represents study cohort with deaths, nonfatal MI, and CHF excluded (1353 subjects). Reproduced with permission from Franklin SS, Gustin WG, Wong ND, Larson MG, Weber MA, Kannel WB, Levy D (1997) Hemodynamic patterns of age-related changes in blood pressure: The Framingham Heart Study. *Circulation* 96:308–315.

With aging and stiffening of central elastic arteries, there is a resulting increase in amplitude and velocity of the incident waves, so that the heart is now impacted from early wave reflection during systole rather than diastole, further adding to increased cardiac afterload. Given the same stroke volume and ejection rate, the resulting early wave reflection will produce a higher SBP, a lower DBP, and therefore a wider PP, but PVR will remain unchanged. In elderly hypertensive patients, in

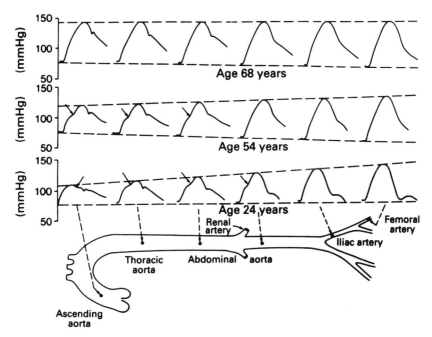

Fig. 10-2. Pressure wave recorded along the arterial tree from the proximal ascending aorta to the femoral artery in three adult subjects ages 24, 54, and 68 yr. In the youngest subject, amplification of the pressure wave increases approx 60% during transmission. By contrast, the oldest subject shows minimal amplification of the pressure wave during transmission. With aging there is a progressive increase in SBP and decrease in DBP. Reproduced with permission from Nichols WW, Avolio AP, Kelly RP, O'Rourke MF (1993) Effect of age and of hypertension on wave travel and reflections. In: O'Rourke MF, Safar ME, Dzau JV, eds. *Arterial Vasodilation: Mechanisms and Therapy,* London: Edward Arnold.

contrast to younger adults, early wave reflection can produce increases in amplitude of PP in the ascending aorta by as much as 40–50%. With this central augmentation, the amplification effect is significantly reduced in subjects ≥50 yr of age and may be eliminated by age 65, so that central and brachial artery PP become almost identical.

The peripheral amplification and central augmentation phenomena secondary to pulse wave propagation and wave reflection have important clinical implications. First, very young adults may present with predominant diastolic hypertension by brachial artery cuff pressure measurements as a result of decreased peripheral amplification of SBP. Second, because central augmentation abolishes peripheral amplification in middle-aged and older subjects, brachial cuff PP can more accurately predict cardiovascular risk than in younger subjects. Third, pharmacologic agents that vasodilate peripheral arteries may largely abolish early wave reflection and central augmentation, thereby reducing central PP by a greater margin than brachial artery cuff PP.

CLINICAL AND PATHOLOGIC RELEVANCE OF INCREASED PP

If arterial stiffness is a risk factor for cardiovascular disease, elevated PP and reduced DBP should be markers of this risk. Considerable evidence now favors the superiority of increased PP and decreased DBP to that of elevated SBP in predicting this risk. In middle-aged and elderly subjects, PP is an independent predictor of left ventricular hypertrophy, aortic atherosclerosis, acute myocardial infarction (MI), stroke, and congestive heart failure (CHF).

Increased PP may be a surrogate marker for several pathologic mechanisms that contribute to the development of cardiac events. A rise in aortic pulsatile load increases left ventricular systolic wall stress, decreases coronary flow reserve, and impairs left ventricular relaxation. A rise in aortic pulsatile load is a major factor in the development of left ventricular dysfunction and hypertrophy. Simultaneously, decreased DBP further compromises the oxygen supply:demand ratio by reducing coronary flow. Finally, a rise in pulsatile shear stress leads to endothelial dysfunction and a greater propensity for coronary artery artherosclerosis. Conversely, a wide PP may simply serve as a marker for diffuse atherosclerosis. Increased pulsatile stress may also be a factor in the rupture of unstable atheromatous plaques leading to acute MI and sudden death. Even after extensive MI, PP remains a potent predictor of future coronary heart disease (CHD) events and the eventual development of CHF.

WHICH BP COMPONENT IS THE BEST PREDICTOR OF PVR, LARGE-ARTERY STIFFNESS, AND HYPERTENSIVE CARDIOVASCULAR RISK?

In the very young adult hypertensive subject, increases in MAP, DBP, and SBP can be surrogate measurements of increased PVR or high cardiac output. Although accelerated or malignant hypertension

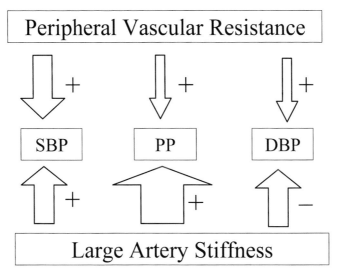

Fig. 10-3. The dual influence of peripheral vascular resistance and large-artery stiffness on components of BP in a young hypertensive subject (upper arrows) and in an elderly hypertensive subject (lower arrows). The width of the arrows depicts the relative magnitude of change in the BP component. The small increase in PP (upper arrow) in a young hypertensive subject is secondary to the stretching of central large arteries from resistance-initiated hypertension. The large increase in PP (lower arrow) in the elderly hypertensive subject is secondary to structural change in central large arteries that increase their stiffness. Increased resistance and large-artery stiffness both increase SBP, but have opposite effects on DBP. See text for details.

generally presents with severe increases in both SBP and DBP, occasionally there is a greater rise in DBP than SBP because of left ventricular dysfunction and/or failure. For example, BP of 190/140 mmHg would suggest a possible urgent or emergent clinical state secondary to accelerated or malignant hypertension. In this uncommon form of acute hypertensive syndrome, the very high DBP is a surrogate measurement of the severe increase in PVR that can rapidly result in organ failure and death in the absence of promptly administered antihypertensive therapy.

In the young adult, an increase in PVR may be associated with a slightly greater increase in SBP than DBP, resulting in a small rise in PP (Fig. 10.3). This is thought to be a functional increase in PP and can be explained by a downstream increase in PVR causing an upstream increase in transmural pressure, which in turn chronically stretches large central arteries and increases their stiffness. With increasing severity of hypertension, SBP may become superior to DBP as a predictor of cardiovascular risk.

In the middle-aged or elderly hypertensive subject, the onset of structural damage leads to further large-artery stiffness so that DBP levels off or falls while SBP continues to rise (Fig. 10.3). Therefore, PP becomes the single best surrogate for large-artery stiffness and the single best predictor of cardiovascular risk when elevated SBP is accompanied by discordantly normal or low DBP. These findings support the concept that cardiovascular events are more related to the pulsatile stress of large-artery stiffness and early wave reflection during systole than the steady-state stress of PVR during diastole.

In summary, the current classification of middle-aged and geriatric hypertension, which uses the rise in SBP or DBP, or both, overemphasizes small-vessel resistance and underestimates the influence of large-artery stiffness. By contrast, increased PP and decreased DBP are superior risk markers of cardiovascular disease because arterial stiffness is represented fully by these components of BP. An elevated PVR can initiate hypertension and is the dominant component of hypertension in the young, but large-artery stiffness and early pulse wave reflection become paramount in the middle-aged and elderly. Therefore, in subjects with identical levels of SBP, those with isolated systolic hypertension are at greater risk for CHD than those with combined systolic/diastolic hypertension.

TREATMENT GOALS

Hypertensive treatment goals must be reexamined in light of the discussed observational findings. The treatment goal may well be SBP reduction in the young and PP reduction in the middle-aged and elderly. Clearly, it is invalid to assume that treatment goals have been achieved with reduction of DBP when systolic hypertension and wide PP persist. There are many unanswered questions that will require careful testing in prospective clinical trials: What level of increased PP requires therapeutic intervention? How does PP risk compare with the current national and international BP staging classification? What should be the treatment goal of PP reduction in order to achieve optimal improvement in cardiovascular morbidity and mortality rates? And what level of therapeutic SBP reduction should be achieved to optimize reduction in PP?

SUGGESTED READINGS

Nichols WW, O'Rourke MF (1998) *McDonald's Blood Flow in Arteries,* 4th ed., London: Arnold, Hodder Headline Group.

Berne RM, Levy MN (1992) *Cardiovascular Physiology,* St. Louis: Mosby Year Book.

Smulyan H, Safar ME (1997) Systolic blood pressure revisited. *J Am Coll Cardiol* 29:1407–1413.

Nichols WW, Nicolini FA, Pepine CJ (1992) Determinants of isolated systolic hypertension in the elderly. *J Hypertens* 10(Suppl. 6):S73–S77.

O'Rourke MF, Kelly RP, Avolio AP (1993) Wave reflection in the systemic circulation and its implications in ventricular function. *J Hypertens* 11:323–337.

Franklin SS, Gustin W, Wong ND, Larson MG, Weber MA, Kannel WB, Levy D. Hemodynamic patterns of age-related changes in blood pressure: The Framingham Heart Study. *Circulation* 96:308–315.

Benetos A, Safar M, Rudnichi A, Smulyan H, Richard JL, Ducimetieere P, Guize L (1997) Pulse pressure: a predictor of long-term cardiovascular mortality in a French male population. *Hypertension* 30:1410–1415.

11 Manual Blood Pressure Measurement—Still the Gold Standard

Why and How to Measure Blood Pressure the Old-Fashioned Way

Carlene M. Grim, RN, MSN, SPDN, and Clarence E. Grim, MS, MD, FACP, FACC

Contents

From: *Hypertension Medicine*
Edited by: M. A. Weber © Humana Press Inc., Totowa, NJ

Key Points

- Hypertension detection, referral, and treatment guidelines are based on blood pressures (BPs) by trained observers using the standardized BP technique recommended by the American Heart Association (AHA) *(1)*.
- All clinical studies of BP use a mercury manometer, because it is the most accurate and reliable instrument available and should always be the primary standard for indirect BP measurement.
- Inaccuracies are the result of equipment error or human observer error. Observer errors include errors in technique and errors related to the subject or patient *(2)*.
- Because of inadequate training and lack of knowledge, BP readings taken in practice today are rarely accurate, precise, or reliable.
- A few simple techniques allow you to detect error and increase accuracy of readings taken in your clinical setting.

Indirect BP measurement is one of the most frequently performed health care procedures. Because BP measurement is a simple procedure, it is taken for granted that all graduates from medical training programs have the ability to record accurate, precise, and reliable BP readings. However, research since the 1960s has shown this assumption to be false. Most health professionals do not measure BP in a manner known to be accurate and reliable. If you doubt this statement, watch as BPs are taken in your own clinical setting to determine whether the guidelines discussed herein are followed, and then examine recorded readings for signs of observer bias. We have published a teaching curriculum that ensures that those who take BP have mastered the knowledge, skills, and behaviors needed to obtain an accurate and reliable BP (see ref. *3* for more details on the training and testing of observers).

BP errors may be equipment related, observer related, or patient related. The two factors that contribute most to poor BP measurement by modern-day observers are lack of depth when teaching the basic skills needed to master BP measurement during professional education; and the growing tendency to rely on, and failure to question, BPs measured by non-mercury devices. Such devices have been repeatedly proven less accurate and reliable than a well-trained observer utilizing a standard mercury manometer, the low-frequency detector of the stethoscope (bell), and the "old fashioned," auscultatory method.

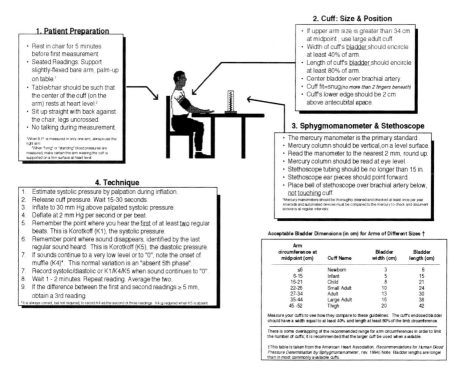

1. Patient Preparation

- Rest in chair for 5 minutes before first measurement.
- Seated Readings: Support slightly-flexed bare arm, palm-up on table.[1]
- Table/chair should be such that the center of the cuff (on the arm) rests at heart level.[2]
- Sit up straight with back against the chair, legs uncrossed.
- No talking during measurement.

When B.P. is measured in only one arm, always use the right arm.
[2]When "lying" or "standing" blood pressures are measured, make certain the arm wearing the cuff is supported on a firm surface at heart level.

2. Cuff: Size & Position

- If upper arm size is greater than 34 cm at midpoint , use large adult cuff.
- Width of cuff's bladder should encircle at least 40% of arm.
- Length of cuff's bladder should encircle at least 80% of arm.
- Center bladder over brachial artery.
- Cuff fit=snug (no more than 2 fingers beneath)
- Cuff's lower edge should be 2 cm above antecubital space.

3. Sphygmomanometer & Stethoscope

- The mercury manometer is the primary standard .
- Mercury column should be vertical,on a level surface.
- Read the manometer to the nearest 2 mm, round up.
- Mercury column should be read at eye level.
- Stethoscope tubing should be no longer than 15 in.
- Stethoscope ear pieces should point forward.
- Place bell of stethoscope over brachial artery below, not touching cuff.

*Mercury manometers should be thoroughly cleaned and checked at least once per year. Aneroids and automated devices must be compared to the mercury to check and document accuracy at regular intervals.

4. Technique

1. Estimate systolic pressure by palpation during inflation.
2. Release cuff pressure. Wait 15-30 seconds.
3. Inflate to 30 mm Hg above palpated systolic pressure.
4. Deflate at 2 mm Hg per second or per beat.
5. Remember the point where you hear the first of at least two regular beats. This is Korotkoff (K1), the systolic pressure.
6. Remember point where sound disappears, identified by the last regular sound heard. This is Korotkoff (K5), the diastolic pressure.
7. If sounds continue to a very low level or to "0", note the onset of muffle (K4)*. This normal variation is an "absent 5th phase".
7. Record systolic/diastolic or K1/K4/K5 when sound continues to "0".
8. Wait 1 - 2 minutes. Repeat reading. Average the two.
9. If the difference between the first and second readings ≥ 5 mm, obtain a 3rd reading.

*It is always correct, but not required, to record K4 as the second of three readings. K4 is required when K5 is absent.

Acceptable Bladder Dimensions (in cm) for Arms of Different Sizes †

Arm circumference at midpoint (cm)	Cuff Name	Bladder width (cm)	Bladder length (cm)
≤6	Newborn	3	6
6-15	Infant	5	15
16-21	Child	8	21
22-26	Small Adult	10	24
27-34	Adult	13	30
35-44	Large Adult	16	38
45-52	Thigh	20	42

Measure your cuffs to see how they compare to these guidelines. The cuff's enclosed bladder should have a width equal to at least 40% and length at least 80% of the limb circumference.

There is some overlapping of the recommended range for arm circumferences in order to limit the number of cuffs; it is recommended that the larger cuff be used when available.

† This table is taken from the American Heart Association, Recommendations for Human Blood Pressure Determination by Sphygmomanometer, rev. 1994) Note: Bladder lengths are longer than in most commonly available cuffs.

Fig. 11-1. Proper BP technique using American Heart Association Guidelines.

Although one's work might require few manual readings, it is necessary to know and understand the principles and steps needed to obtain accurate indirect auscultatory BPs to verify any automated device. This chapter provides tools to assess the quality of BP measurement in your setting and suggestions for implementing a system of quality assurance. It is likely that patients you care for will be healthier once you adopt these methods (Fig. 11.1).

OBSERVER ERRORS: CORRECT INTERPRETATION OF KOROTKOFF SOUNDS

When asked what they were taught about how to measure BP, most professionals state that they were told only to record the first and last sounds heard. Accurate measurement is a simple procedure that most people can learn in a few hours with repeated practice. However, accurate measurement requires knowledge of the Korotkoff sounds as well as knowledge and performance of the steps required to control factors that can alter BP readings. Accurate measurement also depends on one's ability to see, hear, coordinate hand and eye movements, interpret sounds, and remember the readings.

Errors are common and may be owing to lack of knowledge, inability to perform the skills necessary to obtain accurate readings, observer bias, poor judgment, and poor interaction with the subject being measured. Eyesight and hearing must be good enough to allow the observer to see the small marks on the manometer and hear the Korotkoff sounds needed to interpret the reading. In addition, he or she must know the current recommendations about which Korotkoff phases determine systolic and diastolic readings.

Hand-eye coordination must be sufficient to release the pressure at the rate of 2 mmHg per beat while counting backward down the scale. The observer must learn to listen for the onset and disappearance of regular sounds, to concentrate in order to remember the systolic until arriving at the diastolic, and to record the reading immediately and accurately.

RECOMMENDATIONS/ALERTS

How Well Do You Measure Up?

Assess your own and others' ability to listen for and interpret Korotkoff sounds using standardized videotapes of recorded BP readings and using a dual or teaching stethoscope to listen and compare readings with a colleague.

When hearing loss is suspected, test acuity and document the results. Persons with documented hearing loss in a range that affects ability to read BPs should not take readings. So-called enhanced stethoscopes do not guarantee readings comparable to those by persons with average hearing, using a standard stethoscope. We have found that it is not possible to set these devices so that those with impaired hearing can reliably obtain accurate readings.

Quality Assurance

Warning signs that readers are not precise and accurate:

- More than 30% of recorded systolics and diastolics end in 0 (terminal digit bias).

continued

- Readings ending in odd numbers. The AHA guidelines recommend reading to the nearest 2 mmHg.
- Readings consistently slightly above or below treatment cutoffs (cutoff bias or knowledge of treatment bias).
- Readings very similar or identical to last recorded reading (previous reading bias).

Assessment Tip

- Common errors occur because people are taught to listen for the first loud, distinct, or strong sound. As a result, they may record single sounds (artifacts or noise) and ignore most soft regular sounds when they occur at the systolic or diastolic level. Before deciding that an observer is unable to hear, make sure he or she knows how to rule out extraneous sounds and is listening for the soft sounds that sometimes occur at the systolic or diastolic levels.
- The usual error is in the range of 8, 10, or 12 mmHg.

Observer Errors: Selecting and Using Equipment

Equipment selection errors include failure to choose the primary standard mercury manometer and lack of a selection of cuffs with bladder sizes to accommodate your patient population in your equipment inventory. Common equipment use errors include failure to choose the correct cuff for a given individual, failure to center the cuff bladder over the brachial artery in the upper inner arm so that pressure is maximally transmitted over the brachial artery during measurement, inflating too slowly, and deflating too quickly. Common reading errors include failure to record systolic and diastolics to the nearest 2 mmHg and a tendency to read only the left or only the right side of the mercury column.

Quality Assurance: BP Equipment

- **Sphygmomanometers:**
  —Set up a maintenance schedule.
  —Clean and check mercury manometers yearly.

continued

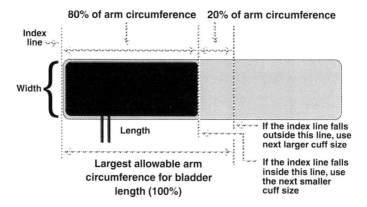

Fig. 11-2. How to check and mark the cuffs used in your setting to ensure that you use the most accurate cuff. Most cuffs made today are not marked correctly according to the AHA guidelines. The width of the cuff should encircle at least 40% of the arm circumference. The markings for the correct length range for any cuff are shown in the figure.

—Check aneroid manometers at purchase and at least every 6 mo.

—Check automated devices for ambulatory and home use at purchase and prior to placing on a given patient.

—Educate staff about how to avoid and what to do in the case of a mercury spill.

• **Stethoscopes:**

—Tubing should be thick and no longer than 15 inches.

—Earpieces should be adjustable and eartips cleaned frequently.

—Chestpiece should have a low-frequency detector—most commonly the bell.

• **Cuffs: mark your cuffs (Fig. 11.2):**

—Make certain large cuffs are available in each work area.

—Mark cuffs with bladder center and appropriate arm circumference.

—Inflation system: replace when tubing/bladder is weak or cracked.

—Large cuffs need large bulbs for proper inflation. (Some prefer large bulbs for all devices.)

—Replace valves and bulbs as needed.

continued

—Wash or clean cuff fabric frequently. We know of no standards or practice for this cleaning interval.

Assessment Tip

• Look for errors in the range of 8, 10, or 12 mmHg. This occurs when the observer releases the pressure too fast, tends to read only one side of the mercury gage, or fails to concentrate enough to remember the reading. When pressure is released at 10 mm/beat, readings can only be to the closest 10.
• **What to do when observers have difficulty hearing blood pressure:**
   —Make sure they palpate to locate the best place to listen over the brachial artery.
   —Check to see that eartips fit and are pointing in the direction of the ear canal.
   —Use a dual stethoscope to check an observer's hearing.
• **Recheck elevated readings on patients with large or muscular arms:**
   —Measure the arm circumference at the midpoint between the olecranon and acromial process and verify cuff size referring to Table 11.1.
   —When in doubt, use the larger cuff.
   —Check to see that the arm and cuff size are recorded in the patient's record.
• **Questionable readings owing to arm size >41 cm and shape: choose the cuff that fits the forearm:**
   —Center the bladder and place the stethoscope over the radial artery.
   —Support the forearm at heart level.
   —If unable to hear, palpate the systolic.
   —In some patients with large and short arms, it is not possible to obtain an accurate BP with a large cuff. In these cases, compare the palpated pressure taken with the large cuff on the upper arm to that taken with an appropriately sized cuff on the forearm. If the palpated systolic pressures are within 10 mm Hg of each other, then the upper arm pressure is reliable. If the forearm is over 10 mm Hg less, then prefer to use the forearm palpated pressures.

Table 11-1
Label Your Cuffs: Acceptable Bladder Dimensions (in cm)
for Arms of Different Sizes

Cuff	AHA Bladder Width (cm)	AHA Bladder Length (cm)	Arm Circumference Midpoint (cm)	Best Available Cuff from Practice Setting (Bladder width should Fit 40% of arm circumference)
Newborn	3	6	≤6	
Infant	5	15	6–15	
Child	8	21	16–21	
Small adult	10	24	22–26	
Adult	13	30	27–34	
Large Adult	16	38	35–44	
Adult thigh	20	42	45–52	

The shaded portion of this table is taken directly from Appendix D of the American Heart Association's "Human Blood Pressure Determination by Sphygmomanometry" and shows ideal cuff bladder sizes for a given arm circumference. Complete the 4th column by measuring the bladders in your cuffs. Make sure you have at least one cuff with a bladder width at least 40% of the arm circumference for each range.

OBSERVER ERRORS: FAILURE TO OBTAIN READINGS THAT ESTIMATE BP OUTSIDE THE OFFICE OR CLINICAL SETTING

The goal of BP measurement in the clinical setting is to get the best estimate of usual BP, a measurement that has been used in the research setting to diagnose and treat increased BP. To accomplish this, one must attempt to control the biological and environmental factors that cause temporary changes in BP and obtain an average reading in the arm with the highest reading.

Positioning

Failure to properly position the patient for seated, standing, and supine readings is a frequent occurrence in the clinical setting. Regardless of the position, the limb wearing the cuff should be resting and supported on a flat surface allowing the center of the cuff to be at the subject's heart level. Inaccurately low readings occur when the cuff is above heart level, and inaccurately high readings occur when the cuff is below heart level. Seated readings require back support. Seat the patient in a straight-back chair, next to a table or desk, with legs uncrossed and feet flat on the floor. Standing readings require that the arm be supported on an inanimate object adjusted, prior to standing, to place the cuff at heart level. Supine readings may require a small support such as a firm pillow to raise the center of the cuff to midchest level. Position yourself and the manometer so that you can easily view the instrument at eye level.

Environment

Whether BPs are taken in an office or an examination room, the environment must be controlled in order to obtain accurate readings. It should be private, quiet, and have good lighting and a comfortable temperature. After measuring and placing the correct cuff on the patient's arm, provide a simple explanation of the procedure and let the patient rest for 5 min prior to taking the first reading.

Patient Instruction Prior to Measurement

- Ask about the following:
  —Exercise within the past hour
  —Intake: prescription and over-the-counter medications, food, and alcohol
  —Need to empty bladder prior to measurement
- Determine cuff size and arm required to obtain an accurate reading. Make sure each person knows the proper cuff size.
- Explain the following:
  —The need to rest quietly for at least 5 min
  —The need to sit straight with legs uncrossed, feet flat on the floor
  —The need for silence during the reading
  —That you will take more than one reading to get an average
  —That you will first feel the pulse to estimate the systolic in order to know how much pressure is needed for an accurate reading

These steps are necessary for good technique. Following these steps will help you hear BP sounds more clearly, decrease patient discomfort, and obtain accurate readings when there is an auscultatory gap.

- **Determining how high to inflate the cuff:**
  - —Prior to listening, estimate the systolic pressure by palpating the brachial or radial artery for pulse obliteration as the cuff is inflated.
  - —Wait 15 s and reinflate to 30 mm Hg above the estimated systolic. Then begin to listen. This is the only way to avoid missing an auscultatory gap.
- **Allowing the arm to rest between readings:**
  - —Listen as you allow the mercury to fall at 2 mm Hg/s.
  - —Remember the first of at least two regular beats (systolic reading).
  - —Control the valve so that the mercury falls at 2 mm Hg/beat until the last regular sound is heard.
  - —Listen for an additional 10–20 mm Hg to confirm disappearance.
  - —Record systolic and diastolic readings.
  - —Wait 1 to 2 min before repeating the reading. This is a good time to take the pulse.
- **Placing the stethoscope:**
  - —Hyperextend and support the patient's elbow while palpating to locate the best listening point over the brachial artery. This is usually just under and to the inside of the biceps tendon. If doing multiple sitting and standing readings, mark the spot for subsequent readings.
  - —Gently rest the bell of the stethoscope over this artery listening point. Make sure the bell is fully in contact with the skin surface on all sides. This can be determined by lightly touching the skin next to the bell. If no sound is heard, the bell needs to be repositioned.
- **Avoiding diastolic errors in the presence of an auscultatory gap:**
  - —When the diastolic is high, listen for an additional 40 mmHg to make certain the Korotkoff sounds do not reappear after a period of silence.

continued

- **Obtaining accurate estimates when the pulse is irregular:**
  —Take more readings to get the best average.
  —Start listening earlier and listen longer.
  —Deflate very slowly.
  —Note on the chart that the pulse is irregular.

When sounds are difficult to hear and you have used accurate technique, try one of these methods to make the sounds louder.[a]

- **Method 1:**
  —Explain what you are going to do and why.
  —Get ready by wearing the stethoscopes' earpieces forward.
  —Support the patient's arm in a raised position above the head for 15 s.
  —Quickly inflate the cuff while the arm is raised and supported to 60 mmHg above the palpated systolic pressure.
  —Quickly and gently lower the arm to the table.
  —Place the stethoscope over the artery.
  —Deflate and listen.
  —Record the reading and that enhancement was used.
- **Method 2:**
  —Explain what you are going to do and why.
  —Ask the patient to pump his or her hand, making a fist 8–10 times after the cuff is inflated.
  —Quickly inflate the cuff while the arm is still resting on the table.
  —Remind the patient to start squeezing.
  —Stop the patient after 8–10 squeezes.
  —Deflate and listen after the patient relaxes his or her arm.
  —Record the reading and that enhancement was used.

[a]Use of enhancement techniques can change the true BP. Use them only when you are sure you have followed good technique and are listening in the best place.

ENSURING THAT THE EQUIPMENT USED BY YOU AND YOUR PATIENTS IS ACCURATE

Accurate equipment is key to good clinical practice. Every clinic should have at least one mercury manometer to use as the primary standard. If the tube is clean, the top of the meniscus is at zero, and the pressure rises and falls quickly and evenly as pressure is changed in the cuff, the manometer is accurate. It is the primary standard for pressure measurement and the same device used for the primary standard at the National Bureau of Standards.

Campaigns to minimize the use of mercury in medical practice in order to minimize the loss of mercury into the environment are taking place throughout the world. You should know that compared to other sources, mercury manometers are not a significant source of mercury released into the environment and that every office should have at least one manometer.

If you use aneroid instruments, someone in your setting must be responsible for regular inspection and repair. Indeed, most research has shown that at least 30% of aneroid devices go out of calibration with age *(4)*. The only way to be certain your aneroid devices are accurate is to check them against a mercury device at regular intervals. This process takes less than 10 min and can also be used to test the accuracy of a patient's home device. If using a Y tube, simply connect the two devices and a bulb and inflate to compare readings. The following method explains how to compare aneroid calibration to an accurate mercury manometer without a Y tube:

1. Remove the aneroid device from the tubing connecting it to the cuff on the mercury device.
2. Take the mercury system cuff and pump enough air into it so that you can squeeze the rolled up cuff, and the pressure in the manometer will rise and fall (approx 10–20 mmHg).
3. Fold over the tubing leading to the bulb and pinch it off to hold the air while you remove the bulb.
4. While continuing to pinch the tubing, replace the bulb with the aneroid device gage.
5. Release the pinched tubing. Now you should be able to squeeze the rolled up cuff to vary the pressure in the mercury and the aneroid gage. You can now "set" the pressure in the mercury manometer to the level of pressure you want to compare on the aneroid. We recommend you start at 200 mmHg and pause to check each device at the levels of pressure used to make medical decisions: 180, 150, 140, 130, 120, 110, 100, 90, and 80. If the aneroid reads greater than ±3 mmHg it should be discarded or returned to the manufacturer for recalibration.
6. Place a sticker with the day's date on the device. Record the results on your equipment inventory or quality control document. Implement a quality assurance system in your office that ensures that all devices are inspected and calibrated every 3 mo.

7. Automated and aneroid devices must be checked regularly against a mercury device. This can be done by using a "Y" tube to connect the two devices to a common inflation bulb. However, some self-inflating devices give an error if they do not detect an oscillating BP signal as the bulb deflates. This can be simulated by gently squeezing the cuff as the pressure decreases, at, say, 60 cycles per minute. Many automated devices slow their deflation rate once systolic BP has been detected.

DO YOU HEAR WHAT I HEAR?—CHECK TO VERIFY ACCURACY DURING ACTUAL MEASUREMENT

After checking the manometer's pressure-registering system against a mercury manometer, you are ready to review the patient's technique and verify accuracy during measurement. We recommend this be done at least every 3 mo:

1. Place the automatic cuff on the arm the patient routinely uses during measurement. It is usually the left arm in right-handed patients because they can operate the device more easily with the right hand. Of course, you need to be certain that the BP in the left arm is the same as that in the right arm.
2. Palpate the brachial artery in the antecubital fossa so that you know where to place the stethoscope to get the best Korotkoff sounds. If the patient's device utilizes an attached stethoscope, place the bell downstream from where it fits over the brachial artery.
3. Have the patient pump the bulb or initiate automatic inflation.
4. Place the bell of your stethoscope over the brachial artery. Listen for the Korotkoff sounds and record the pressure you read from their electronic monitor display. Then note the pressure the automatic device recorded of the patient. Repeat this three times and compute the average and then the average by the automated device. If the average of the readings differs by more than 5 mmHg, this device is not accurate and should be discarded or returned to the manufacturer.

HOME BPs BY THE PATIENT OR ANOTHER PERSON

Research has demonstrated that patients who take their own BP are more likely to stay in treatment and have better control *(5)*. The Sixth Joint National Committee on the Prevention, Detection, Evaluation and Treatment of High Blood Pressure recommends that patients take their own BP. If the patient can hear and operate an aneroid device we prefer to use this method. The patient is taught using a videotape and individual instruction *(6)*. The principles and techniques of self-measurement are the same as described elsewhere in this chapter. We ask patients to obtain a small calendar record book in which to record their pressure and pulse. If diabetic they can record their glucose readings there as well. The goal BP and the medication regimen are recorded in this book at each visit. Patients are also asked to record their questions for discussion at the next visit.

Once informed and able to perform accurate readings patients can be managed over the Internet. After they send a record of their readings and the medications they are taking, questions can be answered and dosage adjustments made by e-mail.

CONCLUSION

1. The accurate and reliable measurement of BP is the key to good BP control.
2. Current evidence documents that correct measurement is almost never done in practice today.
3. The major reason for the failure to perform this critical medical skill in a manner required to obtain an accurate measurement is the failure of the education system to train medical professionals adequately.
4. To ensure accurate measurement the equipment must be accurate. The primary standard is the mercury manometer and it must be used to calibrate other devices.
5. The observer must be able to hear the sounds accurately. This can easily be tested with a dual stethoscope or standardized videotape testing.
6. A quality assurance program can easily be implemented in your practice setting using the methods described.
7. Methods to check patient devices are easy to perform in the office setting using a mercury manometer.
8. Schools teaching BP measurement should follow the AHA guidelines to minimize differences in techniques and readings by graduates.

REFERENCES

1. Perloff D, Grim CM, Flack J, Frolich ED, Hill M, McDonald M, Morgenstern BZ (1993) Recommendations for human blood pressure determination by sphygmoma-nometry. *Circulation* 88:2460–2470.
2. Bruce NG, Shaper AG, Walker M, Wannamethee G (1988) Observer bias in blood pressure studies. *J Hypertens* 6:375–380.
3. Grim CM, Grim CE (1995) A curriculum for the training and certification of blood

pressure measurement for health care providers. *Can J Cardiol* 11(Suppl. H):38H–42H.

4. Bailey RH, Knaus VL, Bauer JH (1991) Aneroid sphygmomanometers: an assessment of accuracy at a university hospital land clinics. *Arch Intern Med* 151:1409–1412.

5. Stahl SM, Kelly CR, Neil PJ, Grim CE, Mamlin J (1984) Effects of home blood pressure measurement on long-term BP control. *Am J Public Health* 74:704–709.

6. Grim CM (1991) *Taking Your Own Blood Pressure: A Skill for Life*, Torrance, CA: Shared Care Research and Education (video).

12 Initial Routine Tests for Diagnosis and Risk Stratification of the Patient with Hypertension

What Is Mandatory?

Tudor Vagaonescu, MD, PhD
and Robert A. Phillips, MD, PhD, FACC

Contents

Arterial hypertension is one of the most frequent causes of doctor's office visits in the United States and in the Western countries. Because the assessment of the hypertensive patient may vary from a simple clinical examination that focuses on the cardiovascular status of the patient to an extensive multisystem evaluation that involves expensive invasive procedures, it is important to understand the rationale behind the various laboratory procedures before ordering them. As part of the initial assessment with history, physical examination, and simple

From: *Hypertension Medicine*
Edited by: M. A. Weber © Humana Press Inc., Totowa, NJ

Table 12-1
Routine Tests for Essential Hypertension

Definitely indicated	Selectively indicated
Serum electrolytes	Home BP monitoring
Creatinine	Ambulatory BP monitoring
Urinalysis	Echocardiogram
Electrocardiogram	
Lipid profile	

laboratory tests including serum electrolytes, creatinine, and an electrocardiogram (Table 12-1), the following questions should be answered (*see* also Fig. 12-1):

1. Is the patient really hypertensive?
2. Is the hypertension essential or secondary?
3. What is the degree of target organ damage (TOD)?
4. What is the cardiovascular risk profile of the hypertensive patient?
5. Are there any associated diseases in the hypertensive patient?
6. How easy is it to control the blood pressure (BP) by diet and/or medication?

The answers to these questions determine whether further workup is necessary. The decision to order a specific test should be individualized to the specific patient and should always follow a thorough clinical assessment of the patient; ordering everything to be thorough, from urinary metanephrines to a magnetic resonance angiogram in a shotgun approach, is poor medical procedure.

ESSENTIAL VS SECONDARY HYPERTENSION

Essential hypertension is the most frequently encountered form of hypertension, occurring in more than 95% of the patients; in the remaining cases a cause of the hypertension, i.e., a secondary cause, can be identified and successfully treated. The patient with essential hypertension presents commonly with an unremarkable clinical examination and often with a family history significant for arterial hypertension. In the patient with newly diagnosed borderline and stage I hypertension, it is extremely helpful to obtain repeated home BPs and/or ambulatory BP monitoring to be certain that the patient does not have "white coat" hypertension and that treatment is necessary. Once treatment is initiated,

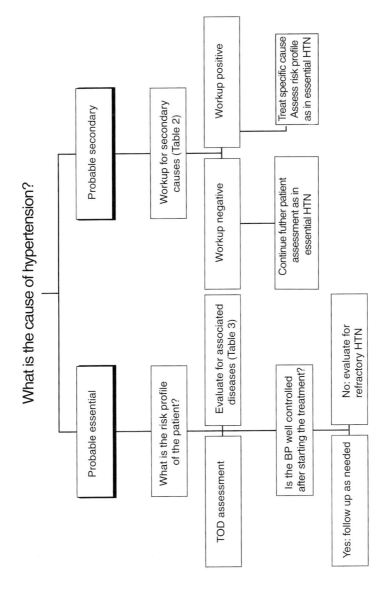

Fig. 12-1. Flow diagram for initial assessment and management of the patient with hypertension.

149

if there is no reason to suspect secondary hypertension and BP can be easily controlled, no further laboratory tests are required for the etiologic diagnosis of the arterial hypertension. Otherwise, laboratory tests should be ordered based on a specific suspected diagnosis (*see* Table 12-2).

ASSESSMENT OF TARGET ORGAN DAMAGE (TOD)

The degree of injury to various organs and systems, i.e., TOD, as a result of elevated BP, should be quantified in every patient. This helps to risk stratify the hypertensive patient and to guide treatment.

Assessment can begin with a funduscopic examination. It is useful to tell the patient during the examination that this is the only "window" that allows direct visualization of hypertension-induced vessel damage. "Copper wiring" and arteriovenous nicking are retinal changes that are specific for arterial hypertension; others may be found in various other diseases such as "cotton wool spots" in diabetes, systemic lupus erythematosus, and autoimmune deficiency syndrome; flame-shaped intraretinal hemorrhages in diabetes, retinal vein occlusion, and blood dyscrasias; and "silver wiring" in diabetes, collagenoses, and arterial occlusive disease. In selected cases such as retinal vein or artery occlusion, or optic disk swelling, the patient should be referred also to an ophthalmologist.

When the history or examination reveals a history of stroke, ischemic transitory attacks, carotid bruits, or abnormal neurologic examination, further noninvasive evaluation of the cerebral circulation is warranted. The cerebrovasculature can be investigated with Doppler flow studies of the extra- and intracranial arteries, ultrasound of the carotid arteries, MRA of the cerebral arteries, and so forth. CT or MRI scans document previous cerebrovascular accident.

Hypertensive heart disease can be assessed by clinical examination that elicits history of dyspnea, heart failure, angina, myocardial infarction (MI), or coronary revascularization and by a physical examination that describes the point of maximal impulse (PMI) and presence or absence of an S_4 or S_3. In all patients with hypertension, an electrocardiogram should be obtained to ascertain the pressure of left atrial and left ventricular hypertrophy (LVH), intraventricular conduction delay, or prior MI. Because regression of left ventricular mass is associated with improved prognosis, it could be argued that a "limited echocardiogram" to measure left ventricular mass should be a routine part of the laboratory evaluation of all patients with hypertension.

Table 12-2
Testing for Secondary Hypertension[a]

Possible secondary cause of hypertension	Clinical hints suggesting condition	Initial testing for condition	Additional testing
Renovascular disease	Age of onset <20 or >50 yr Smoking history Atherosclerotic vascular disease Abdominal bruit Severe, accelerated, or malignant hypertension ACEI-induced reversible creatinine elevation	Captopril-enhanced isotopic nephrogram Duplex sonography (renal arteries) MRA (renal arteries)	Renal arterogram
Renoparenchymal disease	Known preexistent renal disease (uni- or bilateral) Chronic renal failure Known use of analgetics Family history of polycystic kidney disease Palpable abdominal mass	Serum creatinine Urine analysis Renal sonography	Renal biopsy
Cushing syndrome	Long-term corticosteroid therapy Truncal obesity with moon facies, buffalo hump Fatigability and proximal muscle weakness Hirsutism Skin striae and ecchymoses	Urinary free cortisol level Dexamethasone suppression test	Adrenal CT/MRI scan ACTH sampling (plasma, inferior petrosal sinus, after CRF stimulation)
Primary hyperaldosteronism	Muscle weakness and fatigue Polyuria and polydipsia	Serum electrolytes Plasma aldosterone ratio (PRA) 24-h urinary potassium and aldosterone	Adrenal CT/MRI scan Aldosterone sampling (adrenal veins)

continued

151

Table 12-2
Continued

Possible secondary cause of hypertension	Clinical hints suggesting condition	Initial testing for condition	Additional testing
Pheochromocytoma	Paroxysms or crisis (sudden onset, headache, profuse sweating, palpitations, apprehension) Orthostatic hypotension Familial history significant for phacomatoses Known thyroid or parathyroid tumor	Urine sample for metanephrines or catecholamines Plasma catecholamines (basal and after clonidine)	Adrenal CT/MRI scan ^{131}I-MIBG test
Coarctation of the aorta	Young age Headache, epistaxis, cold extremities and claudication with exercise Femoral pulses diminished and delayed when compared with the radial, brachial, or carotid pulses Arterial pulsations in the posterior intercostal spaces Ejection murmur at the LSB and in the interscapular area Difference in BP between upper and lower extremities	Chest X-ray ECG	MRI Aortic (and coronary) angiography

[a]ACEI, angiotension converting enzyme inhibitor; MRA, magnetic resonance angiogram; CT, computed tomography; MRI, magnetic resonance imaging; ACTH, adrenocorticotropic hormone; CRF, corticotropin releasing factor; PRA, plasma renin activity; ECG, electrocardiography; LSB, left sternal border; MIBG, mono-iodo-benzylguanidine.

The kidney involvement in hypertension can be assessed by serum creatinine and urine analysis that measures microalbuminuria or low degree of proteinuria in the absence of cells or casts as markers of an active renal disease.

EVALUATION OF OTHER CARDIOVASCULAR RISK FACTORS

Arterial hypertension is the leading cause for LVH and congestive heart failure and is a major risk factor for atherosclerosis. During the initial work-up of the hypertensive patient, one should also assess the cardiovascular risk profile. The following necessary information can be obtained from the clinical examination:

1. Family history significant for coronary artery diseases in a first-degree female relative under age 65 or a first-degree male relative under age 55.
2. Presence of diabetes mellitus, dyslipidemia, or smoking.
3. Body mass index.
4. Known cardiovascular disease.
5. Previous MI, angina, stroke, or transient ischemic attack.
6. Peripheral arterial disease.
7. Sedentary lifestyle, dietary habits, ability to cope with stress.

The following laboratory tests also provide necessary information:

1. Fasting blood sugar.
2. Lipid profile that consists of total cholesterol, triglycerides, low-density lipoprotein cholesterol and high-density lipoprotein cholesterol.

Homocysteine, Lp (a), and fibrinogen levels are tests that may emerge in the early part of the twenty-first century as routine risk factors.

It is controversial whether determination of plasma renin activity (PRA) (normalized for the urinary sodium) should be part of the routine risk assessment. There is good evidence that elevated PRA is an independent predictor of future ischemic heart disease that is independent of smoking history, glucose level, or cholesterol. However, perhaps because the PRA level has not yet been incorporated into standard risk formula, such as the Framingham risk score, it is not standard practice to obtain this laboratory test. In addition, some advocate that a plasma renin level may streamline antihypertensive selection. However, choosing initial drug therapy based on age and race is at least as effective as that based on a renin profile.

Table 12-3
Testing for Diseases Associated with Arterial Hypertension

Associated disease	Clinical clues	Initial test
Diabetes mellitus	Polyuria, polydipsia, weight loss despite polyphagia	Fasting blood sugar, glycosylated hemoglobin Urine analysis
Hyperuricemia	Arthritis, kidney stones	Serum uric acid Urine analysis
Obstructive sleep apnea	Disruptive snoring, excessive daytime hypersomnolence and fatigue, upper body obesity	Sleep studies
Atherosclerosis	History of cardiovascular disease	Fasting lipid profile Fibrinogen?, Lp (a)?, homocysteine?

ASSOCIATED DISEASES IN HYPERTENSIVE PATIENTS

Hypertension can present as an isolated disease or it can be accompanied by other diseases, such as diabetes mellitus, obesity, gout, and atherosclerosis. If the clinical examination and initial routine laboratory tests present enough clues to suggest the presence of these diseases, further testing is warranted (*see* Table 12-3).

RESISTANT ARTERIAL HYPERTENSION

Optimal control of BP is as follows:

1. Below 140/90 mmHg in patients with uncomplicated hypertension.
2. Below 130/80 mmHg in the patient with hypertension and diabetes mellitus.
3. Below 125/75 mmHg in hypertensive patients with renal insufficiency and proteinuria in excess of 1 g/24 h.

In patients who remain above these goals despite adherence to a triple drug regimen that includes a diuretic and near maximal doses of medications, one should reassess the patient for resistant hypertension. Many patients with resistant hypertension have normal BP on ambulatory or home BP monitoring and require no additional medications.

CONCLUSION

The evaluation of the hypertensive patient relies mainly on the history and clinical examination. Routine tests (*see* Table 12-1) are recommended to assess the TOD and the risk profile of the patient. Home BP and/or ambulatory monitoring should be performed in borderline or stage I hypertensive patients. Optional tests should be ordered in selected patients, after an initial thorough clinical examination suggests a possible curable cause of the arterial hypertension or for a better risk factor stratification of the particular hypertensive patient. Some of the tests may be repeated in the follow-up of the hypertensive patient if, after clinical reassessment, they are considered to be helpful in providing better BP control

SUGGESTED READINGS

Izzo JL Jr, Black HR, eds. (1999) *Hypertension Primer*, 2nd ed. The Council on High Blood Pressure Research, American Heart Association.

The Sixth Report of the Joint National Committee on Prevention, Detection, Evaluation, and Treatment of High Blood Pressure (1997) *Arch Inter Med* 157:2413–2446.

Williams GH (1998) Hypertensive vascular disease. In: Fauci AS, Braunwald E, Isselbacher KJ, et al., eds. *Harrison's Principles of Internal Medicine, 14th ed.*, New York: McGraw-Hill, pp. 1380–1394.

Black HR (1998) Approach to the patient with hypertension. In: Goldman L, Braunwald E, eds. *Primary Cardiology*, Philadelphia: WB Saunders, pp. 129–143.

Frohlich ED (1996) Hypertension and hypertensive heart disease. In: Chizner MA, ed. *Classic Teachings in Clinical Cardiology: A Tribute to W. Proctor Harvey*, Cedar Grove, NJ: Laennec Publishing, pp. 1249–1274.

Kaplan NM (1998) *Clinical Hypertension*, 7th ed., Baltimore: Williams & Wilkins.

Krakoff LR (1995) *Management of the Hypertensive Patient*, New York: Churchill Livingstone.

Phillips RA and Diamond JA (1999) Non-invasive modalities for evaluating the hypertensive patient: focus on left ventricular mass and ambulatory blood pressure monitoring. *Prog Cardiovasc Dis* 41:397–440.

13 When to Suspect Secondary Hypertension

Donald G. Vidt, MD

CONTENTS

A thorough history and physical examination together with selected, office-based laboratory studies are recommended in the evaluation of each new patient with hypertension (Table 13-1). This initial evaluation is designed to assess the presence or absence of target organ damage and cardiovascular disease, to identify other cardiovascular risk factors or comorbid conditions that may have an impact on the prognosis and selection of therapy, and to provide valuable clues to other secondary causes of hypertension. When preliminary examination affords no clues, an extensive search for secondary and possibly curable causes of hypertension is unproductive, unnecessarily costly, and, on occasion, may be hazardous. This chapter does not address the problem of alcohol excess, which represents the most common cause of reversible hypertension in our society, or oral contraceptive therapy, which may be associated with significant hypertension in a small number of women. Table

From: *Hypertension Medicine*
Edited by: M. A. Weber © Humana Press Inc., Totowa, NJ

Table 13-1
Routine Laboratory Studies Recommended Prior to Initiating Therapy[a]

Urinalysis
Complete blood count
Blood chemistries
  Potassium
  Sodium
  Creatinine
  Fasting glucose
  Total cholesterol
  High-density lipoprotein cholesterol
Electrocardiogram (12-lead)

[a]Data from ref. 11.

Table 13-2
Clues to Secondary Hypertension from Initial Evaluation

Medical history	Excludes most cases of pheochromocytoma
Physical examination	Excludes coarctation of the aorta and Cushing syndrome
Complete blood count	Excludes polycythemia and other unrelated diseases
Urinalysis	Excludes most cases of significant renal parenchymal disease
Creatinine or blood urea nitrogen (BUN)	Excludes renal insufficiency
Electrolytes (serum potassium)	Excludes most cases of primary aldosteronism

13-2 summarizes the information to be gained from the initial clinical evaluation regarding selected secondary causes of hypertension, and this information is discussed further in this chapter.

COARCTATION OF THE AORTA

While coarctation of the aorta may cause left ventricular failure in early life, adults with coarctation are usually asymptomatic with the problem uncovered during a search into the etiology of hypertension (1). As a result, the medical history may be of little help in suggesting the presence of a coarctation unless suspected in association with other congenital malformations such as bicuspid aortic valve, patent ductus or ventricular septal defect, and mitral valve abnormalities.

The most common location for the coarctation is just distal to the origin of the left subclavian artery. Occasionally the coarctation is proximal to or involves the origin of the left subclavian artery and may be missed if blood pressures (BPs) are not checked in both upper extremities and at least one lower extremity. Absent or reduced pulses in the lower extremities, together with lower BP in the legs than in the arms, are obviously valuable clues to diagnosis. Typically, systolic pressures in the arms are similar and significantly higher than the systolic pressure in either leg, and systolic pressures are elevated dispro-portionately to the diastolic pressure, resulting in a wide pulse pressure and bounding pulses proximal to the coarctation. On precordial exami-nation, a thrill may be observed in the suprasternal notch area, and visible or palpable pulsations over the intercostal arteries in the posterior thorax are observed. On auscultation, bruits may be heard over the intercostal arteries, and if a chest X-ray were obtained, notching along the inferior border of the ribs and an absent aortic knob may be seen.

CUSHING'S SYNDROME

The astute clinician may pick up on a history of recent change in facial appearance and considerable weight gain, together with complaints of weakness, muscle wasting, peripheral bruising, and impotence, and in women, amenorrhea and hirsutism. On physical examination, the typical features include truncal obesity, moon face, plethora, and typical pur-plish skin stria *(2)*. On screening laboratory studies, glucose intolerance or frank diabetes mellitus may be noted and, occasionally, neutrophilia with relative lymphocytopenia. A history of recent pathologic fracture of a rib or vertebra may be obtained.

PHEOCHROMOCYTOMA

Nearly all tumors produce symptoms or signs related to excessive production and release of catecholamines, and, therefore, the medical history provides valuable clues to diagnosis *(3)*. A history of symptom-atic episodes or "spells" including headache, palpitations, pallor, and profuse perspiration, together with unusual lability of BP or occasional presentation as accelerated or malignant hypertension, are observed *(4)*. A history of multiple endocrine neoplasia (MEN) type II, in associa-tion with pancreatic islet cell tumors, neurofibromatosis, or von Hippel–Lindau disease, and medullary carcinoma of the thyroid gland or para-thyroid disease can be most valuable to diagnosis. It is critical to characterize these spells relative to onset, precipitating activities, sever-ity, and duration, which should be repetitive and predictable.

On examination the hypertension may be persistent or intermittent, and, rarely, hypotension may be a presenting feature in patients secreting predominantly epinephrine or dopamine. Approximately 90% of tumors occur within the adrenal glands, and with larger tumors, a midline abdominal mass may be observed. A palpable thyroid or parathyroid mass occasionally may be found in the presence of a MEN type II syndrome. Screening laboratory studies are of little assistance except for the possible presence of abnormal glucose tolerance.

PRIMARY ALDOSTERONISM

Hypokalemia, whether spontaneous or provoked, provides the best clue to the presence of primary aldosteronism. One must remember, however, that normal serum potassium concentrations may be observed in upward of one third of cases (5). In the normokalemic group, moderate to severe hypokalemia may be induced even by today's smaller doses of diuretics. Also, consider the diagnosis in any patient presenting with resistant hypertension. A history of inordinate weakness, periodic paralysis, or paresthesias, often noted in older textbooks, is rarely observed. Similarly unusual is the finding on physical examination of a positive Chvostek's and/or Trousseau's signs. In the absence of hypokalemia primary aldosteronism masquerades well as essential hypertension and is easily overlooked on initial evaluation.

RENOVASCULAR DISEASE

Renovascular hypertension may affect as many as 30% of patients presenting to academic specialty clinics for resistant hypertension. A thorough initial evaluation and a high index of suspicion will often identify clinical clues suggestive of renovascular hypertension (Table 13-3). By identifying patients at higher risk, subsequent screening tests can be both more predictable and cost-effective (6,7).

Fibromuscular dysplasias predominate in younger females in whom the finding of a continuous epigastric bruit is highly suggestive of the diagnosis. In patients over age 55, two thirds of the cases are attributable to atherosclerosis. The finding of hypertension, azotemia, cigarette smoking, and evidence of extensive vascular disease are all highly suggestive of the diagnosis. The clinical history and presentation may suggest consideration of other etiologies including Takayasu's arteritis, renal thrombosis or emboli, trauma, radiation, or occasionally extrinsic

Table 13-3
Clinical Clues to Presence of Renovascular Hypertension

Abrupt onset of hypertension age <30 or >55 yr
Accelerated/malignant hypertension (grade 3 or 4 retinopathy)
Hypertension refractory to a triple-drug regimen
Hypertension and diffuse vascular disease (carotids, coronary, peripheral
    vascular)
Systolic-diastolic epigastric bruit
Hypertension and unexplained renal insufficiency
Renal insufficiency induced by angiotensin-converting enzyme inhibitor
    therapy

lesions such as retroperitoneal fibrosis or neurofibromatosis. If these clinical clues are not apparent on initial evaluation, it would seem inappropriate to pursue additional diagnostic testing as part of the initial evaluation.

RENAL PARENCHYMAL DISEASE

Patients with renal parenchymal disease usually present with renal insufficiency, proteinuria, or hematuria *(8)*. Renal parenchymal disease is a common secondary cause of hypertension although often not reversible. The aforementioned clinical clues are easily detected with a carefully performed urinalysis and simple screening tests of renal function such as a serum creatinine or BUN determination. Proteinuria found by dipstick should always be confirmed with sulfosalicylic acid because the dipstick detects only albumin whereas sulfosalicylic acid precipitates any urinary protein, including light chains present in dysproteinemic states. When proteinuria is observed, 24-h urine for quantitative protein should be obtained because proteinuria > 150 mg/24 h represents significant proteinuria. Renal ultrasound studies are often helpful in diagnosis and renal biopsy may occasionally be required.

Hypertension, often of moderate to severe degree, usually accompanies renal parenchymal disease, particularly when renal insufficiency is present. It must be remembered that initial, significant reductions in creatinine cleareance may not be reflected by changes in the serum creatinine or BUN concentrations. In an average size adult, a serum creatinine >1.5 mg/dL may reflect a 40% loss of clearance function; in an older patient, a serum creatinine >1.4 mg/dL may reflect a similar loss of renal function.

THYROID AND PARATHYROID DISORDERS

Thyroid dysfunction, both hyperthyroidism and hypothyroidism, can associate with hypertension particularly in older patients *(9)*. Thyroid dysfunction and renovascular disease represent the most common forms of reversible secondary hypertension observed in hypertensive individuals over age 60. The mechanisms of hypertension may provide valuable clinical clues in these disorders. Thyrotoxic patients have a hyperdynamic hypertension and high cardiac output seen predominantly as an elevated systolic blood pressure. Hypothyroid patients, on the other hand, have a high prevalence of primarily diastolic hypertension, and this can be a valuable clue in the elderly, in whom primary diastolic hypertension is most unusual.

Easily performed thyroid function tests provide the clues to diagnosis, with an elevated blood thyroxin level and a suppressed serum thryoid-stimulating hormone (TSH) level being the hallmarks of hyperthyroidism. These values are of course reversed in patients with hypothyroidism.

Hypercalcemia is associated with an increased incidence of hypertension, and hyperparathyroidism is a common cause of hypercalcemia *(10)*. Most patients with primary hyperparathyroidism are asymptomatic, and a cursory history and physical examination do not provide specific indications for this disorder. The clinical diagnosis is strongly supported by the finding of hypercalcemia together with an increased serum parathyroid hormone value. The side effects of hypercalcemia such as polyuria, polydipsia, renal calculi, peptic ulcer disease, and hypertension may offer diagnostic clues.

MEN syndromes that may associate with pheochromocytoma and/ or hyperparathyroidism are an important exception. A finding of a thyroid nodule, thyroid mass, or cervical lymphadenopathy should suggest the possibility of a medullary thyroid carcinoma.

CONCLUSION

Valuable clinical clues to the presence of secondary forms of hypertension may be provided by a thorough initial evaluation of the hypertensive patient. Appropriate referral of patients will depend on the availability of additional screening studies when indicated and subspecialty expertise. Table 13-4 summarizes additional screening studies that can

Table 13-4
Studies to Establish Diagnosis of Secondary Hypertension[a]

	Additional screening studies	Diagnosis/localization
Coarctation of the aorta	Chest X-ray	2D-echocardiogram Aortagram MRI
Cushing's syndrome	Dexamethasone suppression test	24-h urinary-free cortisol CT Radioimmune assay of plasma ACTH
Pheochromocytoma	Plasma catecholamines Urinary catecholamines, metanephrine, VMA Clonidine suppression test	Plasma catecholamines Urinary catecholamines, metanephrine, VMA Clonidine suppression test *Preceding to help establish diagnosis, plus:* CT MRI (extraadrenal tumor) MIBG scan
Primary aldosteronism	Plasma aldosterone:plasma renin activity ratio	Aldosterone excretion rate during salt loading Adrenal CT

continued

Table 13-4
Continued

	Additional screening studies	Diagnosis/localization
Renovascular hypertension	Captopril renography Renal duplex sonography MRI	Renal angiography Renal vein renin ratio
Renal parenchymal disease	24-h urine protein, creatinine Renal ultrasound	Iothalamate GFR Renal biopsy
Thyroid disease	TSH Serum thyroid hormone level Serum calcitonin level	Hyper: $\downarrow$ TSH $\uparrow$ thyroid level Hypo: $\uparrow$ TSH $\downarrow$ thyroid level Medullary thyroid CA; $\uparrow$ calcitonin
Hyperparathyroidism	Serum calcium Serum phosphorous Serum PTH level	Hypercalcemia Hypophosphatemia $\uparrow$ PTH level

[a]VMA, vanillic mandelic acid; MRI, magnetic resonance imaging; CT, computed tomography; ACTH, adrenocorticotropic hormone; MIGB, I[131] meta-iodobenzyl-guanidine iothalamate[131]; GFR, glomerular filtration rate; CA, calcium; PTH, parathyroid hormone.

be of particular value when a secondary cause of hypertension is suspected, and also lists more definitive studies required for diagnosis and localization.

REFERENCES

1. Serfas D, Borow KM (1983) Coarctation of the aorta: anatomy, pathophysiology, and natural history. *J Cardiovasc Med* 8:575.
2. Kaye TB, Crapo L (1990) The Cushing syndrome: an update on diagnostic tests. *Ann Intern Med* 112:434–444.
3. Manger WM, Gifford RW Jr (1977) *Pheochromocytoma.* New York: Springer-Verlag.
4. Bravo EL (1991) Pheochromocytoma: new concepts and future trends. *Kidney Int* 40:544–556 (clinical conference).
5. Melby JC (1991) Diagnosis of hyperaldosteronism. *Endocrinol Metab Clin North Am* 20:247–255.
6. Mann SJ, Pickering TG (1992) Detection of renovascular hypertension. State of the Art: 1992. *Ann Intern Med* 117:845–853.
7. National High Blood Pressure Education Program (NHBPEP) Working Group (1996) 1995 Update of the working group reports on chronic renal failure and renovascular hypertension. *Arch Intern Med* 156:1938–1947.
8. Moore MA (1993) Renal parenchymal disease: evaluation. In: Izzo JL, Black HR, eds. *Hypertension Primer,* 3rd ed., Dallas: American Heart Association, pp. 265–267.
9. Streeten DH, Anderson GH Jr, Howland T, Chiang R, Smulyan H (1988) Effects of thyroid function on blood pressure: recognition of hypothyroid hypertension. *Hypertension* 11:78–83.
10. Richards AM, Espiner EA, Nicholls MG, Ikram H, Hamilton EJ, Maslowski TA (1988) Hormone, calcium and blood pressure relationships in primary hyperparathyroidism. *J Hypertens* 6:747–752. (published erratum appears in *J Hypertens* 1988; 6(11):ii).
11. Joint National Committee (1997) The sixth report of the Joint National Committee on the Prevention, Detection, Evaluation and Treatment of High Blood Pressure (JNC-VI). *Arch Intern Med* 157:2413–2446.

14 Evaluation of Renal Function and Proteinuria

Ira W. Reiser, MD
and Jerome G. Porush, MD

CONTENTS

When evaluating renal function, the clinician is oftentimes asked to estimate the glomerular filtration rate (GFR) and to determine whether the ability of the kidney to dilute and concentrate, acidify the urine, or function as a barrier to the excretion of protein is impaired. This chapter reviews each of these integral functions of the kidney and provides the clinician with a useful and practical approach to their assessment.

GLOMERULAR FILTRATION RATE

Glomerular filtration rate (GFR), a measure of the functional renal mass, is the rate at which an ultrafiltrate of the plasma is formed by the glomeruli. Ideally, a substance that is unbound by serum proteins, freely permeable through the glomerular capillaries, and not reabsorbed, secreted, metabolized, or synthesized by the renal tubules is best suited for measuring the GFR. The GFR is determined by the urinary clearance

From: *Hypertension Medicine*
Edited by: M. A. Weber © Humana Press Inc., Totowa, NJ

of such a substance, expressed as milliliters/minute or liters/24 h, and derived by calculating the urinary excretory rate of the substance (the product of the urinary concentration of the substance [U] and urine flow rate [V]) divided by the plasma concentration of the substance (P), or by determining the plasma clearance of such a substance over time (the rate at which the substance is removed from the plasma).

Inulin, an uncharged fructose polymer, fulfills the aforementioned criteria and is the gold standard by which other markers of GFR are judged (1). Unfortunately, the use of inulin is impractical in clinical medicine because it requires that laboratory facilities be capable of measuring inulin, and necessitates either a constant infusion with timed and complete urine collections for determination of urinary clearances or multiple plasma samples to determine its plasma clearance following a single injection.

Creatinine, an endogenous product of muscle cells, is not protein bound and is freely filtered at the level of the glomerulus (2). Because the daily generation of creatinine in normal subjects consuming a stable diet is fairly constant, the serum creatinine (Scr) concentration has been used as a substitute for inulin in estimating GFR. The use of the Scr as a marker for GFR, however, has many shortcomings (2,3). Although primarily produced by muscle, approx 30% of the daily creatinine pool is derived from ingested meat. Thus, muscle mass (which declines after age 30), creatinine generation (which is reduced in renal failure), and diet, in addition to urinary clearance, may affect the Scr concentration (2,3). Furthermore, unlike inulin, creatinine is secreted by the proximal tubule of the nephron, which may constitute 10–40% of the total creatinine in the urine of normal subjects and up to 50–60% in subjects with renal disease (2,3). Tubular secretion of creatinine may be inhibited with many commonly used medications (cimetidine, ranitidine, trimethoprim, triamterene, amiloride, and probenecid), and although the GFR is unchanged the Scr will increase as a result of the diminished total renal clearance of creatinine (2). Finally, the methodology by which creatinine is measured may also result in either spuriously low or high Scr concentration levels because of the presence of substances that may alter the accuracy of the assay (2). In addition, regardless of the method chosen to measure creatinine, a wide range of variability exists among simultaneously repeated measurements within the same subject (2). Thus, an increase in the measured Scr from 0.7 to 1.0 mg/dL (both within the normal range) may reflect a significant diminution in renal function (~30%) or may only reflect assay variability. Because of these limitations, the Scr may be variably independent of the absolute renal

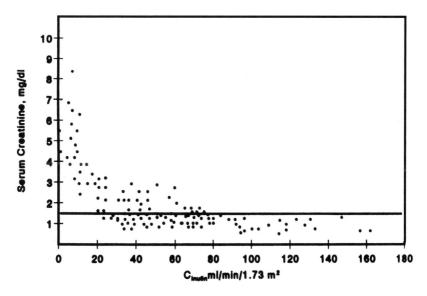

Fig. 14-1. Relationship between inulin clearance and the serum creatinine concentration in subjects with glomerular disease. The upper limit of normal for the serum creatinine concentration (1.4 mg/dL) is represented by the horizontal line (Reproduced with permission from Levey AS [1990] Measurement of renal function in chronic renal disease. *Kidney Int* 38:171).

function, and as shown in Fig. 14-1, which illustrates the relationship between the Scr and inulin clearance, the Scr may remain within the normal range despite a decrement in the GFR of 60% or greater.

The determination of a creatinine urinary clearance (Ccr) will provide a better estimate of the GFR than the Scr alone. Ccr is usually determined by measuring the total creatinine excreted during a finite period of time (generally 24 h) and obtaining a single Scr at the end of the collection period or averaging two values taken prior to and after the completion of the urine collection. Because of the contribution from tubular secretion to the total creatinine excretion, the relationship between the true GFR, as determined by inulin clearance, and Ccr will not be linear *(2–5)*. Difficulties with obtaining either complete or accurately timed urine collections may limit the accuracy of a Ccr. Thus, the adequacy of a collection should be determined and may be done so by comparing the amount excreted with the amount anticipated for a subject based on his or her daily production of creatinine *(2)*. Men generally excrete 28– (age/6) mg(kg·d) of creatinine and women 22– (age/9) mg(kg·d). It is also possible to estimate the Ccr for any given Scr when a steady state of creatinine balance exists. The most widely used formulas, devised by Cockcroft and Gault (6), are as follows:

$$Ccr = \frac{(140-age) \times Weight\ (kg)}{Scr\ (mg/dL) \times 72} \quad (for\ men)$$

$$Ccr = \frac{(140-age) \times Weight\ (kg)}{Scr\ (mg/dL) \times 85} \quad (for\ women)$$

These formulas will overestimate Ccr when the body weight is significantly greater than the lean body mass, and, because they are derived from the Scr, the same problems exist as already outlined regarding its relationship with the true GFR as measured by inulin.

Urea, an end product of protein metabolism, is synthesized in the liver, and following its generation is primarily excreted by the kidney. Although of small molecular weight, unbound by serum proteins, and uncharged and freely filtered at the glomerulus, the kidney's handling of urea (in the absence of advanced renal failure, i.e., GFR < 20 mL [min · 1.73 m²]) is greatly dependent on the rate of urine formation (7–9). Following its filtration, approx 40–50% of the filtered load of urea is reabsorbed by the proximal tubule regardless of the state of hydration. It is at the level of the medullary collecting duct (the site at which antidiuretic hormone [ADH] exerts its action) that the state of hydration influences urea handling. In the setting of antidiuresis (presence of ADH), urea permeability is increased in this nephron segment, resulting in only 35–40% of the total filtered urea load being excreted, whereas during states of water diuresis (absence of ADH), urea permeability is negligible and may result in an excretion of 50–60% of the filtered urea load. Aside from the state of hydration, the blood urea nitrogen (BUN) is also dependent on both nitrogen load and metabolism (10). An increase in the BUN may be observed with an increase in the total nitrogen load such as with increased protein intake, enhanced catabolism (infection, trauma), or suppression of anabolism (as observed with corticosteroid or tetracycline adminstration). By contrast, a lower BUN will be noted whenever there is a reduction in catabolic rate or dietary protein intake (10). Finally, the BUN will be lower in the presence of severe parenchymal liver disease and myxedema because urea generation is reduced. For these reasons, the BUN is a poor marker of GFR. However, despite these shortcomings, the BUN may be clinically helpful in diagnosing renal insufficiency owing to volume contraction, renal ischemia, acute glomerulonephritis, and early obstructive uropathy because these conditions are associated with a reduced urine flow rate and may result in a disproportionate increase in the BUN/Scr ratio (normally 10–15) to two to three times normal *(10)*. Several radioactive and nonradioactive agents are available to measure GFR. The radionuclides most frequently used are ^{125}I-iothalamate (and ^{131}I-iothalamate), diethylenetriaminepenta-acetic acid (DTPA) chelated to ^{99m}technetium and ethylenediaminetetraacetic acid (EDTA) chelated to ^{51}Cr *(11)*. These agents are almost entirely cleared by glomerular filtration and, although not as accurate as inulin, are frequently used because of the ease, accuracy, and reproducibility of their measurement. With these agents, the GFR may be obtained with either standard urine clearances (requiring timed urine and plasma collections) or by the rate at which the radioactive tracer disappears from the plasma over a 2- to 6-h period (generally requiring more than one timed plasma specimen) following a bolus or SC injection of the radioactive agent *(11,12)*. The plasma clearance of each radioactive isotope is not as accurate as the renal clearance (exceeding renal clearance by 10–15 mL/min), and, in general, the plasma clearance will overestimate GFR. Nevertheless, this method of measuring GFR is the most commonly used. Direct renal scintigraphic measurement of the radioisotope in the 1- to 3-min interval following its administration will also allow a determination of the GFR because the renal uptake of these radionuclides is directly proportional to GFR *(13)*. Although advantageous because it is quick and easy to perform (there is no need for blood or urine collection) and the percentage of contribution of each kidney to the total GFR may be obtained, it is the least accurate method utilizing radionuclides. To obviate the need for radioactive agents, the renal and plasma clearance of nonradioactive iothalamate and the plasma clearance of nonionic iodinated contrast media (primarily iohexol) have been used *(14–18)*. The plasma clearances of both have been shown to be reliable and reproducible, and to correlate well with simultaneously obtained plasma clearances of ^{51}Cr EDTA over a wide range of GFR.

EVALUATION OF THE KIDNEY'S ABILITY TO DILUTE AND CONCENTRATE URINE

To discern the cause of abnormal water homeostasis frequently encountered in clinical medicine, an assessment of the kidney's capacity to either dilute or concentrate the urine is required. The urine's osmolality (which is directly proportional to the number of particles in the urine), specific gravity (the weight of the urine as compared with an equal volume of distilled water), and refractive index (the ratio of the speed of light through air to that of light through urine) have all been used to assess the concentration of random urine samples *(19)*. Because osmolality, unlike either the specific gravity or refractive index, is unaffected by the size, charge, and density of the particles, it is the most accurate of the three measurements. With high urine concentrations of protein, glucose, or exogenous solutes such as mannitol and radiocontrast material, the determination of the urine's specific gravity or refractive index will be increased compared with that of a simultaneously obtained urine osmolality. In the absence of these substances, however, the correlation between specific gravity or refractive index and osmolality is quite good. Because these measurements reflect only the degree of dilution or concentration of the urine at one specific moment in time, other methods are required to assess the kidney's ability to handle a water load or to determine the maximal concentrating capacity of a subject.

An indirect method of quantifying the diluting capacity may be made by determining free water clearance (CH_2O), the hypothetical volume of urine that is excreted free of solute *(20,21)*. CH_2O, which is dependent on the osmotic load that must be excreted, the minimal achievable urine osmolality, the presence or absence of ADH and the GFR, may be derived from the following formula:

$$CH_2O = V - C_{osm} \quad \text{or} \quad V - (U_{osm} \times V)/P_{osm}$$

in which V is the urine volume, C_{osm} is the urine osmolar clearance, U_{osm} is the urine osmolality, and P_{osm} is the plasma osmolality. When the capacity to handle a water load is exceeded, retention of water and dilution of the fluid spaces of the body will result. For example, if two subjects with similar plasma osmolalities (300 mOsm) and identical osmolar loads to excrete (600 mOsm) but differing minimal achievable urine osmolalities (150 vs 50 mOsm/kg H_2O) are compared, the subject with the higher urine osmolality will be able to excrete his or her osmotic load in 4 L of urine ($150 \times 4 = 600$) and have a CH_2O of 2 L, whereas the other subject's osmotic load could be excreted in 12 L of urine ($50 \times 12 = 600$) and have a CH_2O of 10 L. In the former subject, water retention and dilution would occur only after the ingestion of 4 L of fluid, whereas in the latter it would require the ingestion of more than 12 L. A more exact assessment of the diluting capacity may be obtained following water loading by determining the rate at which the water load is excreted and measuring the minimum urine osmolality attained. The need for formal assessment, however, is rarely necessary in clinical medicine because it may be discerned that a defect in the

Table 14-1
Anticipated Response to Fluid Deprivation Followed by
Vasopressin in Patients with Hypotonic Polyuria[a]

	Urine osmolality after dehydration (mOsm/kg H₂O)	Change in urine volume and osmolality following vasopressin given after dehydration
Normal	>900	No further change.
Complete DI	<200	Urine volume is reduced and osmolality increased markedly, but does not approach normal maximal osmolality.
Partial DI	<500	Urine volume is reduced and osmolality is increased by 20–30%.
Nephrogenic DI	<300	Urine volume is unchanged; osmolality remains low.
Compulsive water drinking	600–800	No further change in urine volume. Osmolality may rise but by <10%.

[a]Reproduced with permission from *Massry & Glassock's Textbook of Nephrology*, 3rd ed., Baltimore: Williams & Wilkins, 1995, p. 1786. DI, Diabetes Insipidus.

kidney's diluting process is already present whenever serum hypotonicity coexists with a urine that is not maximally dilute.

Although a random urine osmolality or specific gravity does not allow one to determine the maximal concentrating ability of a subject, an osmolality >800 mOsm/kg H₂O or a specific gravity >1.020, in the absence of those solutes that may falsely increase these measurements, implies that the urine concentrating capacity is normal. The need for formally assessing the kidney's concentrating ability becomes important, however, when evaluating a subject with polyuria *(21–23)*. Polyuria that results from an osmotic diuresis is isoosmolar and will have a total urinary solute excretion exceeding the usual 500–800 mOsm/d seen in normal subjects, whereas subjects with diabetes insipidus (complete central, partial central, nephrogenic) and psychogenic polydipsia will be characterized by polyuria with low urine osmolalities. As depicted in Table 14-1, the response to fluid restriction (approx 12–16 h with a 3% loss of body weight) and exogenous vasopressin will help distinguish between these various causes of dilute polyuria. The diagnostic yield of fluid deprivation is further enhanced by measuring plasma ADH levels (drawn prior to exogenous vasopressin administration).

CLINICAL ASSESSMENT OF RENAL ACIDIFICATION

Reclamation of bicarbonate (HCO_3^-) and hydrogen ion (H^+) secretion (predominantly in the form of ammonium ion [NH_4^+] in the urine) by the kidney constitute the normal renal response to an acid load. It is generally thought that a defect in the urinary acidification process exists whenever the urine pH is found to be "inappropriately" high (>5.5); however, this is not always the case *(24)*. In subjects who are chronically academic, ammoniagenesis has been primed, and as a result, an excess of ammonia (NH_3) relative to H^+ exists in the distal nephron. Consequently, the urinary concentration of NH_4^+ increases and the urine pH will be high *(24)*. Normal subjects rendered acutely acidotic, by contrast, will have an excess of H^+ secretion compared with NH_3 in this nephron segment and, as a result, will have a low urine pH until ammoniagenesis has been established *(24)*. Therefore, the urine pH alone is not a sufficient parameter for uncovering a defect in renal acidification, and other tests are needed.

In view of the foregoing, determining the amount of NH_4^+ excreted by the kidney will allow a clinician to distinguish between extrarenal and renal causes of metabolic acidosis *(25–27)*. Extrarenal causes will result in urine NH_4^+ concentrations > 100 m*M*/L, whereas renal causes will be associated with low NH_4^+ concentrations (usually <40 m*M*/L). The amount of NH_4^+ in the urine may be estimated by calculating the urine anion gap ([$Na^+ + K^+$] – Cl^-). Because urinary Cl^- is the major anion that accompanies NH_4^+ in the urine (the exception being when there is an increase in unmeasured non-Cl^- anions such as ketones), the presence of a negative urine anion gap implies significant NH_4^+ excretion, whereas a positive gap implies little excretion and an abnormality in the renal acidification process. Because the amount of NH_4^+ excreted when the urine anion gap is zero is approx 80 m*M*/L (representing the excretion of NH_4^+ with sulfates, phosphates, and organic anions), a urine anion gap of −60 will reflect the excretion of approx 140 m*M*/L of NH_4^+. The amount of NH_4^+ excretion, however, will be underestimated whenever umeasured anions (i.e., ketones) accompany NH_4^+; this possibility should be suspected whenever a significant urine osmolar gap exists (the difference between the actual and the calculated urine osmolality).

When confronted with a nonanion gap metabolic acidosis of renal origin (urinary NH_4^+ excretion <40 m*M*/L), the algorithm illustrated in Fig. 14-2 will allow the practitioner to unravel the cause of the renal acidification defect. Although this algorithm serves as a useful tool, it

APPROACH TO RENAL TUBULAR ACIDOSIS

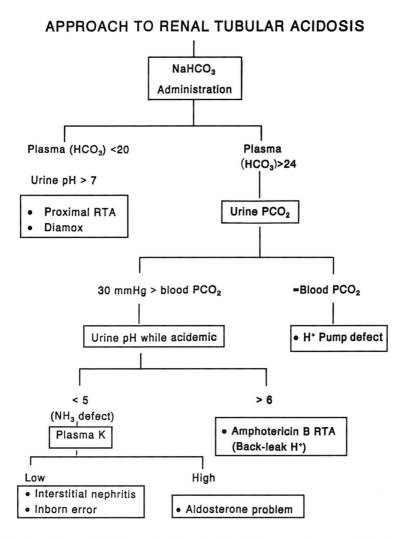

Fig. 14-2. A useful clinical algorithm for identifying the urinary acidification defect in a subject with a nonanion gap metabolic acidosis of renal origin. (Reproduced with permission from Goldstein MB, Levin A [1989] Insights derived from the urine in acid-base disturbances. *AKF Nephrol Lett* 6:22).

must be remembered that patients may on occasion have mixed defects (as may be seen in those with severe tubulointerstitial disease) in which both H^+ secretion and ammoniagenesis are impaired. In these cases, a low urine pH (<5.3), an abnormal urine to blood P_{CO_2}, and a low NH_4^+ excretory rate may all be observed.

EVALUATION OF PROTEINURIA

Normally <150 mg of protein is excreted per day, and levels greater than this require further investigation *(28,29)*. When evaluating a subject with proteinuria, it is useful to determine the kind of protein being excreted, as well as the setting in which it occurs.

Proteinuria may be categorized as being of glomerular, tubular, or overflow in origin *(28)*. Glomerular proteinuria results from the abnormal filtration of macromolecules (i.e., albumin) across the glomerular capillary wall, and is the only type of proteinuria that may be detected by urine dipstick. Low molecular weight proteins, such as β_2-microglobulin, amino acids, and immunoglobulin light chains, are normally filtered at the glomerulus and then reabsorbed by the proximal tubules of the kidney. The excretion of these low molecular weight proteins is termed *tubular proteinuria* and results whenever there is a disruption in the reabsorptive process. When the production of low molecular weight proteins (primarily immunoglobulin light chains) is excessive and the normal capacity for their tubular reabsorption is surpassed, overflow proteinuria results.

Proteinuria may be characterized as being transient (intermittent), orthostatic (postural), or persistent *(28,29)*. Transient proteinuria is the most common of the three types and may be seen in the absence of renal disease. Transient increases in protein excretion may be observed with heavy exercise, fever, congestive heart failure, and emotional stress, and are probably induced by a reduction in renal plasma flow through the effects of angiotensin II or norepinephrine on glomerular hemodynamics *(28,29)*. Orthostatic proteinuria is characterized by increased protein excretion while upright but normal protein excretion while recumbent *(28,29)*. Although the exact cause is unknown, it too may be the result of neurohormonal activation or transient changes in glomerular permeability. Transient and orthostatic proteinuria are generally benign conditions, and the latter may resolve over time *(29–32)*. By contrast, persistent proteinuria is more often the result of an underlying renal or systemic illness.

The amount of proteinuria being excreted may be assessed both qualitatively and quantitatively *(33)*. The urine dipstick detects albumin but not light chains, and is positive when protein excretion exceeds 300 mg/d; thus, it will not be positive in the presence of microalbuminuria. Although useful as a qualitative measure of protein excretion, the urine dipstick is affected by urine concentration (dilute or concentrated urines will underestimate or overestimate, respectively, the amount of proteinuria), and false-positive results may result in the presence of highly buffered alkaline urines, phenazopyridine (pyridium), or gross hematuria *(33)*. Unlike the urine dipstick, mixing an aliquot of urine with sulfosalicylic acid (SSA) will detect the presence of all proteins in the urine. The resultant turbidity may be graded and the protein concentration estimated as follows: trace turbidity, 1–10 mg/dL; 1+ turbidity (turbidity through which print can be read), 15–30 mg/dL; 2+ turbidity (the presence of a white cloud without precipitate through which a black line on a white blackground can be seen), 40–100 mg/dL; 3+ turbidity (the presence of a white cloud with a precipitate through which black lines on a white background cannot be seen), 150–350 mg/dL; and 4+ turbidity (flocculent precipitate), >500 mg/dL *(33)*. False-positive results with SSA may be caused by radiocontrast agents, tolbutamide, sulfonamides, high-dose penicillin, or cephalosporin antibiotics, and strongly alkaline urine may produce a false-negative result *(33)*. The standard method for quantifying protein excretion is usually accomplished by measuring the protein excretion in a 24-h urine collection. Although precise, it may be cumbersome and inconvenient to perform, and at times inaccurate because of incomplete collections. Because of these difficulties, the protein:creatinine (milligram/milligram) ratio in a random urine has been used as an alternative to a 24-h urine collection *(34,35)*. A close correlation has been shown to exist between this ratio and the daily protein excretion in grams/day (i.e., a ratio of 2.0 would equal a 2 g/d protein excretion). Although not exact, it does provide the clinician with a semiquantitative measure to classify the degree of proteinuria in any particular subject. Figure 14-3 depicts a clinical approach to a subject found to have proteinuria on urinalysis.

As stated, the standard urine dipstick is insensitive for detecting microalbuminuria. Microalbuminuria is the earliest clinical sign of diabetic nephropathy, and may be an important marker of atherosclerosis and early cardiovascular mortality in those subjects with hypertension *(36–39)*. Microalbuminuria is present whenever the excretion of albumin is found to be between 30 and 300 mg/d (20–200 µg/min). Although screening for microalbuminuria may be done either with timed urine collections or by determining the albumin concentration in a random urine sample, the gold standard for detection is still a 24-h urine collection. The calculation of the albumin:creatinine ratio in a random urine specimen may minimize the effect of urine volume on the albumin concentration and provide a useful alternative for detecting microalbuminuria since it correlates well with those determined by 24-h urine collections *(40)*. When this ratio exceeds 30 mg/g (or 0.03

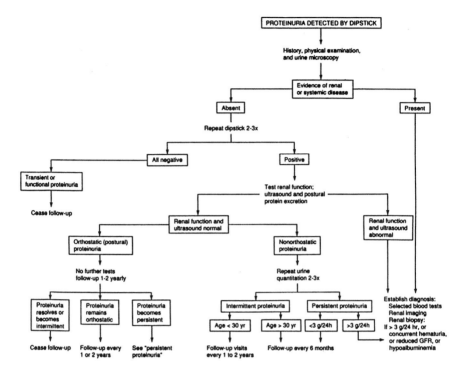

Fig. 14-3. A clinical approach to a subject with proteinuria detected by urine dipstick. (Reproduced with permission from Bernard DB, Salant DJ [1995] Clinical approach to the patient with proteinuria and the nephrotic syndrome. In Jacobson HR, Striker GE, Klahr S, eds. *The Principles and Practice of Nephrology,* 2nd ed., St. Louis: Mosby Year Book).

mg/mg), it suggests that the albumin excretion is >30 mg/d and that microalbuminuria is present. Transient increases in albumin excretion and microalbuminuria may be observed in the presence of fever, exercise, heart failure, and poor glycemic control *(36,41).* Thus, prior to screening for microalbuminuria, care must be taken to ensure that none of these factors exist.

REFERENCES

1. Smith HW (1951) The reliability of inulin as a measure of glomerular filtration. In: *The Kidney: Structure and Function in Health and Disease,* New York: Oxford University Press, pp. 231–238.
2. Levey AS, Perrone RD, Madias NE (1988) Serum creatinine and renal function. *Annu Rev Med* 39:456–490.

3. Levey AS (1990) Nephrology forum: measurement of renal function in chronic renal disease. *Kidney Int* 38:167–184.
4. Bauer JH, Brooks CS, Burch RN (1982) Clinical appraisal of creatinine clearance as a measurement of glomerular filtration rate. *Am J Kidney Dis* 2:337–346.
5. Shemesh D, Golbetz H, Kriss JP, et al. (1985) Limitation of creatinine as a filtration marker in glomerulopathic patients. *Kidney Int* 28:830–838.
6. Cockcroft DW, Gault MH (1976) Prediction of creatinine clearance from serum creatinine. *Nephron* 16:31–41.
7. Moller E, McIntosh JF, Van Slyke DD (1928) Studies on urea excretion: relationship between urine volume and the rate of urea excretion by normal adults. *J Clin Invest* 6:427–.
8. Lassiter WE, Gottschalk CW, Mylle M (1961) Micropuncture study of net transtubular movement of water and urea in non-diuretic mammalian kidney. *Am J Physiol* 200:1139–.
9. Lassiter WE, Mylle M, Gottschalk CW (1964) Net transtubular movement of water and urea in saline diuresis. *Am J Physiol* 206:669–.
10. Dossetor JB (1966) Creatininemia versus uremia: the relative significance of blood urea nitrogen and serum creatinine concentrations in azotemia. *Ann Intern Med* 65:1287–1299.
11. Perrone RD, Steinman TI, Beck GJ, et al. and the modification of diet in renal disease study (1990) Utility of radioisotopic filtration markers in chronic renal insufficiency: simultaneous comparison of 125I-Iothalamate, 169Yb-DTPA, 99mTc-DTPA, and inulin. *Am J Kidney Dis* 16:224–235.
12. Rehling M, Rabol A (1989) Measurement of glomerular filtration rate in adults: accuracy of five single-sample plasma clearance methods. *Clin Physiol* 9:171–182.
13. Blaufox MD (1991) Procedures of choice in renal nuclear medicine. *J Nucl Med* 32:1301–1309.
14. Lundqvist S, Hietala SO, Groth S, et al. (1997) Evaluation of single sample clearance calculations in 902 patients: a comparison of multiple and single sample techniques. *Acta Radiol* 38:68–72.
15. Nilsson-Ehle P, Grubb A (1994) New markers for the determination of GFR: iohexol clearance and cystatin C serum concentration. *Kidney Int* 46(Suppl. 47):S17–S19.
16. Rocco MV, Buckalew VM Jr, Moore LC, et al. (1996) Capillary electrophoresis for the determination of glomerular filtration rate using nonradioactive iohexol. *Am J Kidney Dis* 28:173–177.
17. Gaspari F, Mosconi L, Vigano G, et al. (1992) Measurement of GFR with a single injection of nonradioactive iothalamate. *Kidney Int* 41:1081–1084.
18. Frennby B, Sterner G, Almen T, et al. (1995) The use of iohexol clearance to determine GFR in patients with severe chronic renal failure—a comparison between different clearance techniques. *Clin Nephrol* 43:35–46.
19. Wolf AV (1962) Urinary concentrative properties. *Am J Med* 32:329–331.
20. Rose BD (1986) New approach to disturbances in the plasma sodium concentration. *Am J Med* 81:1033–1040.
21. Harrington JT, Cohen JJ (1973) Clinical disorders of urine concentration and dilution. *Arch Intern Med* 131:810–825.
22. Miller M, Dalakost T, Moses AM, et al. (1970) Recognition of partial defects in antidiuretic hormone secretion. *Ann Intern Med* 73:721–729.
23. Tryding N, Berg B, Ekman S, et al. (1988) DDAVP test for renal concentration capacity: age-related reference intervals. *Scand J Urol Nephrol* 22:141–145.

24. Richardson RMA, Halperin ML (1987) The urine pH: a potentially misleading diagnostic test in patients with hyperchloremic metabolic acidosis. *Am J Kidney Dis* 10:140–143.

25. Batlle DC, Hizon M, Cohen E, et al. (1988) The use of the urinary anion gap in the diagnosis of hyperchloremic metabolic acidosis. *N Engl J Med* 318:594–599.

26. Halperin ML, Richardson RMA, Bear RA, et al. (1988) Urine ammonium: the key to the diagnosis of distal renal tubular acidosis. *Nephron* 50:1–4.

27. Arruda JAL, Kurtzman NA (1980) Mechanisms and classification of deranged distal urinary acidification. *Am J Physiol* 239:F515–F523.

28. Rose BD (1988) Isolated Proteinuria and Hematuria, in *Manual of Clinical Problems in Nephrology*. Boston: Little Brown, pp. 130–132.

29. Robinson RR (1980) Isolated proteinuria in asymptomatic patients. *Kidney Int* 18:395–406.

30. Poortmans JR (1985) Postexercise proteinuria in humans: facts and mechanisms. *JAMA* 253:236–240.

31. Springberg PD, Garrett LE Jr, Thompson AL Jr, et al. (1982) Fixed and reproducible orthostatic proteinuria: results of a 20-year follow-up study. *Ann Intern Med* 97:516–519.

32. Rytand DA, Spreiter S (1981) Prognosis in postural (orthostatic) proteinuria: forty to fifty-year follow-up of six patients after diagnosis by Thomas Addis. *N Engl J Med* 305:618–620.

33. Rose BD (1987) *Pathophysiology of Renal Disease,* 2nd ed, New York: McGraw-Hill, pp. 11–16.

34. Ginsberg JM, Chang BS, Matarese RA, et al. (1983) Use of single voided urine samples to estimate quantitative proteinuria. *N Engl J Med* 309:1543–1546.

35. Schwab SJ, Christensen RL, Dougherty K, et al. (1987) Quantitation of proteinuria by the use of protein-to-creatinine ratios in single urine samples. *Arch Intern Med* 147:943–944.

36. American Diabetes Association (1994) Consensus development conference on the diagnosis and management in patients with diabetes mellitus. *Diabetes Care* 17:1357–1361.

37. James MA, Fotherby MD, Potter JF (1995) Screening tests for microalbuminuria in non-diabetic elderly subjects and their relation to blood pressure. *Clin Sci* 88:185–190.

38. Damsgaard EM, Froland A, Jorgensen OD, et al. (1990) Microalbuminuria as predictor of increased mortality in elderly people. *BMJ* 300:297–300.

39. Yudkin JS, Forrest RD, Jackson CA (1988) Microalbuminuria as predictor of vascular disease in non-diabetic subjects: Islington Diabetes Survey. *Lancet* 2:530–533.

40. Nathan DM, Rosenbaum C, Protasowicki VD (1987) Single-void urine samples can be used to estimate quantitative microalbuminuria. *Diabetes Care* 10:414–418.

41. Mogensen CE, Vestbo E, Poulsen PL, et al. (1995) Microalbuminuria and potential confounders: a review and some observations on variability of urinary albumin excretion. *Diabetes Care* 18:572–581.

15 Ambulatory Blood Pressure Monitoring

David H.G. Smith, MD

CONTENTS

EQUIPMENT
INSTRUCTIONS FOR THE PATIENT
WHEN SHOULD AMBULATORY BP MONITORING BE
CONSIDERED?
AN APPROACH TO INTERPRETING AMBULATORY
BP RESULTS
REFERENCES

The US-based Sixth Joint National Committee on the Prevention, Detection, Evaluation and Treatment of High Blood Pressure (JNC VI) *(1)* and the World Health Organization International Society of Hypertension (WHO-ISH) *(2)* agree that ambulatory blood pressure (BP) monitoring is a valuable tool in assessing hypertension. Not only is it helpful in affirming the diagnosis of hypertension, but it can also provide useful information regarding prognosis and treatment efficacy of the hypertensive disease process.

The principal advantage of ambulatory BP monitoring over office-derived BPs is that ambulatory BP monitoring provides a time series of BPs measured in the patient's own environment. This includes measurements taken not only during sleep or wakefulness but also away from the influences of the clinical office. Yet despite this advantage, ambulatory BP monitoring is not readily used in hypertension clinics. There are two reasons for this. First, third-party payers do not usually cover the procedure, leaving the physician or the patient to foot the

From: *Hypertension Medicine*
Edited by: M. A. Weber © Humana Press Inc., Totowa, NJ

Table 15-1
Ambulatory BP Monitoring Devices Fulfilling USAAMI or
BHS Specifications

Manufacturer	Model
SpaceLabs	SL90202, SL90207, SL90209
AND	TN2440, TN2421
QietTrack	—
NISSEI	D240
Profilemet	—
CH DRUCK	—

bill. Second, most physicians have difficulty in interpreting the results of ambulatory BP. The aim of this chapter is to provide the guidelines for a rational approach to the interpretation of the ambulatory BP monitoring printout.

EQUIPMENT

The ambulatory BP monitor consists of a pump and an arm cuff. An appropriately sized BP cuff should be selected and placed comfortably on the patient's upper arm. It is advisable to select the nondominant arm because this will diminish excessive movement during the measurements of the 24-h procedure. Inflation of the cuff is driven by a small battery-operated air pump carried in a pouch supported by either the patient's belt or a separate shoulder strap. The device is programmed to automatically measure BP at intervals ranging from every 15 to 30 min. Recorded BPs are stored in the unit and are downloaded to a computer device on conclusion of the monitoring period. Of the more than 43 available devices for measuring ambulatory BP monitoring, one should choose a monitor that complies with the protocol for accuracy and performance established by the United States Association for the Advancement of Medical Instrumentation (USAAMI) or the British Hypertension Society (BHS). Table 15-1 provides a partial list of such devices.

INSTRUCTIONS FOR THE PATIENT

Make sure that the patient feels comfortable when the cuff is applied. It should not fit too tightly but should fit snuggly in order to avoid any

Table 15-2
Current Recommendations for Clinical Use of Ambulatory BP Monitoring

	JNC VI	WHO-ISH
ABPM endorsed indications	Yes	Yes
Evaluation of white coat hypertension	Yes	Yes
Evaluation of labile BP	Yes	Yes
Suspicion of hypotensive episodes	Yes	Yes
Investigation of resistant hypertension	Yes	Yes
Autonomic dysfunction	Yes	No

excessive rotation or movement up and down the upper arm. The cuff should not be removed during the monitoring period. To obtain clinically accurate readings, it is important to instruct the patient to pursue activities generally representative of a typical day with the exception of abstaining from formal exercise routines or bathing (because this requires removal of the device). More important, if not excessively inconvenient, monitoring should also be performed on a typical workday. In addition, the patient should be informed regarding the frequency of measurements. During the hours the patient is awake, inflation of the cuff is preceded by a soft tone, which is an indication to the patient that the cuff will commence inflation in 5 s. Without unduly interrupting his or her current activity, the patient should try to minimize any excessive movement of the arm to which the BP cuff is applied. The patient should also carry a diary to record any unusual activities or symptoms so that they can be correlated with the BP printout. This may be helpful when exploring symptoms such as flushing, palpitations, dizziness, headaches, or syncope. Finally, the patient should be encouraged to retire for the night and to rise in the morning at the customary hour. When monitoring is completed, the cuff is removed and the device is connected to a computer or other printer device, which generates the printout result.

WHEN SHOULD AMBULATORY BP MONITORING BE CONSIDERED?

Both the US JNC VI and the WHO-ISH advocate the use of ambulatory BP monitoring in the diagnosis and management of hypertension in the clinical situations given in Table 15-2.

White Coat Hypertension

A high index of suspicion for white coat hypertension should exist when a patient reports on discrepancies between BPs measured in the clinic and elsewhere (such as at home or the local pharmacy). White coat hypertension is also more likely to occur when the patient is highly dependent on a favorable medical examination outcome in order to pursue a chosen career or to gain employment. People with anxious and hyperactive personalities may also be vulnerable. Remember, though, that the existence of any evidence of hypertensive target organ damage (such as hypertensive retinopathy, left ventricular hypertrophy, or proteinuria) precludes a diagnosis of white coat hypertension.

Labile Hypertension

Labile hypertension is manifested by conflicting and fluctuation office BP readings—sometimes elevated, sometimes normal. This is usually more of a problem among the elderly and in assessing systolic BP.

Hypotensive Episodes

Complaints from the patient regarding light headaches, dizziness, vertigo, and syncope may sometimes be related to overzealous treatment of hypertension. It is in these situations that the temporal association of recorded BPs to symptoms documented on a diary card is most useful.

Resistant Hypertension

In cases of resistant hypertension, ambulatory BP monitoring can also be useful because even when a firm diagnosis of hypertension has been established, some treated patients can still exhibit elements of a white coat effect. Typically, readings are high in the office but much lower when measured at home, and the dilemma is whether to increase the antihypertensive medication or to leave the treatment unchanged. Also, refractory hypertension in the face of a loss of the natural diurnal variation of BP should raise concerns regarding secondary hypertension.

Autonomic Dysfunction

Ambulatory BP monitoring can be useful in diagnosing autonomic dysfunction when the recorded BPs and heart rates lose their diurnal pattern of higher BPs during the daytime and lower BPs during sleep and the nighttime.

AN APPROACH TO INTERPRETING
AMBULATORY BP RESULTS

The ambulatory BP monitoring report consists of several pages, all of which can provide useful information when perused for a few minutes. In general, the report consists of a patient information page; summary pages of the 24-h, daytime, nighttime, and 1-h averaged BP periods; a listing of each recording obtained during the monitoring period along with a date and time stamp; a similar listing of instances in which the device attempted but failed to obtain measurements; and various graphic displays relating collected BPs and heart rates to time of day. What follows is an approach to the interpretation of each of these segments of the report.

Summary Page

The summary page is the most useful place to begin interpreting BP results, although often it is the last page of the BP monitoring report (Fig. 15-1). The 24-h mean provides the average of all BPs measured during the monitoring period. Because BPs are generally lower during sleep, a normal 24-h ambulatory BP mean is a little lower than the normal office BP level of <140/90 mmHg. Normal values of ambulatory BP continue to be a matter of debate, but a cutoff 24-h mean BP of 130/85 mmHg is generally consistent with most published guidelines. BP in excess of these values is compatible with a diagnosis of hypertension.

Next, scrutinize the daytime and nighttime mean BPs. During the daytime hours (defined as the period of most active awake activity for the patient—usually between 6 AM and 6 PM), BP is higher and the cutoff between normal and abnormal is usually set at the conventional office BP cutoff of 140/90 mmHg. By contrast, the nighttime mean BP is lower, with values in excess of 125/75 mmHg, indicative of hypertension. Another source of contention is in determining what time periods constitute day and night. Some investigators prefer fixed time periods (as just suggested) whereas others prefer to relate time periods for day and night to the actual time the patient was awake or asleep

SUMMARY

	MIN	MEAN	MAX	STD
Systolic	111 (1-11:08)	145	199 (1-04:38)	18.77 mmHg
Diastolic	45 (1-20:08)	62	88 (1-14:08)	11.25 mmHg
MAP	61	89	124	13.70 mmHg
Heart Rate	58	72	94	6.50 BPM

Percent of Systolic Readings above period limits: 64.2%
Percent of Diastolic Readings above period limits: 0.0%

Percent of time Systolic was above period limits: 64.9%
Percent of time Diastolic was above period limits: 0.0%

SUMMARY PERIOD: 6:00 to 18:00

	MIN	MEAN	MAX	STD
Systolic	111 (1-11:08)	141	183 (1-07:08)	17.27 mmHg
Diastolic	49 (1-26:48)	63	88 (1-14:08)	11.40 mmHg
MAP	61	89	124	15.68 mmHg
Heart Rate	63	73	94	6.67 BPM

Percent of Systolic Readings > 140 mmHg   40.5%
Percent of Diastolic Readings >   90 mmHg   0.0%

Percent of time Systolic >   140 mmHg   31.7%
Percent of time Diastolic>   90 mmHg   0.0%

SUMMARY PERIOD: 18:00 to 6:00

	MIN	MEAN	MAX	STD
Systolic	117 (1-18:28)	149	199 (1-04:38)	20.46 mmHg
Diastolic	45 (1-20:08)	61	78 (1-19:08)	10.81 mmHg
MAP	69	88	109	10.87 mmHg
Heart Rate	58	69	82	5.99 BPM

Percent of Systolic Readings > 120 mmHg   93.9%
Percent of Diastolic Readings > 80 mmHg   0.0%

Percent of time Systolic >   120 mmHg   93.9%
Percent of time Diastolic >   80 mmHg   0.0%

Fig. 15-1. A typical summary page of an ambulatory BP report.

during the monitoring period. Until further research resolves this issue, choose one method consistently.

Determining the differences between the daytime and nighttime mean values may be of value both prognostically and diagnostically. Nighttime values should be between 10 and 20% less than the daytime values. This indicates that BP is falling adequately at night, which is consistent with the normal diurnal variation in BP. Day-night differences in this range confer "dipper" status to the patient, which is prognostically favorable (3). Differences less than 10% indicate a nondipping status, which can be associated with an increased tendency toward the development of hypertensive end-organ damage such as hypertensive retinopathy, left ventricular hypertrophy, and proteinuria. Furthermore, the absence of normal dipping may be consistent with secondary hypertension or autonomic dysfunction and is therefore a good marker for the need of further work-up *(4)*. Alternatively, dipping in excess of 20%, especially in the elderly, may also be detrimental and contribute to watershed or lacunae cerebral infarcts *(5)* as well as anterior ischemic optic neuropathy, an increasingly important cause of deteriorating vision among the elderly population and closely correlated with excessive dipping *(6)*. Overzealous antihypertensive therapy is one correctable factor contributing to excessive dipping *(7)*. Remember, though, that of the three mean values on the summary page the overall 24-h mean ranks highest in importance in terms of diagnosing hypertension.

Also located on the summary page are measures of systolic and diastolic load. These represent the percentage of BPs in excess of either 140/90 mmHg for the daytime period and 120/80 mmHg for the nighttime period. Although even normotensive patients have some measurements in excess of these ranges, it is advisable to keep the loads as low as possible. Their value in assessing hypertensive status based on ambulatory BP monitoring does not supersede that of the 24-h mean but can be useful in evaluating efficacy of therapy or worsening hypertension—especially when repeated ambulatory BP monitorings are obtained over time.

BP Listings Page

The BP listings page is simply a chronological record of all BPs recorded during the monitoring period. It is most useful for the temporal correlation of BP with symptoms recorded in the patient's diary. For example, a quick scan of the listing can uncover paroxysms of hypertension or tachycardia, episodes of hypotension, or hypertensive readings recorded only at the start and end of the monitoring period (i.e., associated with visits to the clinic), and are strongly indicative of white coat hypertension. Patients usually enjoy reviewing this list with the physician and correlating their BPs with various activities during the monitoring period. This can also be a valuable educational exercise for patients and is particularly gratifying when the results of therapy are appreciated.

A review of the listing when the monitor has failed to obtain a reading gives an indication of the quality of the monitoring. Ideally, more than 75% of measurements should result in a BP value, and there should not be any periods in excess of 2 h in which no usable data have been collected. Monitorings for which many of the attempted measurements result in failure need to be repeated because the remaining BPs may not be truly representative of the patient's BP pattern.

Graphic Displays of Data

Usually three displays of the data are presented. Two are line graphs of the BPs and heart rates recorded as a function of time (one plots every reading and the other depicts the data averaged for each hour of the monitoring period). The third may be a frequency histogram of the ranges of systolic and diastolic BPs recorded during the monitoring period. These graphic displays are mainly useful in rapidly evaluating the degree to which BP boundaries are violated and are useful reinforcements to the patient. They are also valuable in determining whether any antihypertensive effects provided by therapy are sustained throughout the dosing interval, especially if once daily medication is being used. The frequency histograms are really a graphic representation of the previously discussed BP loads.

Final Considerations

Although the amount of data generated by ambulatory BP monitoring can be intimidating to the uninitiated, a systematic approach to the data and pages of the report provides a great deal of valuable information quickly. Too often, reviewers are unduly focused on the need for cutoffs between normal and abnormal when, ultimately, the real value of ambulatory BP monitoring lies in its repeated use and data trends over time. An underappreciated value of ambulatory BP monitoring is its value in reinforcing for the patient the appropriate diagnosis of hypertension or normotension, and patients are generally quite appreciative of a brief review of the data with their physician.

REFERENCES

1. The Joint National Committee on Prevention Detection, Evaluation and Treatment of High Blood Pressure and the National High Blood Pressure Education Program Coordinating Committee (1997) The sixth report of the Joint National Committee on Prevention, Detection, Evaluation, and Treatment of High Blood Pressure. *Arch Intern Med* 157:2413.

2. The 1999 World Health Organization—International Society of Hypertension Guidelines for the management of hypertension (1999) *Hypertension* 17:151–183.
3. Ohkubo T, Imai Y, Tsuji I, et al. (1997) Relation between nocturnal decline in blood pressure and mortality: the Ohasama Study. *Am J Hypertens* 11:1201–1207.
4. Hany S, Baumgart P, Frielingsdorf J, et al. (1987) Circadian blood pressure variability in secondary and essential hypertension. *J Hypertens* 5(Suppl. 5):S487–S489.
5. Shimada K, Kawamoto A, Matsubayashi K, et al. (1990) Silent cerebrovascular disease in the elderly: correction with ambulatory pressure. *Hypertension* 16:692–699.
6. Hayreh SS, Zimmerman MB, Podhajsky P, et al. (1994) Nocturnal arterial hypotension and its role in optic nerve head and ocular ischemic disorders. *Am J Ophthalmol* 117:5603–5624.
7. Raccaud O, Waeber B, Petrillo A, et al. (1992) Ambulatory blood pressure monitoring as a means to avoid over treatment of elderly hypertensive patients. *Gerontology* 38:99–104.

16 Arterial Compliance in Hypertension

G.E. McVeigh, MD and Li Lan Yoon, MD

CONTENTS

THE ARTERIAL CIRCULATION AND ARTERIAL
COMPLIANCE
BLOOD PRESSURE AND ARTERIAL COMPLIANCE
REFERENCES

The arterial circulation represents a branching system of conduits that conduct blood from the heart to the capillaries, where exchange of nutrients and waste products occurs between tissue cells and the blood. The large arteries are distensible and act as an elastic reservoir storing part of the energy of cardiac contraction that maintains pressure and flow during diastole when the heart is not ejecting blood. The smallest arteries and arterioles are the sites of greatest hemodynamic resistance and act in conjunction with precapillary sphincters to form a variable resistance that controls the rate of blood flow to the tissues. An arterial system composed of elastic conduits and high-resistance terminals constitutes a hydraulic filter that converts the intermittent output from the heart into steady capillary flow. A compromise is reached between the heart and the systemic circulation to provide optimal coupling so that the left ventricle can supply the minimum amount of blood necessary for tissue metabolism at the least cost of energy to the body and still be able to adapt quickly to the wide range of metabolic demands imposed on it.

From: *Hypertension Medicine*
Edited by: M. A. Weber © Humana Press Inc., Totowa, NJ

THE ARTERIAL CIRCULATION AND
ARTERIAL COMPLIANCE

Arterial blood vessels are complex three-dimensional structures whose components differ in mechanical, biochemical, and physiologic characteristics *(1)*. The endothelium represents a single monolayer of cells and possesses little tensile strength but can alter the mechanical behavior of arterial blood vessels through the production and release of vasoactive substances that influence vascular tone and structure. The arterial media bears most of the tensile strain of the blood vessels. The relative proportions of its constituents—elastin, smooth muscle, and collagen—as well as the thickness of the media vary considerably between blood vessels, according to their type, site, and physiologic function. As the outermost layer of the arterial blood vessel, the tunica adventitia contains a large number of collagen fibers that can also influence mechanical properties of the vessels.

The pressure in all systemic arteries fluctuates; the source of the fluctuation is the pumping action of the heart. The systolic and diastolic pressures, as traditionally measured by sphygmomanometry, represent the limits of the pressure fluctuations during the cardiac cycle. This measurement provides only a limited amount of information about the cardiovascular system. More information about the interaction of the heart and systemic circulation may be obtained by measuring the mean arterial pressure (MAP) and considering the systolic blood pressure (SBP) and diastolic blood pressure (DBP) at the upper and lower limits of periodic oscillations about the mean pressure. The MAP can be obtained by integrating the area under the pulse pressure (PP) contour or approximated by adding one third of the PP to the diastolic pressure. The MAP depends only on the cardiac output and the peripheral resistance. The arterial PP, defined as the difference between SBP and DBP, is a function of the stroke volume, the pattern of left ventricular ejection, and arterial compliance. Further additional information about the interaction between the heart and the arterial system can be obtained by analysis of the total BP curve that provides information about steady-state and pulsatile phenomena in the circulation.

Arterial compliance is defined as a change in area, diameter, or volume for a given change in pressure and is dependent on vessel geometry in addition to the mechanical properties of the vessel wall

(2). Arterial wall properties differ in different vessels, differ in the same vessel at various distending pressures, and differ with the activation of smooth muscle in the vessel wall. Although no single descriptor of arterial physical characteristics can completely describe the mechanical behavior of the vasculature, arterial compliance represents the best clinical index of the buffering function of the arterial system. Changes in the mechanical behavior of blood vessels manifested by reduced arterial compliance can influence growth and remodeling of the left ventricle, large arteries, small arteries, and arterioles. Clearly arterial blood vessels can no longer be considered as passive conduits to deliver blood to peripheral tissues in response to metabolic demands. Instead they should be viewed as biophysical sensors that respond to hemodynamic and neurohumoral stimuli that influence the tone and structure of blood vessels. Figure 16-1 outlines the pathophysiologic consequences of a reduced arterial compliance.

A wide variety of techniques, both direct and indirect, have been employed to assess the compliance characteristics of arteries in health and disease (Table 16-1). Previous studies indicate that patients with documented vascular disease or with a history of vascular events tend to have less compliant arteries than control subjects *(3)*. Furthermore, an excess of risk factors for the future development of vascular disease may also be associated with a less compliant arterial circulation. Thus, a reduced arterial compliance may provide an index of early arterial damage that could predispose to the development of major vascular disease. At present, diagnostic procedures are aimed at assessing the extent and severity of vascular disease after the development of symptoms or when morbid events occur. At this stage the disease process is already well advanced. The diagnostic challenge must be to detect abnormal structure and function in the vascular system prior to the development of symptoms and signs of disease. In this regard, a reduced arterial compliance may precede the development of cardiovascular disease and act as a risk factor, or occur as a consequence of established cardiovascular disease and represent a marker for its presence.

Increased peripheral vascular resistance is regarded as the hemodynamic hallmark of sustained hypertension. This measure has been used to estimate vascular adaptations in response to disease in arterial blood vessels and to monitor the hemodynamic effect of drug interventions. The resistance calculation reflects a reduction in capillary density and

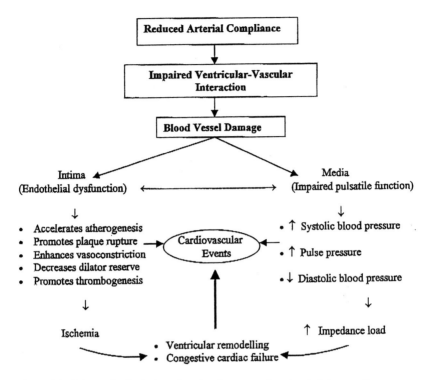

Fig. 16-1. Schematic depiction showing how a reduced arterial compliance may promote blood vessel damage and predispose to premature clinical events.

changes in the wall thickness:lumen ratio of the media in small arteries and arterioles. It ignores pressure fluctuations occurring in the aorta and its major branches, where the compliance characteristics of the vessel wall provide the vital buffering function required to smooth pulsatile outflow from the heart.

Recent evidence suggests that the altered vascular architecture described in small arteries may in large part be owing to a remodeling process rather than growth. Intuitively, changes in small-artery remodeling and growth would be expected to influence the compliance characteristics of these vessels in addition to increasing resistance to blood flow. Regarding the large arteries, hypertension can be viewed as an accelerated form of aging. The pathologic changes that occur in the aortic wall and the associated aortic dilatation and wall thickening occur at an earlier age if BP is elevated. These degenerative changes will not influence the resistance to steady blood flow but will significantly influence the pulsatile pressure load on the heart. Thus, changes in the

Table 16-1

Methods Used to Estimate Arterial Compliance[a]

Methods	Advantages	Limitations	Information provided
Direct			
Angiography	Evaluation of aortic segments	Expensive, invasive	Regional aortic compliance
Magnetic resonance imaging	Noninvasive, not limited by acoustic window, can examine multiple segments	Expensive, remote site of BP measurement	Regional aortic compliance
TTE/TEE	TTE noninvasive, reasonable availability	Expensive, TTE limited by acoustic window, operator-dependent techniques, TEE invasive	Regional aortic compliance
Transcutaneous ET/IVUS techniques	Transcutaneous technique noninvasive, reproducible	Operator dependent, IVUS invasive, remote site of BP measurement with ET	Regional compliance of peripheral arteries
Plethysmographic techniques	Noninvasive, clinical research application	Remote site of BP measurement	Compliance of vascular bed under cuff
Indirect			
Stroke volume:PP ratio	Noninvasive	Needs measure of stroke volume and brachial BP	Total arterial compliance
Pulse wave velocity	Noninvasive, reasonable availability, reproducible	Limited to larger arteries, errors owing to wave reflections	Segmental arterial compliance
Fourier analysis of pressure and flow waveforms	Standard technique, reproducible	Expensive, invasive	Total arterial compliance
Pulse contour analysis	Noninvasive, reproducible	Measurement of stroke volume	Total arterial compliance

[a] IVUS, intravascular ultrasound; TTE, transthoracic echocardiography; TEE, transesophageal echocardiography; ET, echo tracking.

physical characteristics of large blood vessels will not only alter BP and in particular the PP, but also cardiac workload and ventricular performance.

BLOOD PRESSURE AND ARTERIAL COMPLIANCE

Hypertension is a major risk factor for cardiovascular morbidity and mortality. Approximately 20–25% of the adult population in Western society has hypertension, and about 70% of these individuals have mildly elevated BPs. The reliability of this measurement in clinical practice and the minor absolute difference between defined normal and abnormal readings in different age groups can present difficulties in deciding who has the disease and who requires treatment. Furthermore, arterial BP, particularly in the mildly elevated range, lacks sensitivity in identifying those individuals at greatest risk of developing vascular events. At present, therefore, many patients are treated to prevent complications that would arise in only a few.

Classification schemes and guidelines have been developed to aid diagnosis, help assess severity, and determine prognosis in patients with hypertension (4). Previous recommendations based on the level of BP alone misclassified individual patients in terms of their risk of developing future vascular events. It must be emphasized that cardiovascular disease progression is a multifactorial process that can vary by a factor of 10-fold, depending on the presence of target organ damage or other traditional cardiovascular risk factors in patients with the same degree of BP elevation. The concept of absolute risk and its importance in modifying decision-making processes have been emphasized in more recent iterations from the Joint National Committee on the diagnosis, treatment, and control of hypertension guidelines. Thus, cost-effectiveness may be improved by optimizing the use of monetary resources for cardiovascular care by limiting exposure of individuals to long-term drug therapy from which they may gain little, if any, benefit.

A reduced large-artery compliance is a well-accepted finding in hypertension, whatever the site and method of measurement. As a more direct measure of vascular damage associated with elevated BP, arterial compliance may be of value in further improving risk stratification in these patients (5). It may also serve as a sensitive parameter to assess the effects of therapeutic interventions on pulsatile arterial function. Emerging data support the concept that the cardioprotective actions of drug interventions may depend, at least in part, on improvement in the compliance characteristics of the arterial circulation. Hypertension is a vascular disease characterized by structural and functional changes in the cardiovascular system. Left ventricular hypertrophy (LVH) and arterial wall thickening of the blood vessels have been well documented in chronic hypertension. To some extent, these cardiovascular structural alterations are a natural physiologic response to high BP and are protective. Nevertheless, it has been suggested that optimal antihypertensive therapy not only normalizes BP but also cardiovascular structure.

Because high BP itself will induce a decrease in arterial compliance, it remains a matter of debate whether the reduction in compliance represents an alteration of wall properties or is merely a consequence of the elevated pressure. Currently, considerable controversy exists as to whether abnormalities in arterial compliance in hypertensive patients represent intrinsic change in the arterial wall or merely a reflection of pressure changes, and whether the changes in compliance are located primarily in the large or small vessels. Several observations suggest that decreased compliance is not solely a mechanical consequence of increased BP. These observations include the finding that compliance is reduced in patients with borderline hypertension and that in patients with established hypertension, compliance estimates are reduced to the same extent regardless of the degree to which the BP is elevated. However, it must be emphasized that a reduced arterial compliance in hypertensive patients has not been a universal finding, and that mechanical alteration in the muscular conduit arteries in particular may not be a prominent feature of the disease.

The therapeutic benefits of antihypertensive drugs on arteries consist of two major effects: the effect owing to the BP lowering and the direct effect of the drug on the vessel wall. Arterial compliance will increase as BP decreases owing to the nonlinear distensibility characteristics of arteries. Most studies cannot differentiate between a compliance change that is the result of a drug effect on BP and the direct effect of the drug on the vessel wall *(6)*. This differentiation is important because a more physiologic therapy, one that benefits pulsatile and nonpulsatile flow, may be of greater clinical benefit than therapy that lowers BP alone. The presence of LVH is known to represent an important complication of established hypertension. Because the association between ventricular hypertrophy and BP elevation is low, it appears that it is not a totally pressure-dependent phenomenon. Furthermore, regression of LVH with drug therapy can occur independent of the decrease in arterial BP. These data suggest that some antihypertensive agents can influence growth and remodeling of the left ventricle independent of their actions on lowering BP. Similar provocative data can be presented for the effects of antihypertensive drugs on the physical characteristics of blood vessels. Clearly, changes in blood vessel structure will affect the compliance characteristics of the blood vessel. To date, there are no longitudinal studies that relate abnormal compliance and drug effects to outcome. Nonetheless, monitoring changes in arterial compliance may provide a better marker for structural and functional changes associated with hypertension and their response to therapeutic interventions than can be achieved by monitoring BP alone.

An understanding of the age- and disease-related physiologic changes that occur in the arterial system is crucial in order to appreciate their influence and the occurrence of cardiovascular diseases and their response to treatment. By providing a direct assessment of abnormal structure and tone in the arterial vasculature, abnormalities in arterial compliance may improve cardiovascular risk stratification and identify individuals with early vascular damage who are predisposed to future vascular events. This hypothesis can be proved only when large groups of patients are evaluated and followed in a longitudinal fashion over time. To achieve this objective, techniques for estimating the compliance characteristics of arterial segments or the arterial circulation in general should be easy to use, robust, reproducible, and noninvasive. With recent advances in technology, this goal is now becoming a reality.

REFERENCES

1. Lee RT, Kamm RD (1994) Vascular mechanics for the cardiologist. *J Am Coll Cardiol* 23:1289–1295.
2. McVeigh GE, Bank AJ, Cohn JN (1995) Vascular compliance. In: Willerson JT, Cohn JN, eds. *Cardiovascular Medicine*, New York: Churchill Livingstone, pp. 1212–1227.
3. Safar ME, Frohlich ED (1995) The arterial system in hypertension: a prospective view. *Hypertension* 26:10–14.
4. The sixth report of the Joint National Committee on Prevention, Detection, Evaluation, and Treatment of High Blood Pressure (1997) *Arch Intern Med* 2157:2413–2446.
5. Franklin SS, Weber MA (1994) Measuring hypertensive cardiovascular risk: the vascular overload concept. *Am Heart J* 128:793–801.
6. Glasser SP, Arnett DK, McVeigh GE, Finkelstein SM, Bank AJ, Morgan DJ, Cohn JN (1997) Vascular compliance and cardiovascular disease: a risk factor or a marker? *Am J Hypertens* 10:1175–1189.

III Principles of Treatment

17 Starting Hypertension Treatment

Setting Targets

Michael A. Weber, MD

Guidelines on when to start antihypertensive treatment have been published recently. The Sixth Joint National Committee on the Prevention, Detection, Evaluation and Treatment of High Blood Pressure (JNC VI) *(1)* and the World Health Organization—International Society of Hypertension *(2)* have provided very similar criteria to assist decision making. Table 17-1 presents the JNC VI recommendations.

The concept is relatively straightforward. Milder forms of hypertension, in patients who do not have other risk factors or evidence of target organ damage, can be managed simply by observation or by institution of lifestyle modifications for 6–12 mo. On the other hand, more severe forms of hypertension, or the presence of other important risk factors or target organ involvement, mandate early prescription of medications. The recommendations shown in Table 17-1 are based partly on the results of clinical end point trials in hypertension, and partly on the opinions of experts in the field. Under these circumstances, the recommendations cannot be regarded as ironclad: there is room for judgment and discretion in clinical decision making. In reality, however,

From: *Hypertension Medicine*
Edited by: M. A. Weber © Humana Press Inc., Totowa, NJ

Table 17-1
Risk Stratification and Treatment[a]

BP stages (mmHg)	Risk group[b]		
	(A) No risk factors; no TOD/CCD	(B) At least one risk factor, not including diabetes mellitus; no TOD/CCD	(C) TOD/CCD and/or diabetes, with or without other risk factors
High normal (130–139/85–89)	Lifestyle modification	Lifestyle modification	Drug therapy[d]
Stage 1 (140–150/90–99)	Lifestyle modification	Lifestyle modification[c]	Drug therapy
Stages 2 and 3 (≥160/≥100)	Drug therapy	Drug therapy	Drug therapy

Adapted from JNC VI with permission.

[a]A patient with diabetes and a BP of 142/94 mmHg plus left ventricular hypertrophy (LVH) should be classified as having stage 1 hypertension with TOD (LVH) and with another major risk factor (diabetes). This patient would be categorized as stage 1, risk group C and recommended for immediate initiation of pharmacologic treatment. Lifestyle modification should be adjunctive therapy for all patients recommended for pharmacologic therapy.

[b]TOD/CCD, target organ damage/clinical cardiovascular disease.

[c]For patients with multiple risk factors, clinicians should consider drugs as initial therapy plus lifestyle modifications.

[d]For those with heart failure or renal disease or diabetes.

because concomitant risk factors are so common in people with hypertension, the majority of patients whose blood pressures (BPs) are consistently 140/90 mmHg or higher are likely to require active treatment.

ARE LIFESTYLE MODIFICATIONS WORTH PURSUING?

Virtually all physicians, as well as the majority of laypeople, know that losing weight or reducing salt intake is helpful in managing hypertension. But most attempts at lifestyle modification are perfunctory, and there remains considerable skepticism about these nonpharmacologic strategies.

In fairness, a critical attitude is justified. In an era of so-called evidence-based medicine, there are few if any data to indicate that lifestyle modifications actually prevent major clinical events or improve survival in hypertensive patients. Another problem is one of practicality. It is truly difficult to achieve and especially to maintain weight loss, and in contemporary times, when so many meals are eaten away from the traditional family setting, it is challenging to adhere to meaningful changes in diet. For this reason, most patients who are told to lose weight or to make other lifestyle changes will be relatively unsuccessful.

Worse yet, when the physician is then compelled to prescribe medications to control BP, this can be seen as a punitive response to the patient's failure and therefore may compromise his or her commitment to the drug therapy. Some physicians have proposed an innovative alternative: start with drug therapy with the aim of controlling BP effectively and rapidly; then offer the patient the opportunity of decreasing or even eliminating the drug therapy by making appropriate lifestyle changes. Regardless of how this is done, there are some important issues to consider.

Obesity

Obesity is now recognized as a cardiovascular risk factor in its own right, and is present in about half of all hypertensive patients. Obesity leads to such abnormalities as LVH, glomerular hyperfiltration and albuminuria, lipid abnormalities, and insulin resistance. Thus, the hypertensive patient with obesity can present a multitude of problems to be addressed and monitored during treatment. Strategies that are effective in reducing weight might have the added benefits of reversing or preventing the other cardiovascular and metabolic abnormalities that accompany obesity. Although weight loss through diet is difficult to achieve and maintain, some new pharmacologic agents have become available that might facilitate successful dieting and have acceptable safety profiles during long-term administration. If effective, this type of strategy could become an important part of managing hypertension. From the BP point of view, it should be remembered that even modest reductions in body weight can produce meaningful antihypertensive effects.

Reduced Sodium Intake

Reducing sodium intake is an area of continuing controversy. It is likely that effective reduction of sodium in the diet can reduce BP in some patients. Unfortunately, long-term outcome studies using this strategy have not yet provided definitive data. One recent trial claimed that sodium reduction, as well as weight reduction or the combination of the two strategies, decreased cardiovascular events in elderly hypertensive patients *(3)*. On the other hand, other investigators have agreed that BP reductions with sodium diets, in general, are modest, and that the resulting stimulatory effects on the sympathetic and renin-angiotensin systems could be counterproductive. Clearly, more research is needed before authoritative guidelines can be issued. Potassium supplementation of the diet has also been recommended as a strategy for BP reduction *(4)*. There is some theoretical support for this approach, but, again, clinical end point data are lacking.

Exercise

Exercise is a strategy that is reasonably effective in reducing BP. An aerobic regimen should be considered as part of the overall hypertension treatment plan. Individuals who exercise regularly are more likely to be motivated to undertake dietary changes, and hence weight loss and possibly sodium reduction may be useful dividends of this approach.

Lipid Disorders

Decreased high-density lipoprotein cholesterol and increased low-density lipoprotein cholesterol are common in hypertension. Abnormalities in lipids can be addressed, to some extent, by appropriate dietary modification. A substantial number of hypertensive patients actually meet the published criteria for treatment with the HMG CoA reductase inhibitors, and the use of these drugs—particularly because they appear to have cardiovascular primary prevention properties in appropriate patients—should be strongly considered.

Smoking

Smoking exaggerates the adverse cardiovascular effects of the other risk factors that tend to cluster in hypertension, and cessation should be a cornerstone of management.

BP TARGETS

Factors concerning the selection of an initial pharmacologic agent for treating hypertension are dealt with elsewhere in this book. Also of interest, however, is the selection of a target BP for each patient. Despite all the attention that has been directed toward effective management of the several risk factors associated with the syndrome of hypertension, it has recently become apparent that BP itself should be a critical target of therapy. JNC VI, e.g., requires that BP be <130/85 mmHg to be regarded as normal; to be optimal, BP should be <120/80 mmHg. As a practical matter, the JNC VI recommends treating BP to below 140/90 mmHg in most hypertensive patients, and to below 130/85 mmHg in patients with concomitant conditions such as renal insufficiency or diabetes mellitus.

The Hypertension Optimal Treatment (HOT) study (5) has strongly influenced aggressive new BP targets. This study examined the impact of differing degrees of BP control on cardiovascular clinical outcomes. In general, best results were observed when BP was reduced to the area of 130/82 mmHg. In vulnerable patients, particularly diabetic hypertensive patients, the final few BP points in this range were important; for example, there were fewer events when diastolic blood pressure (DBP) was reduced to 82 mmHg than when it was reduced only to the mid-80s. Two other important points were revealed by the HOT study. First, quality of life was highest in those patients whose BPs were most markedly reduced. This should help put to rest fears that intensive treatment of hypertension produces excessive side effects. Second, multiple drugs, in many cases three or more, were required to achieve the BP targets. The following conclusion can be drawn: if physicians attempt to achieve aggressive BP goals, they can do so in the majority of hypertensive patients, and even if this requires multiple drugs, there does not appear to be a quality of life penalty.

Similar findings have emerged from other studies. In a trial in patients with already existing renal insufficiency—admittedly a minority of hypertensive patients—optimal prevention of events was achieved at a BP of approx 125/75 mmHg *(6)*. Another recent study, the United Kingdom Prospective Diabetes Study, has also shown the clinical end point benefit of aggressive BP reduction in hypertensive patients with diabetes. In fact, this study's investigators claimed that reaching target BP goals may be more important than the issue of which type of antihypertensive agent should be used as the basis of treatment *(7)*.

One other point should be mentioned. There has been concern among some clinicians about the so-called J-curve phenomenon in which excessive reduction of DBP is thought to increase rather than decrease the probability of major cardiac events. The basis for this concern is that because filling of the coronary circulation occurs by backflow during diastole, excessive reduction in diastolic pressure could result in decreased blood supply to the myocardium. Several recent studies, however, have focused on whether or not there is any excess risk associated with large reductions in the DBP. To date, there does not appear to be evidence to suggest any particular risk with this strategy, and it seems that many more hypertensive patients are hurt by inadequate reduction in BP than by excessive reduction.

HOW WELL IS BP BEING CONTROLLED?

Although the diagnosis and management of hypertension in the United States is probably better than in any other country in the world, according to the National Health and Nutrition Examination Survey, barely one quarter of hypertensive patients in the United States have their BPs controlled to the recommended level of 140/90 mmHg *(8)*. This critical issue is discussed in greater detail elsewhere in this book. When the question arises about why we are not doing a better job of controlling BP, most physicians state that they believe the problem lies with poor patient compliance. To be sure, this is a problem, and much research needs to be done to understand why hypertensive patients, who clearly are at risk of devastating strokes and other cardiovascular events, so inconsistently adhere to their treatment.

But, much of the blame also can be attributed to physicians. A recent study from the Veterans Affairs system has indicated that physicians appear to be reluctant to enforce the changes in therapy necessary to achieve optimal BP control *(9)*. Indeed, there appears to be a need to understand why physicians, even when the importance of effective BP control is clearly understood, are so reluctant to take the necessary steps to provide the full measure of treatment that patients require.

If reaching target BP goals is so important, how can it be achieved? First, it is important to prescribe drugs in their full dose. With modern drugs, including angiotensin-converting enzyme inhibitors, angiotensin receptor blockers, and even calcium channel blockers, maximum doses can be given in most patients without significant side effects. Second, it must be understood that achieving meaningful target BP goals will require multiple drugs. Fixed combination products are sometimes a useful solution to this issue because they provide the convenience and cost savings associated with providing two drugs in one pill or capsule.

Large-scale clinical trials have shown that patients are willing to take multiple drugs to achieve goal BPs, particularly if they know that preventing strokes and other serious outcomes is the real objective of treatment. It should also be acknowledged that there are patients whose BPs are truly difficult to control. New types of pharmacologic agents will be an important answer to this problem, and physicians must continue to encourage development of new therapies that will allow the achievement of effective care for all hypertensive patients.

REFERENCES

1. Joint National Committee (1997) The sixth report of the Joint National Committee on prevention, detection, evaluation and treatment of high blood pressure. *Arch Intern Med* 157:2413–2446.
2. Guidelines Subcommittee (1999) 1999 World Health Organization—International Society of Hypertension Guidelines for the Management of Hypertension. *J Hypertens* 17:151–183.
3. The Trials of Hypertension Prevention Collaborative Research Group (1997) Effects of weight loss and sodium reduction intervention on blood pressure and hypertension incidence in overweight people with high-normal blood pressure: The Trials of Hypertension Prevention, phase II. *Arch Intern Med* 157:657–667.
4. Whelton PK, He J, Cutler JA, et al. (1997) Effects of oral potassium on blood pressure: meta-analysis of randomized controlled clinical trials. *JAMA* 277:1624–1632.
5. Hansson L, Zanchetti A, Carruthers SG, et al. (1998) Effects of intensive blood pressure lowering and low dose aspirin in patients with hypertension: principal

results of the Hypertension Optimal Treatment (HOT) randomized trial. HOT Study Group. *Lancet* 351:1755–1762.

6. Bakris GL (1998) Progression of diabetic nephropathy: a focus on arterial pressure level and methods of reduction. *Diabetes Res Clin Pract* 39(Suppl.):S35–S42.

7. UK Prospective Diabetes Study Group (1998) Tight blood pressure control and risk of macrovascular and microvascular complications in type 2 diabetes: UKPDS.38.BMJ 317:703–713.

8. Burt VL, Whelton PK, Roccella EJ, et al. (1995) Prevalence of hypertension in the US adult population: results from the Third National Health and Nutrition Examination Survey 1988–1991. *Hypertension* 25:305–313.

9. Berlowitz DR, Ash AS, Hickey EC, et al. (1998) Inadequate management of blood pressure in a hypertensive population. *N Engl J Med* 339:1957–1963.

18 Choosing the First Agent

Matthew R. Weir, MD

Hypertension is an asymptomatic disease that we frequently render symptomatic with our recommended lifestyle modifications and antihypertensive therapy. This alteration of an asymptomatic disease into a symptomatic one likely explains the inadequate current hypertension treatment and control rates. Nonadherence to prescribed therapy is one of the most serious problems we face in clinical practice. The source of this problem relates to inadequate education, a poor physician/patient relationship, and a lack of understanding of the pathophysiology contributing to hypertension. The statistics of nonadherence and inadequate control rates are alarming. The most recent data from the National Health and Nutrition Examination Survey 3 (Phase II) show that only

From: *Hypertension Medicine*
Edited by: M. A. Weber © Humana Press Inc., Totowa, NJ

one in four Americans has blood pressure (BP) control to a level of 140/90 mmHg or less *(1,2)*. Even more surprising is that only 50% of patients who are treated actually achieve this level of BP control. In fact, there has been a steady erosion in hypertension control rates over the past 10 yr. Thus, current strategies are not working.

Historically, physicians have been taught to keep the treatment of hypertension simple. Once behavioral modification efforts have proven unsuccessful, the physician should start with a single agent and titrate it sufficiently in order to control BP. Unfortunately, in the majority of cases, higher doses of individual agents result in an increased risk of adverse events. Thus, rather than a symptomatic improvement in the condition, symptoms develop that encourage the patient to be noncompliant. More recent effort has focused on studying the use of lower doses of two or more medications in order to facilitate better BP reduction yet avoid adverse events associated with higher doses of the individual drugs.

More intensive reduction in BP is also an area of growing interest, as numerous outcome clinical trials demonstrate the benefits of lower systolic blood pressure (SBP) and diastolic blood pressure (DBP) in reducing the risk for stroke, congestive heart failure, myocardial infarction (MI), and the rate of progression of renal disease *(3,4)*. In their sixth report, the Joint National Committee stressed the importance of controlling BP to 130/85 mmHg, or less, particularly in patients with diabetes, target organ disease, or renal insufficiency. Consequently, it is unlikely that there will be a single therapeutic agent that provides sufficient efficacy and tolerability that it can be used in many patients as successful monotherapy. Our future approaches to the treatment of hypertension will rest largely with the optimal combination of two or more drugs to more intensively lower BP yet avoid the hazards of higher dose monotherapy. Ultimately, this may prove to be the key strategy. Note, however, that no two patients are alike. Adverse events are not uncommon and may vary substantially between patients, not only for different drugs but also for different doses of medications. Pathophysiologic explanations for hypertension remain unidentified although abnormalities of the renin-angiotensin system, the sympathetic nervous system (SNS), and salt and water handling by the kidney are leading candidates. Consequently, pharmacologic strategies must consider targeting one or all of these possible contributing factors.

The purpose of this chapter is to highlight some of the key factors the physician must consider when choosing the first agent, while also realizing that in the vast majority of patients a second and possibly even

Table 18-1
Consideration for Initial Therapy in Older Patients

Pathophysiology	Desirable pharmacologic approach[a]
Decreased vascular compliance and ↑ PVR	Use a vasodilator (e.g., HCTZ, ACEI, ARB, CCB, α-blockers).
Isolated systolic hypertension and wider pulse pressure	Use HCTZ.
Reduction of cardiovascular baroreflex function with blood lability	Avoid sympatholytics and volume depletion.
Orthostatic hypotension	Consider using short-acting meds (<8 h duration) at bedtime during recumbency.
Reduced metabolic capability	Adjust all medications for renal/hepatic function—start at half dose.
Prostatic hypertrophy (BPH)	Use prostatic urethral dilation (α-blockers).

[a]ACEI, ACE inhibitor; ARB, angiotensis type 1 receptor blocker; BPH, Benigen prostatic hypertrophy; PVR, peripheral vascular resistance.

a third agent will be required. The first agent may then be viewed as the starting point on which subsequent therapies will be added depending on the patient's underlying demographic variables and comorbid medical conditions. This chapter also highlights my own personal opinions with regard to optimal starting points in different types of patients.

CONSIDERATIONS FOR INITIAL THERAPY IN OLDER PATIENTS (TABLE 1)

With aging there is a substantial decrease in vascular compliance and an increase in peripheral vascular resistance *(5,6)*. This results in a wider pulse pressure (PP) with an increase in SBP and a decrease in DBP. Frequently, there is an associated reduction in cardiovascular baroreceptor reflex function and greater BP lability, orthostatic hypotension, reduced left ventricular compliance and function, and impaired renal blood flow *(5)*.

An ideal starting point in older patients would be a vasodilator. I believe that the ideal "conditioning" agent is a low dose of hydrochlorothiazide (HCTZ) approx 12.5 mg. This dose improves the blood vessels' response to other commonly used drugs. Low doses of diuretics are extremely well tolerated and have a very low risk for causing

abnormalities in glycemic control, potassium homeostasis, and cholesterol metabolism. They have been shown to be particularly effective
in controlling SBP. Diuretics primarily control BP through a reduction
in peripheral vascular resistance. At the beginning of treatment, they
induce very mild volume contraction. The biologic half-life of diuretics
extends for many months, far beyond their pharmacologic half-life.

Other initial pharmacologic approaches would include other vasodilator classes such as an angiotensin-converting enzyme (ACE) inhibitor,
an angiotensin type 1 receptor blocker, a calcium channel blocker
(CCB), or an α-blocker. These drugs are also safe and effective and
well tolerated particularly when used in lower doses. In particular, the
ACE inhibitor and the angiotensin type 1 receptor blocker can be
titrated effectively without a substantial increase in adverse events.
CCBs and α-blockers are much better tolerated in the lower half of
their dosing range. CCBs are quite effective even in the face of a
high-salt diet, perhaps owing to their renal vasodilatory effects and an
intrinsic ability to facilitate natriuresis. α-Blockers may have a particular advantage in elderly males in facilitating prostatic urethral relaxation
and improving urinary stream.

Whatever drugs are chosen, slow, careful titration is recommended,
preferably not more frequently than every 3 mo, in order to gain more
intensive control of both SBP and DBP. In many patients, it has taken
them 30–40 yr to develop hypertensive vascular disease. Physicians
should not try to correct that in a matter of weeks. The use of lower
doses of more drugs appears to be ideal in these types of patients,
particularly when one of those drugs is a low-dose thiazide diuretic.

If orthostasis is present, shorter-acting medications dosed at night
may provide an ideal approach. One also needs to remember to adjust
medications for renal and hepatic dysfunction, which is also more
common in older hypertensive patients.

CONSIDERATIONS FOR INITIAL THERAPY BASED ON GENDER (TABLE 2)

Men and women appear to benefit equally with more intensive control
of BP in reducing the risk for cardiovascular end points (7,8). Men
appear to have decreased resting heart rate, longer left ventricular
ejection fraction time, and increased PP when stressed, compared with
women. Women tend to have reduced total peripheral resistance and
greater blood volume compared with men. Women have a lesser

Table 18-2
. Consideration for Initial Therapy

Pathophysiology	Desirable pharmacologic approach[a]
Men have ↓ resting HR, longer LVEF time, ↑ stressed pulse. pressure compared to women	Use vasodilator (e.g., HCTZ, ACE inhibitor, ARB, CCB).
Women have ↓ TPR and ↑ blood volume compared to men.	Use vasodilator, heart rate reduction, less need for diuresis (HCTZ, ACE inhibitor, ARB, β-blocker, CCB).
Postmenopausal women more frequently have CAD with atypical chest pain.	Use an antianginal; reduce heart rate (β-blocker, CCB).
Osteoporosis.	Antagonize calciuria (HCTZ).
Pregnancy.	Avoid teratogenic drugs (ACE inhibitor, ARB). Avoid drugs that may delay labor (CCB). Avoid drugs that may cause ureteroplacental insufficiency (loop diuretics). Optimal choices: alphamethyldopa, hydralazine, β-blocker.
Women report more pedal edema with CCB and cough with ACEI than men.	Adjust medications if these symptoms are present.

[a]CAD, coronary artery disease; HR, heart rate; LVEF, left ventricular ejection factor; TPR, total peripheral resistance.

likelihood of coronary disease before menopause. However, once menopause occurs, women rapidly develop coronary disease and more frequently present with atypical chest pain *(9)*. Osteoporosis is also more frequent in women in the postmenopausal period.

The choice of an initial therapy should be based on the need for vasodilation as well as treatment of attendant comorbidities. Vasodilators such as HCTZ, ACE inhibitors, angiotensin type 1 receptor blockers, and CCBs are reasonable choices. Many patients will require two or more of these drugs classes in order to facilitate more intensive BP reduction. With concomitant coronary disease, an approach to lower antianginal heart rate with a β-blocker or nondihydropyridine CCB could be used. In patients with diabetes and or renal disease, ACE inhibitors, angiotensin type 1 receptor blockers, or nondihydropyridine CCBs could be used alone or in combination.

Women should avoid the use of drugs such as ACE inhibitors and angiotensin type 1 receptor blockers in pregnancy because of their

Table 18-3
Considerations for Initial Therapy in African-American Patients

Pathophysiology	Desirable pharmacologic approach
High peripheral vascular resistance with associated reduction in cardiac output	Use a vasodilator (e.g., HCTZ, ACE inhibitor, CCB, ARB).
Salt sensitivity	Use natriuresis (HCTZ, ACE inhibitor, ARB, CCB).
Variable blood volume (perhaps greater in some patients relative to ↑ PVR)	Use natriuresis, diuresis (HCTZ; if creatinine >2.0, loop diuretic).

possible teratogenic effects. Similarly, CCBs may delay labor. Optimal choices would remain alphamethyldopa, hydralazine, or a β-blocker under these circumstances. In women with osteoporosis, HCTZ is the ideal agent because it antagonizes calciuria and facilitates bone mineralization *(10)*. Women note more pedal edema with CCBs and a cough with ACE inhibitors compared with men. These differences in side effects may be less apparent if lower doses of these medications are employed, particularly in concert with other medications. Despite underlying pathophysiologic differences between genders, there do not appear to be any specific differences in response rates to commonly used antihypertensive drugs.

CONSIDERATIONS FOR INITIAL THERAPY IN AFRICAN-AMERICAN PATIENTS (TABLE 3)

African-American hypertensive patients present at an earlier age and more commonly have greater degrees of BP elevation compared with their Caucasian counterparts *(11)*. They also develop target organ damage (TOD) sooner and have a greater proclivity for hypertensive renal insufficiency *(12)*. Because these patients are younger and have greater BP elevation, they frequently pose therapeutic dilemmas. How to avoid side effects yet provide needed BP reduction requires careful effort. Lower doses of two or more drugs are frequently necessary.

In African Americans diuretics and CCBs have been demonstrated to possess more robust antihypertensive properties in lower doses than other drugs *(13,14)*. These agents are preferable starting points to which could be added drugs that block the renin-angiotensin system in order

Table 18-4
Considerations for Initial Therapy in Obese Hypertensive Patients

Pathophysiology	*Desirable pharmacologic approach*
Hyperdynamic circulation	Reduce HR and sympathoadrenal outflow (β-blocker).
Increased PVR	Use vasodilation (e.g., HCTZ, ACE inhibitor, ARB, CCB).
Salt sensitivity	Use natriuresis (HCTZ, ACE inhibitor, ARB, CCB).
Expanded plasma volume	Use diuresis.

not only to potentiate reduction in BP but also reduce the likelihood of TOD, particularly to the heart and kidneys. Because African Americans frequently have elevated peripheral vascular resistance, BP salt sensitivity associated with a subtle increase in vascular volume, and more target organ disease, multiple drug therapy is of increased importance.

Because many African-American patients are also younger, it is even more necessary to explain fully the rationale behind treatment and to focus on therapeutic strategies that do not impair quality of life. This is another reason that lower doses of more drugs may be an ideal therapeutic strategy given younger age, greater risk for hypertensive vascular disease, and inherent salt sensitivity.

CONSIDERATIONS FOR INITIAL THERAPY IN OBESE HYPERTENSIVE PATIENTS

Obese hypertensive patients tend to have a hyperdynamic circulation, increased peripheral vascular resistance, expanded plasma volume, and greater sensitivity to the influence of dietary salt to raise BP *(15,16)*. Therapeutic strategies targeted to these specific abnormalities are desirable. A β-blocker may be helpful in diminishing sympathoadrenal outflow. Vasodilators such as HCTZ, ACE inhibitors, angiotensin type 1 receptor blockers, and CCBs are suitable for reducing peripheral vascular resistance. A thiazide diuretic, ACE inhibitor, angiotensin type 1 receptor blocker, or CCB may be helpful for facilitating natriuresis *(17,18)*. If expanded plasma volume is clinically present, a diuretic would be the ideal drug with which to start. Otherwise, the choice of a first agent could be any of the previously listed agents. More often

Table 18-5
Considerations for Initial Therapy in Patients with Heart Disease

Pathophysiology	Desirable pharmacologic approach
Angina	Reduce heart rate and use antianginal therapy (reduce HR 10–20% or to 60–65 bpm).
LVH	Reduce SBP (HCTZ, β-blocker, ACE inhibitor, CCB, ARB). Avoid nonspecific vasodilator or therapies that result in reflex ↑ HR.
Systolic dysfunction	Reduce afterload and use natriuresis (ACE inhibitor, HCTZ, ARB). Sympathetic inhibitor → β-blocker (carvedilol, others?).
Diastolic dysfunction	Improve myocardial compliance, reduce HR, avoid volume depletion (β-blocker, CCB, avoid loop diuretics).
MI	Reduce heart rate (β-blocker, ACE inhibitor if left ventricular dysfunction).

than not, multiple drug therapy will be required in order to facilitate BP reduction to levels <130/85 mmHg. This is frequently desirable in obese hypertensive patients simply because of their frequent comorbid risks and cardiovascular risk clustering. Drug therapies that are inherently metabolically neutral are ideal in this regard, such as the ACE inhibitor, angiotensin type 1 receptor blocker, CCB, or α-blocker.

CONSIDERATIONS FOR INITIAL THERAPY IN PATIENTS WITH HEART DISEASE

Control of heart rate is an important factor in patients with ischemic heart disease. The vast majority of coronary artery perfusion occurs during diastole. Hence, pharmacotherapy that increases heart rate could lower the threshold for an ischemic event, whereas pharmacotherapy that reduces heart rate can diminish that likelihood. For this reason, if concomitant antihypertensive and anti-ischemic therapy is required, a heart rate–lowering β-blocker or nondihydropyridine CCB would be ideal. If a hypertensive patient has had a recent MI, then a heart rate–lowering β-blocker should be employed.

In patients with left ventricular hypertrophy (LVH), it is important to note that intensive BP reduction is the most important factor for reducing LVH regardless of the pharmacotherapy employed. SBP reduction reduces left ventricular strain. Ideally, HCTZ, ACE inhibitors, angiotensin type 1 receptor blockers, and CCBs should be used. There may be some benefits for specific antagonism of the renin-angiotensin system in reducing LVH, as has been suggested in some clinical studies. If heart rate reduction were also necessary, either a β-blocker or a nondihydropyridine CCB blocker would be ideal. This is frequently necessary if there is associated diastolic dysfunction. To improve myocardial compliance, it is necessary to facilitate ventricular relaxation and reduce heart rate *(19,20)*; β-blockers and CCBs are well suited for this. It is important to avoid nonspecific vasodilator therapies that may result in a reflex increase in heart rate. This reflex response may incite myocardial hypertrophic changes and explain why drugs such as hydralazine and minoxidil have not been proven to be useful in reducing LVH despite their antihypertensive properties. Additionally, it is also necessary to avoid volume depletion, which can compromise preload to the heart and result in a reflex increase in heart rate. This is important to avoid in patients with LVH and diastolic dysfunction because it may impair cardiac output.

In patients with systolic dysfunction and an ejection fraction <30%, pharmacotherapy that offers afterload and preload reduction and natriuresis are ideal. Volume control may be necessary, but it is hazardous to cause volume depletion because this may precipitate hypotension and functional renal insufficiency and cause an abrupt drop in cardiac output. Thiazide diuretics are preferred, and only loop diuretics should be employed in the presence of recalcitrant edema or renal insufficiency (serum creatinine >2.0 mg/dL). ACE inhibitors are the ideal preload and afterload reducing agents. ACE inhibitors provide definite survival advantages in patients with systolic heart failure *(21)*. More recent data suggest that metoprolol and cavedilol may also provide morbidity and mortality benefits in conjunction with ACE inhibitor therapy *(22)*. This may be related to inhibition of the activity of the SNS. The angiotensin type 1 receptor blocker losartan also demonstrated a survival benefit in a short-term clinical study *(23)*.

CONSIDERATIONS FOR INITIAL THERAPY IN PATIENTS WITH RENAL DISEASE (TABLE 6)

Patients with renal disease frequently have increased blood volume and increased peripheral vascular resistance. Excess blood volume is

Table 18-6
Considerations for Initial Therapy in Patients with Renal Disease

Pathophysiology[a]	Desirable pharmacologic approach[a]
Increased blood volume (common in glomerular diseases)	Reduce blood volume (loop diuretic, avoid HCTZ if creatinine >2.0).
Decreased blood volume (common in tubular diseases)	Possibly use salt supplementation.
Increased peripheral vascular resistance	Use a vasodilator (ACE inhibitor, CCB, ARB, α-blocker, minoxidil).
Proteinuria	Reduce proteinuria (ACE inhibitor, ARB, NDCCB) (BP systolic ≤125 mmHg).
Diabetes with proteinuria	Control BP and glycemia (ACE inhibitor, NDCCB?, ARB?) (BP systolic ≤125 mmHg).

[a]All medications adjusted according to renal function. NDCCB, nondehydropyridine calcium channel blocker.

more common in glomerular diseases. Patients with primary renal tubular disorders may present with a salt-losing nephropathy and diminished blood volume. If there is an abnormality in blood volume, it should be corrected. Volume overload will more likely be responsive to a loop diuretic, particularly if the serum creatinine is >2.0 mg/dL. Vasodilator therapy is ideal in conjunction with diuretic therapy. ACE inhibitors, CCBs, angiotensin type 1 receptor blockers, α-blockers, and even nonspecific vasodilators such as hydralazine or minoxidil can be helpful.

Clinical trial data demonstrate the need for more intensive BP reduction particularly in patients with diabetes, proteinuria (>1 g/d), or those who are of African-American descent (24). An SBP of 125 mmHg or less is ideal. Consequently, most patients with hypertension and renal disease will require a minimum of three medications, if not more. Preferably, lower doses should be employed in order to avoid toxicity and particularly so with agents that are primarily excreted by the kidney.

In patients with more than 1 g of protein/d in the urine, whether associated with diabetes or not, more intensive BP reduction is required. There is evidence in clinical trials that ACE inhibitors, because of their effects of reducing both BP and proteinuria, may provide an advantage over other commonly used antihypertensive therapies in delaying progression of renal disease in patients with proteinuric nephropathy *(24)*. Angiotensin type 1 receptor blockers also appear to provide similar reductions in both BP and proteinuria as does the ACE inhibitor. However, long-term studies of these drugs to demonstrate similar renal protective effects have not been completed. However, these drugs, like the ACE inhibitors, remain excellent choices in patients with kidney disease. Nondihydropyridine CCBs also have additive antihypertensive and antiproteinuric effects with ACE inhibitors, and may be an ideal strategy in many patients *(25)*. It is also important to realize that reducing dietary salt intake potentiates both the antihypertensive and antiproteinuric properties of ACE inhibitors and nondihydropyridine CCBs and should be routinely employed as an adjunct therapy in all patients with renal disease.

CONCLUSION

The initial choice of the medication in the treatment of hypertension should always be in conjunction with efforts at behavioral modification including reduced dietary salt intake, cessation of smoking, reduced alcohol intake, reduced saturated fat intake, regular exercise, and obtainment of ideal body weight. There is no ideal first-choice agent. Demographic factors and comorbid issues must be assessed with the well-recognized need of more intensive BP reduction. It is also important to realize that the majority of patients will require two or more drugs in order to achieve the lower recommended level of BP now recognized as being beneficial in reducing morbidity and mortality. Lower doses of two or more drugs also provide an improved opportunity to reduce BP, utilize possible synergy between the agents, and reduce the likelihood of dose-dependent adverse events associated with higher doses of the individual monotherapies. Traditional strategies for controlling BP using single agents titrated to their full extent has not been shown to be practical or effective in controlling BP over prolonged periods. Consequently, new approaches need to be adopted. Using lower doses of more medications with the initial choice being directed toward identified pathophysiology contributing to hypertension and specific demographic variables and associated comorbid events may be the ideal long-term strategy.

REFERENCES

1. Burt VL, Cutler JA, Higgins M, et al. (1995) Trends in the prevalence, awareness, treatment, and control of hypertension in the adult US population: data from the health examination surveys, 1960 to 1991. *Hypertension* 26:60–69.
2. Joint National Committee on Prevention, Detection, Evaluation, and Treatment of High Blood Pressure (1997) The Sixth Report of the Joint National Committee on Prevention. *Arch Intern Med* 157:2413–2446.
3. Hansson L, Zanchetti A, Carruthers SG, et al. (1998) Effects of intensive blood pressure lowering and low-dose aspirin in patients with hypertension: principal results of the Hypertension Optimal Treatment (HOT) randomized trial. *Lancet* 351:1755–1762.
4. United Kingdom Prospective Diabetes Study Group (1998) Tight blood pressure control and risk of macrovascular and microvascular complications in type 2 diabetes: UKPDS 38. *BMJ* 317:703–712.
5. Applegate WB, Sowers JR (1996) Elevated systolic blood pressure: increased cardiovascular risk and rationale for treatment. *Am J Med* 101(Suppl. 3A):3S–9S.
6. Messerli FH (1986) Osler's maneuver, pseudohypertension, and true hypertension in the elderly. *Am J Med* 80:906–910.
7. Hanes DS, Weir MR, Sowers JR (1996) Gender considerations in hypertension, pathophysiology and treatment. *Am J Med* 101(Suppl. 3A):10S–21S.
8. Gueyffier F, Bouititie F, Boissel JP, et al., for the INDANA investigators (1997) Effect of antihypertensive drug treatment on cardiovascular outcomes in women and men: a meta-analysis of individual patient data from randomized, controlled trials. *Ann Intern Med* 126:761–767.
9. Douglas PS, Ginsburg GS (1996) The evaluation of chest pain in women. *N Engl J Med* 334:1311–1315.
10. Morton DJ, Barrett-Connor EL, Edelstein SL (1994) Thiazides and bone mineral density in elderly men and women. *Am J Epidemiol* 139:1107–1115.
11. Burt VL, Whelton P, Roccella EJ, et al. (1995) Prevalence of hypertension in the US adult population: results from the third National Health and Nutrition Examination Survey, 1988–1991. *Hypertension* 25:305–313.
12. Klag MJ, Whelton PK, Randall BL, Neaton JD, Brancati FL, Stamler J (1997) End-stage renal disease in African-American and white men: 16-year MRFIT findings. *JAMA* 277:1293–1298.
13. Weir MR, Chrysant SG, McCarron DA, et al. (1998) Influence of race and dietary salt on the antihypertensive efficacy of an angiotensin-converting enzyme inhibitor or a calcium channel antagonist in salt-sensitive hypertensives. *Hypertension* 31:1088–1096.
14. Saunders E, Weir MR, Kong BW, et al. (1995) A comparison of the efficacy and safety of a β-blocker, a calcium channel blocker, and a converting enzyme inhibitor in hypertensive patients. The Trandolapril Multicenter Study Group. *Hypertension* 26:124–130.
15. Bakris GL, Weir MR, Sowers JR (1996) Therapeutic challenges in the obese diabetic patient with hypertension. *Am J Med* 101(Suppl. 3A):33S–46S.
16. Messerli FH, Christie B, Decarvalho JGR, Aristimuno GG, Suarez D, Dreslinski GR, Frohlich ED (1981) Obesity and essential hypertension: hemodynamics, intravascular volume, sodium excretion and plasma renin activity. *Arch Intern Med* 141:81–89.

17. Romero JC, Raij L, Granger JP, et al. (1987) Multiple effects of calcium entry blockers on renal function in hypertension. *Hypertension* 10:140–151.
18. Redgrave J, Rabinowe S, Hollenberg NK, et al. (1985) Correction of abnormal renal blood flow response to angiotensin II by converting enzyme inhibition in essential hypertensives. *J Clin Invest* 75:1285–1290.
19. Bonow RO, Dilsizian V, Rosig DR, et al. (1985) Verapamil-induced improvement in left ventricular diastolic filling and increased exercise tolerance in patients with hypertrophic cardiomyopathy: short- and long-term effects. *Circulation* 72:853–864.
20. Cuocolo A, Sax FL, Brush JE, et al. (1990) Left ventricular hypertrophy and impaired diastolic filling in essential hypertension: diastolic mechanisms for systolic dysfunction during exercise. *Circulation* 81:978–986.
21. Garg R, Yusuf S, for the collaborative group on ACE inhibitor trials (1995) Overview of randomized trials of angiotensin-converting enzyme inhibitors on mortality and morbidity inpatients with heart failure. *JAMA* 273:1450–1456.
22. Packer M, Bristow MR, Cohn JN, et al., of the U.S. carvedilol heart failure study group (1996) The effect of carvedilol on morbidity and mortality in patients with chronic heart failure. *N Engl J Med* 334:1349–1355.
23. Pitt B, Segal R, Martinez FA, et al., for the ELITE study investigators (1997) Randomized trial of losartan versus captopril in patients over 65 with heart failure (Evaluation of Losartan in the Elderly Study, ELITE). *Lancet* 349:747–752.
24. Weir MR, Dworkin LD (1998) Antihypertensive drugs, dietary salt and renal protection: how long should you go, and with which therapy? *Am J Kid Dis* 31:1, 2.
25. Bakris GL, Weir MR, DeQuattro V, McMahon EF (1998) Effects of an ACE inhibitor/calcium antagonist combination on proteinuria in diabetic nephropathy. *Kidney Int* 54:1283–1289.

19 Managing an Inadequate Response to the First Agent

Changing Doses or Drugs, Adding Drugs

L. Michael Prisant, MD, FACC, FACP

CONTENTS

Less than 50% of patients respond to the initial choice of antihypertensive therapy. Some consideration should be given as to why the blood pressure did not achieve the intended goal to the selected medication. There are several approaches to managing an inadequate response to the first agent. These include changing the dose or the drug and adding drugs.

PRELIMINARY CONSIDERATIONS

Several questions should be asked when a patient has not responded adequately to initial antihypertensive drug therapy. Is the drug an appropriate drug for initial therapy? Is this an appropriate drug given the patient's demographics? Is the timing of blood pressure measurement for the drug's duration appropriate? Is the patient adherent to drug

From: *Hypertension Medicine*
Edited by: M. A. Weber © Humana Press Inc., Totowa, NJ

therapy? Is there a drug interaction that is preventing the hypotensive agent from being effective? Is the patient consuming an excess amount of sodium?

Inappropriate Initial Therapy

Some drugs are inappropriate for the initial therapy of hypertension. Direct vasodilators (e.g., hydralazine and minoxidil) are never used as initial antihypertensive therapy. Sympathetic activation and reflex tachycardia leads to rapid tolerance to these drugs by causing sodium and water retention. Peripheral-acting sympathetic drugs such as reserpine and α_2-stimulants (i.e., methyldopa, clonidine, guanabenz, guanfacine) may be initially effective, but volume-related pseudotolerance will develop. Finally, loop diuretics (i.e., bumetanide, ethacrynic acid, and furosemide) are inappropriate therapy for patients who have normal renal function because of their short duration of action; thiazide diuretics are more effective. By contrast, for patients who have abnormal renal function, loop diuretics are appropriate with abnormal renal function.

Demographics

Failure to take into account demographics may also explain the inadequate response to a first agent. In general, hypertension in African Americans is more responsive to monotherapy with the diuretics and calcium antagonists than to angiotensin-converting enzyme (ACE) inhibitors, angiotensin receptor blockers, and β-blockers. This observation only applies to group data and not individual patients. When a diuretic is added to the less effective drugs, there is no difference in the efficacy in African-Americans vs Caucasians. Gender and age do not alter drug responsiveness.

Drug Duration and Timing of BP Measurement

If there is a mismatch between the pharmacologic duration of the antihypertensive agent and the timing of BP measurement, there may be an apparent lack of drug effectiveness. This can be avoided by choosing drugs that are long-acting with at least 50% of peak effect remaining at the end of 24 h and being aware of the pharmacokinetics of the chosen drug.

Adherence

Poor adherence to antihypertensive therapy is an important factor for the low BP control rate of 27% in the United States *(1)*. However, patient adherence to a drug regimen may be difficult to assess. Clues to noncompliance are suggested by a lack of knowledge about the drugs or dosing, failure to keep appointments, evasive answers to direct questions concerning compliance, and complaints about cost or side effects *(2)*. To improve patient adherence to drug therapy, national guidelines recommend the following *(1):*

1. Communicate clearly with the patient.
2. Establish the goal of antihypertensive therapy.
3. Reduce BP gradually to minimize adverse effects.
4. Educate the patient about hypertension and involve him or her in the treatment.
5. Keep care inexpensive and simple, and integrate pill taking into routine activities of daily living.
6. Prescribe medications according to pharmacologic principles favoring long-acting formulations.
7. Stop unsuccessful therapy and try a different approach.

Noncompliance seems to be related to the costs of the drugs, level of education, regimen complexity, and side effects of the drug *(1)*.

Drug Interactions

Many drugs interfere with the efficacy of antihypertensive agents: corticosteroids, monoamine oxidase inhibitors, nonsteroidal anti-inflammatory drugs (NSAIDs), tricyclic antidepressants, oral contraceptives, and sympathomimetic medications (e.g., phenylephrine, phenylpropanolamine *(3)*. NSAIDs deserve special emphasis because they are so easily obtained as over-the-counter drugs. These drugs attenuate the antihypertensive effects of most antihypertensive drugs. I generally try acetaminophen, salsalate, or sulindac because these agents are less likely to cause sodium retention.

Excessive alcohol remains an important drug that is associated with higher BP levels. Ethanol may be an important secondary cause of hypertension. It may make the patient refractory to single or multiple drugs *(3)*. It also appears to independently cause hemorrhagic strokes even after its hypertensive effects are considered.

Sodium Excess

Although all patients do not necessarily benefit from sodium restriction, excess sodium intake may be responsible for an inadequate response to a drug *(3)*. Failure to restrict sodium intake may negate the effectiveness of ACE inhibitors and angiotensin receptor blockers; however, calcium antagonists may be more resistant to a high sodium intake. A simple approach is to check a 24-h urine sodium sample. Excretion of >120 meq of sodium in 24 h reflects a failure to restrict salt intake. Remember that 85% of sodium intake is added in the processing or preparation of food.

CHANGING THE DRUG DOSE

Once the causes of an inadequate response to therapy have been excluded, one is left with the possibility of increasing the dose of the drug (titration), changing drugs (substitution), or adding additional drugs (combination). When antihypertensive therapy is initiated with a single agent, begin with low doses and titrate the dose upward after 4–6 wk if BP is not controlled. Shorter intervals of titration can result in unnecessary additional medication and untoward symptoms.

A drug can be titrated to its highest recommended dose; however, dose-dependent side effects have the potential for limiting titration to the maximum dose *(4)*. For example, when going from a low dose to a medium dose of a dihydropyridine calcium antagonist, peripheral edema may develop. Lethargy sometimes occurs as the dose of β-blockers or α_2-stimulants is increased. Constipation and atrioventricular conduction time increase with higher doses of verapamil. The metabolic side effects of diuretics become more prominent with higher doses. Thus, with upward titration, one has to strike a balance between achieving BP control and increasing side effects.

CHANGING THE DRUG

There are two reasons for considering changing initial drug therapy. First, if a patient experiences side effects on a low or medium dose of a drug, it is reasonable to substitute another drug from a different class. Second, an incomplete antihypertensive response on a single drug at medium or higher dose may be a reason to try another drug *(5)*. Attempting to find a single drug to normalize BP by testing each drug class is referred to as sequential monotherapy. Although it is appealing to find a single drug that will attain goal BP, one could go through each class of first-line antihypertensive drugs and still not achieve BP control. The disadvantage of sequential monotherapy is a prolonged duration of multiple medication attempts. This has the potential for creating a loss of confidence in the physician and may result in the patient seeking another physician to manage his or her care.

Remember that only 27% of hypertension patients currently have their BP under control. Unless the patient has only marginally elevated BP, it is unlikely that BP control cannot be achieved by fully titrating a drug or substituting another drug.

ADDING DRUGS

Adding drugs or combination drug therapy should be considered for those patients who have an incomplete therapeutic response to an initial agent. Fixed-dose combination with low-dose diuretics is also considered appropriate initial drug therapy *(6,7)*. However, not all drugs may be used in combination. Adding an ACE inhibitor to a β-blocker, an α_2-stimulant to an α_1-blocker, or a β-blocker to an α_2-stimulant is not additive *(8)*. Also, it is not wise to combine a loop diuretic and a thiazide diuretic for patients who have normal renal function to avoid volume depletion and major electrolyte disturbances. Diuretics are additive to all agents including the second-line drugs, such as α_2-stimulants and reserpine. There continues to be controversy about whether diuretics and calcium antagonists are additive; however, several studies support their effectiveness in combination *(9,10)*. Figure 19-1 gives possible combinations of first-line drugs.

The main advantage of combining different drugs is potentiation of hypotensive effects. Fixed-dose combination products have the additional advantage of simplifying the dosing regimen, improving compliance, and lowering the dispensing cost *(11,12)*. The disadvantages of fixed-dose combination are the use of undesirable agents, the abandonment of monotherapy, the potential loss of dosing flexibility, and the inability to determine the cause of adverse reactions.

The combination of a diuretic with a β-blocker, an ACE inhibitor, or an angiotensin II receptor blocker overcomes the disadvantage of these agents for lower efficacy in African-Americans. If low-dose

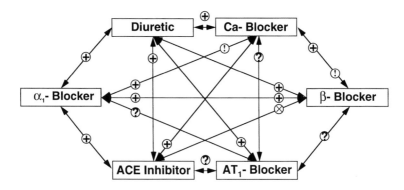

Fig. 19-1. Possible drug combinations of first-line agents. Ca-Blocker, calcium channel blocker; ACE, angiotensin-converting enzyme; AT_1, angiotensin receptor blocker; +, drugs are additive; !, caution is indicated in combining drugs; ?, inadequate data for using these drugs in combination; x, this combination is not additive. (Reprinted with permission from the October 1, 1997, issue of *American Family Physician,* Copyright © American Academy of Family Physicians. All rights reserved.)

diuretics (6.25 or 12.5 mg hydrochlorothiazide) are used in combination with a second agent, then there is a lower probability of metabolic side effects *(13).* The combination of a β-blocker and a low-dose diuretic has been shown to be as effective or more effective than other agents without increased side effects *(14).*

Recently, a new group of combination agents has become available in which an ACE inhibitor is combined with a calcium antagonist *(15–18).* This combination avoids a negative metabolic profile of full-dose diuretics and attenuates the dihydropyridine peripheral edema. Also the combination of verapamil and an ACE inhibitor may be associated with less proteinuria than an ACE inhibitor alone and may be proven to be renoprotective *(19).*

Under special circumstances, adding certain drugs may be useful not only in lowering BP but controlling other problems. Using a dihydropyridine calcium antagonist with a β-blocker is effective for angina. An ACE inhibitor and a diuretic are considered first-line therapy for hypertension with systolic heart failure; however, a combination of angiotensin receptor blocker and diuretic is a reasonable alternative. For the hypertensive patient with either hyperkinetic cardiomyopathy or hyperkinetic heart syndrome, cautiously using a β-blocker and a nondihydropyridine calcium antagonist (verapamil or diltiazem) is reasonable.

Failure to achieve BP control with the combination of three rational drugs, which includes a diuretic, requires applying the preliminary considerations discussed previously as well as the suspicion of a secondary cause of hypertension. If nonadherence is a concern, I ask the patient to bring his or her medications to the clinic in the morning, observe the patient swallowing the pills, and measure his or her blood pressure throughout the day and the following morning. Referral to a hypertension specialist may be needed.

CONCLUSION

When managing an inadequate BP response to an appropriate antihypertensive drug, the physician should consider the possible known causes for the lack of a response. If no cause is found, the physician is left with the possibility of changing the drug dose (titration), changing the drug (substitution), or adding drugs (combination) to the initial therapy. There is a high probability that adding drugs will be necessary. If combination therapy is chosen, there is the option of using rational multiple agents to achieve controlled BP or fixed-dose combination agents. Patients appreciate fixed combinations because it saves them money and simplifies their life. Achieving target BP control with the fewest side effects while reducing morbidity and mortality is the goal of therapy.

ACKNOWLEDGMENT

I gratefully appreciate the excellent secretarial support by Brooke Weir.

REFERENCES

1. The Sixth Report of the Joint National Committee on Prevention, Detection, Evaluation, and Treatment of High Blood Pressure (1997) *Arch Intern Med* 157(21):2413–2446.
2. Gifford RW, Tarazi RC (1978) Resistant hypertension: diagnosis and management. *Ann Intern Med* 88:661–665.
3. Setaro JF, Black HR (1992) Refractory hypertension. *N Engl J Med* 327:543–547.
4. Fagan TC (1994) Remembering the lessons of basic pharmacology. *Arch Intern Med* 154(13):1430, 1431.

5. Brunner HR, Ménard J, Waeber B, et al. (1990) Treating the individual patient: considerations on dose, sequential monotherapy and drug combinations. *J Hypertens* 8:3–11.

6. Prisant LM, Weir MR, Papademetriou V, et al. (1995) Low-dose drug combination therapy: an alternative first-line approach to hypertension treatment. *Am Heart J* 130(2):359–366.

7. Moser M, Prisant LM (1997) Low-dose combination therapy in hypertension. *Am Fam Phys* 56(5):1275–1282.

8. Sutton JM, Bagby SP (1992) Nontraditional combination pharmacotherapy of hypertension. *Cleve Clin J Med* 59:459–468.

9. Burris JF, Weir MR, Oparil S, Weber M, Cady WJ, Stewart WH (1990) An assessment of diltiazem and hydrochlorothiazide in hypertension: application of factorial trial design to a multicenter clinical trial of combination therapy. *JAMA* 263(11):1507–1512.

10. Prisant LM, Carr AA, Nelson EB, Winer N, Velasquez MT, Gonasun LM (1989) Isradipine vs propranolol in hydrochlorothiazide-treated hypertensives: a multicenter evaluation. *Arch Intern Med* 149(11):2453–2457.

11. Prisant LM, Doll NC (1997) Hypertension: the rediscovery of combination therapy. *Geriatrics* 52:28–38.

12. Oster JR, Epstein M (1987) Fixed-dose combination medications for the treatment of hypertension: a critical review. *J Clin Hypertens* 3(3):278–293.

13. Neutel JM (1996) Metabolic manifestations of low-dose diuretics. *Am J Med* 101(3A):71S–82S.

14. Prisant LM, Neutel JM, Papademetriou V, DeQuattro V, Hall WD, Weir MR (1998) Low-dose combination treatment for hypertension versus single-drug treatment—bisoprolol/hydrochlorothiazide versus amlodipine, enalapril, and placebo: combined analysis of comparative studies. *Am J Ther* 5:313–321.

15. Applegate WB, Cohen JD, Wolfson P, Davis A, Green S (1996) Evaluation of blood pressure response to the combination of enalapril (single dose) and diltiazem ER (four different doses) in systemic hypertension. *Am J Cardiol* 78(1):51–55.

16. DeQuattro V, Lee D, Messerli F (1997) Efficacy of combination therapy with trandolapril and verapamil SR in primary hypertension: a 4 × 4 trial design. The Trandolapril Study Group. *Clin Exp Hypertens* 19(3):373–387.

17. Frishman WH, Ram CV, McMahon FG, et al. (1995) Comparison of amlodipine and benazepril monotherapy to amlodipine plus benazepril in patients with systemic hypertension: a randomized, double-blind, placebo-controlled, parallel-group study. The Benazepril/Amlodipine Study Group. *J Clin Pharmacol* 35(11):1060–1066.

18. Morgan TO, Anderson A, Jones E (1997) Comparison and interaction of low dose felodipine and enalapril in the treatment of essential hypertension in elderly subjects. *Am J Hypertens* 5:238–243.

19. Epstein M, Bakris G (1996) Newer approaches to antihypertensive therapy: use of fixed-dose combination therapy. *Arch Intern Med* 156(17):1969–1978.

20 Rationale for Low-Dose Combination Therapy in Cardiovascular Risk Management

Joel M. Neutel, MD
and David H.G. Smith, MD

Data from recent studies have reconfirmed the importance of aggressive blood pressure (BP) control in protecting hypertensive patients from target organ damage. However, surveys performed to assess the adequacy of hypertension control in the United States have demonstrated that only one quarter of hypertensive patients are controlled at a level of 140/90 mmHg. If the currently recommended goals of 130/85 mmHg are applied, the controlled number is much less. Thus, our current approaches to the management of hypertension are failing in the most fundamental goals of treating hypertension. It is therefore crucial that we reassess the currently recommended approaches to hypertension to determine what changes need to be made in order to improve control rates.

From: *Hypertension Medicine*
Edited by: M. A. Weber © Humana Press Inc., Totowa, NJ

An exciting alternative to the stepped-care approach to the management of hypertension is the use of low-dose combination therapy as first-line treatment or much earlier in the course of treatment. The purpose of this chapter is to discuss reasons for poor control rates among hypertensive patients and to demonstrate that low-dose combination therapy may provide a solution to many of our current problems associated with inadequate BP control.

REASONS FOR INADEQUATE BP CONTROL

Data from the National Health and Nutritional Examination Survey (NHANES) have demonstrated that only 27.6% of hypertensive patients in the United States have adequate BP control when using 140/90 mmHg as the goal *(1)*. If the goal for treating hypertension is lowered to 130/85 or 120/80 mmHg, as recommended by the Joint National Committee, in their sixth report, particularly for patients with associated cardiovascular risk factors, the percentage of controlled patients is significantly lower—despite the availability of more than 70 drugs for the management of hypertension *(1)*. Thus, it is clear that the vast majority of hypertensive patients are inadequately controlled for hypertension. It is therefore not surprising that our treatment has not achieved the predicted reduction in coronary artery disease (CAD). There are several factors that contribute to inadequate BP control, which can be corrected by the selection of treatment in the management of hypertension.

Patient Compliance

Patient compliance remains the most important cause of inadequate BP control. Recent surveys have demonstrated that at 1 yr, <30% of patients are still taking their antihypertensive medication. Although there are multiple factors that influence patient compliance, including education, socioeconomic status, and cost, the factors that are most important are side effect profile and convenience of dosing schedule.

SIDE EFFECT PROFILE

The side effects associated with antihypertensive agents remain the most important cause of poor patient compliance. It is crucial and almost always possible to find drugs or drug combinations that can be well tolerated by individual patients, and a concerted effort should be made by physicians to find the "right drugs." It should be remembered that almost all the side effects associated with antihypertensive agents are dose dependent, and utilizing smaller doses of various drugs may alleviate the side effects. Also, various surveys have demonstrated that, for various reasons, patients frequently report side effects to their physicians (particularly impotence) but respond by stopping their medication or taking it irregularly. Patients should be specifically questioned to determine whether their drugs are well tolerated.

CONVENIENCE

It has now been clearly demonstrated that antihypertensive agents dosed twice a day are taken less readily than those dosed once a day *(2)*. Physicians should make a concerted effort to treat hypertensive patients with once-a-day agents. However, it is important to use drugs that have true 24-h efficacy. It has been shown that the risk of nonembolic stroke and of myocardial infarction peaks in the early morning, which coincides with the rapid surge of BP that occurs during arousal (typically between 6 AM and noon) *(3)*. It seems likely that adequate BP control during this period is very important. Antihypertensive drugs, taken once daily in the morning, that do not provide 24-h efficacy may leave patients uncontrolled at a time they are most at risk of developing cardiovascular events. The duration of action of a particular antihypertensive drug can be assessed in the clinical setting by measuring BP at trough of the drug. Patients should omit taking their medication on the morning of the clinic visit so that BP is measured at 24–26 h into the dosing interval. If BP is controlled, the drug is working for 24 h; if not, it should be substituted or dosed twice a day.

Difficulty in Achieving BP Control with Monotherapy

Studies have shown that with any class of antihypertensive drug, the response rate ranges between 30 and 60% *(4)*. The remaining patients will require two or more drugs to achieve BP control. This is not surprising, because hypertension is a multifactorial disease in which multiple systems interact and contribute to the increase in BP. Thus, agents interrupting only one of these systems will fail or will provide inadequate control in a significant proportion of patients. Combining two complementary agents, which interrupt two physiologic pathways, improves the response rates to 75–90% *(4)*. The remaining patients will require three or more drugs in order to achieve BP control.

Lower BP Goals

Data from the MRFIT *(5)* study and from the Hypertension Optional Treatment (HOT) *(6)* study have demonstrated that lower BPs are associated with fewer cardiovascular events. This finding is particularly true in diabetic hypertensive patients *(6,8–10)*. Furthermore, it has been shown in patients with renal insufficiency and proteinuria that the greatest renoprotective effects occur in patients with lower BPs. For these reasons, the Joint National Committee has now classified a BP of 140/90 mmHg as high normal and regards a BP of 130/85 mmHg as normal. In patients with CAD, a BP of 120/80 mmHg should be the goal and 125/75 mmHg in diabetic patients with diabetic nephropathy. Thus, if only 27.5% of hypertensive patients are controlled at a BP of 140/90 mmHg, these numbers are substantially lower at the new BP goals.

Reluctance to Titrate Antihypertensive Medication

In a study performed in 11,613 hypertensive patients in Europe, it was shown that only 37% were adequately controlled by their own physicians' standards for BP control *(7)*. Sixty-three percent were being treated and had inadequate control. When the study assessed what action was taken by physicians in response to the inadequate BP control, it was found that in 82% of cases no action was taken. In the remaining 18% the dose was increased, the drug was changed, or a second drug was added. The main reasons physicians gave for their reluctance to change the regimen were their concerns about increased side effects with increased dose; adverse metabolic consequences, higher cost, and patient resistance to polypharmacy and/or higher doses.

This would suggest that the best "shot" at controlling hypertension is the "first shot" because there seems to be resistance by physicians (in many cases for good reason) to titrate medication. In addition, patients are more likely to be compliant with their medication if they achieve adequate control early in the course of treatment (when they perceive that the drug is really working and achieving good BP control).

RATIONALE FOR THE STEPPED-CARE APPROACH

The stepped-care approach for the management of hypertension is currently the suggested and generally accepted approach to the management of hypertension *(11)*, despite the fact that 50% or more of patients will not be controlled by nonpharmacologic treatment or step 1 of the stepped-care approach *(4)*. The rationale for the stepped-care approach is based on the belief that compared with combination therapy, monotherapy is more convenient, better tolerated, less expensive, and allows more simple identification of side effects if they occur. These assumptions are not entirely correct.

First, several low-dose combination formulations (Table 20-1) are now available as a single pill taken once-a-day. This makes them no more or less convenient than monotherapy. Second, of the approx 50% of patients who respond to monotherapy, about 60–70% require the highest recommended dose to achieve control *(12)*. Because side effects are dose dependent, these patients are at a greater risk of developing side effects. Patients taking low-dose combination agents may have equal or better BP control with fewer side effects because complementary agents in combination will provide the desired BP reduction at lower doses (because of the additive effect on BP), but with few side effects because of the lower doses. Third, two-drug therapy may be the most expensive way of treating hypertension because it involves the cost of titration, two co-payments, two dispensing fees, and the cost of two drugs. High-dose monotherapy also may be expensive because of titration costs, laboratory testing, and visits for increased side effects, and if two tablets are required to achieve the desired dose, the cost is double (in most cases). Low-dose combination therapy requires less titration, one co-payment, one dispensing fee, and a drug price that is typically less than if the two components were used as separate agents. Also it should be remembered that the cost of treating hypertension is not simply the cost of the drug, but includes the cost of the office visits, laboratory testing, visits for adverse events, and costs associated with the consequences of poor compliance and the problems associated with unhappy patients. Finally, the side effects that are typically associated with our modern antihypertensive agents are usually drug specific. It is as simple to stop a combination agent drug because of an adverse event and use another drug as it is to stop monotherapy. Thus, the main reasons for advocating the stepped-care approach for the treatment of hypertension may not apply, particularly with the development of low-dose combination agents as an alternative form of treatment.

Table 20-1
Low-Dose Combination Drugs for Hypertension[a]

Drug class	Approved for initial therapy	Trade name
Beta Adrenergic blockers/diuretics		
Bisoprolol fumarate (2.5, 5, or 10 mg)/HCTZ	Bisoprolol (2.5 mg)/HCTZ (6.25 mg)	Ziac
ACE inhibitors/diuretics		
Benazepril hydrochloride (5, 10, or 20 mg)/HCTZ (6.25, 12.5 or 25 mg)		Lotensin HCT
Captopril (25 or 50 mg)/HCTZ (12.5 mg)	Captopril (25 mg)/HCTZ (15 mg)	Capozide
Enalapril maleate (5 or 10 mg)/ HCTZ (12.5 or 25 mg)		Vaseretic
Lisinopril (10 or 20 mg)/HCTZ (12.5 or 25 mg)		Prinzide, Zestoretic
Angiotensin II receptor antagonists/diuretics		
Losartan potassium (50 mg)/HCTZ (12.5 mg)		Hyzaar
Valsartan (80 mg)/HCTZ (12.5 mg)		Diovan/HCT
Calcium channel blockers/ACE inhibitors		
Amlodipine besylate (2.5 or 5 mg)/ benazepril hydrochloride (10 or 20 mg)		Irbesartan (150/ 300 mg) HCTZ (12.5 mg) Avelide Lotrel
Diltiazem hydrochloride (180 mg)/ enalapril maleate (5 mg)		Teczem
Felodipine (5 mg)/enalapril maleate (5 mg)		Lexxel
Verapamil hydrochloride (extended release) (180 or 240 mg)/ trandolapril (1, 2, or 4 mg)		Tarka

[a]HCTZ, hydrochlorothiazide; ACE, angiotensin-converting enzyme.

BENEFITS OF LOW-DOSE COMBINATION THERAPY

The concept behind low-dose combination therapy is to combine two complementary antihypertensive agents in order to achieve an additive effect on BP reduction, but have fewer side effects because

Table 20-2
Advantages of Low-Dose Combination Therapy

Effectively reduces BP
Effective over 24 h with once-a-day dosing
Higher response rates
Fewer side effects
Fewer adverse metabolic effects
Less expensive than multiple-drug therapy

Table 20-3
Mean Changes in Diastolic BP with a Low-Dose Combination
vs Its Components[a]

Treatment	Mean decrease in diastolic BP (mmHg)[b]	Response rate (%)
Placebo	—	15.8
Amlodipine (5 mg)	8.6	67.5
Benazepril (20 mg)	7.0	53.3
Amlodipine (5 mg)/benazepril (20 mg)	13.9	87.0

[a]Adapted from ref. 13.
[b]Placebo subtracted.

of the ability to achieve BP control with small doses of each of the agents (Table 20-2).

Efficacy

Studies using low-dose combination agents have demonstrated that the use of small doses of complementary antihypertensive agents results in additive reductions in BP frequently greater than larger doses of the component agents (12,13). The greater efficacy occurs as a result of interruption of two or more physiologic mechanisms contributing to the increase in BP, thus producing greater reduction in BP than could be achieved with a more complete block (utilizing high-dose monotherapy) of one pathway (Table 20-3). Furthermore, because studies have shown that physicians are reluctant to titrate antihypertensive medication, agents that produce BP control (with fewer side effects) early in the treatment of hypertension have a greater likelihood of achieving BP control.

Response Rate

Only about 50% of hypertensive patients will respond to any particular class of antihypertensive agent *(4)*. In some subgroups of hypertensive patients, response rates may be much lower than 50% with particular agents, e.g. ACE inhibitors in African-American patients. Adding a second complementary agent significantly increases response to >75% and may equalize rseponse across various patient subgroups, as is seen when adding a small dose of diuretic to an ACE inhibitor or an angiotensin receptor blocker *(4)* (Table 20-3). The use of lower-dose combination drugs thus frequently simplifies the treatment of hypertension in that all subgroups are more likely to respond to these agents.

Adverse Events

Low-dose combination therapy provides the ability to achieve both safety and efficacy. Frequently, the doses of monotherapy that can be used are limited by an associated increase in dose-dependent side effects that has an adverse effect on efficacy. However, the side effect profile of many of the newer low-dose combination agents is at least equal to and sometimes better than that seen with placebo. For example, the side effect profile of the combination of an ACE inhibitor and a calcium channel blocker (CCB) is frequently better than similar doses of each of the components used as monotherapy *(13)*. Peripheral edema is a common side effect of CCBs and occurs as a result of the vasodilatation produced by CCBs, which occurs predominantly in the arterial system, with very little effect on the venous system. These result in increased capillary hydrostatic pressure and the development of a capillary leak syndrome with resultant peripheral edema. ACE inhibitors cause vasodilatation in both the arterial and venous systems. Thus, adding an ACE inhibitor to a CCB results in venous dilatation. The venous dilatation decreases the pressure in the capillary bed, and the combination results in less edema than does a similar dose of the CCB given as monotherapy.

Interestingly, cough is the one antihypertensive-related side effect that is not dose dependent. Therefore, the incidence of cough is similar in the combination of an ACE inhibitor and a CCB as it is when an ACE inhibitor is given alone as monotherapy.

Duration of Action

Studies using ambulatory BP monitoring have demonstrated that low-dose combination agents maintain adequate BP control throughout the dosing interval if the correct agents are utilized in the combination. The reductions in BP will parallel each of the component agents throughout the dosing interval at a consistently lower BP.

Cost

The issue of cost is much more complex with combination therapy than initially realized. It is possible that, in some instances, low-dose combination therapy may be cheaper than high-dose monotherapy or multiple dose therapy.

Metabolic Effects

Several studies have shown that antihypertensive drug–related meta-bolic effects (e.g., hypokalemia, hypoglycemia, and increased low-density lipoprotein cholesterol) are also dose dependent. When given in small doses, drugs such as diuretics and β-blockers may have a slightly beneficial effect on glucose and lipid metabolism, even though at higher doses they may have negative effects on these metabolic parameters *(12)*.

COST OF TREATING HYPERTENSION

The true cost of treating hypertension is not simply the cost of the antihypertensive medication but, rather, includes the costs of office visits, laboratory tests, office visits to deal with adverse events, the cost of poor patient compliance, and the mortality and morbidity associated with inadequate BP control. Multiple office visits for titration to achieve adequate BP control are frequently associated with significant cost in the management of hypertension. Similarly, drugs that require multiple laboratory tests to assess electrolytes and metabolic parameters may also be associated with significant cost. The costs associated with high-dose monotherapy may frequently be higher than realized. The use of high-dose monotherapy have the costs associated with titration, the potential of side effects associated with high-dose therapy, and frequently the cost of two tablets or capsules, which will double the treatment cost. Multiple drug therapy is also quite expensive because it includes the cost of two agents, two copayments, and two dispensing fees, as well as the costs of titration. Low-dose combination therapy is frequently less expensive than multiple drug therapy, requires only one copayment and one dispensing fee, and often requires fewer office visits to achieve adequate BP control. Although it is generally believed that the cost of using combination therapy is higher than any other form of antihypertensive therapy, when carefully compared to other modalities of treatment, it frequently may be cheaper.

OUTCOME DATA

There are now several studies indicating that the protective effect of low-dose combination therapy may be greater than that seen with higher-dose monotherapy. This is probably related to the fact that lower BPs are achieved with combination therapy than with monotherapy, and that BPs have a significant protective effect in terms of cardiovascular outcome. The HOT study demonstrated that patients in the <80 mmHg group had a lower cardiovascular mortality than patients in the <90 mmHg group (6). This was particularly true in the diabetic patients. Perhaps the most important data derived from the HOT study is that when guided by a protocol, physicians can achieve adequate BP control. The second most important piece of information is that although adequate BP control was achieved, it was extremely difficult to achieve it with a single drug, and between two thirds and three quarters of the patients in this study required two or more antihypertensive drugs to achieve the target BP (6).

Data from the Fosinopril Versus Amlodipine Cardiovascular Events Randomized Trial (14) demonstrated that diabetic hypertensive patients treated with an ACE inhibitor had fewer cardiovascular events than those patients treated with a CCB. However, the patients treated with a combination of an ACE inhibitor and a CCB had fewer cardiovascular events than those treated with the ACE inhibitor alone. This finding would suggest that ACE inhibitors are indicated in diabetic hypertensive patients and that they have a protective effect. However, the combination of an ACE inhibitor and a CCB, probably as a result of the lower BPs, have an even greater protective effect on cardiovascular outcome than ACE inhibitors alone. In a study comparing the renoprotective effects of an ACE inhibitor as monotherapy to a combination of an

ACE inhibitor and a CCB in patients with diabetic nephropathy, it was shown that the ACE inhibitor as monotherapy had a protective effect on the kidney and reduced proteinuria, and that the combination of the ACE inhibitor and CCBs had an even greater renoprotective effect with greater reductions in proteinuria (15). This further reduction in proteinuria is also probably related to the great BP reduction seen in the patients with combination therapy.

There are thus multiple benefits to low dose combination therapy which may simplify the treatment of hypertension and provide greater blood pressure control.

LOW-DOSE COMBINATION DRUG ARMAMENTARIUM

There are multiple low-dose combination agents available for use in hypertensive patients, including complementary drugs. To achieve a first-line indication in the treatment of hypertension, low-dose combination agents have to demonstrate in studies that they are more effective in reducing BP than each of the components and that they have a side effect profile that is better than each of the component drugs. All available low-dose combination agents are more effective in reducing BP than each of their component agents. However, most of the available combination agents (with the exception of bisoprolol/HCTZ and captopril/HCTZ) have been given a second-line indication only because they have a side effect profile similar to one of their respective component agents even if they are better than the second component agent. For example, with a combination of an ACE inhibitor and a CCB, the combination generally has a side effect profile slightly better than that of the CCB because of a lower incidence of peripheral edema, but has a side effect profile similar to the ACE inhibitor (because cough is not a dose-dependent side effect) and, thus, has been given a second-line indication. Table 20-1 gives available low-dose combination agents. Low-dose combination drugs should be distinguished from "fixed dose" combination drugs, which combine two agents at each of their highest recommended doses in one tablet for convenience. This usually does not have the desired impact on the side effect profile because higher doses are included in these combinations. Low-dose combination drugs produce additive hypotensive effects, but because they comprise submaximum dose agents, the side effect profile is frequently much better than that seen with higher doses of monotherapy.

CONCLUSION

For many years, combination therapy was considered an option only late in the course of the management of hypertension. The current approach to the management of hypertension has clearly not been as effective as anticipated *(16,17)*. The anticipated reduction in the incidence of CAD among hypertensive patients has not been seen. Also, the control rates of hypertensive patients, as demonstrated by NHANES, are disturbingly low. For these reasons, it is important that alternative modalities for the treatment of hypertension be considered. Low-dose combination therapy provides a very attractive choice either for first-line treatment in hypertension or for earlier use in the course of treating hypertensive patients. In addition, it may provide a means of improving efficacy, increasing patient compliance, and perhaps improving control rates among hypertensive patients. And, improved control rates may result in greater reductions in CAD disease among hypertensive patients.

REFERENCES

1. Burt VI, Cutler JA, Higgins M (1995) Trends in the prevalence, awareness, treatment and control of hypertension in the US population data from the Health Examination Surveys, 1960 to 1991. *Hypertension* 26:60.
2. Sica DA (1994) Fixed dose combination antihypertensive drugs: do they have a role in rational therapy? *Drugs* 48:16.
3. Muller JE, Stone PH, Turi ZG (1985) Circadian variation in the frequency of onset of acute myocardial infarction. *N Engl J Med* 313:1315.
4. Chobanian AV (1987) Effects of beta blockers and other antihypertensive drugs on cardiovascular risk. *Am J Cardiol* 59:S1.
5. National High Blood Pressure Education Program Working Group (1983) *Arch Intern Med* 153:186–193.
6. Hansson L, Zanchetti A, Carruthers SG, et al. (1998) Effects of intensive blood pressure lowering and low-dose aspirin in patients with hypertension: principal results of the Hypertension Optimal Treatment (HOT) randomized trial. *Lancet* 351:1755–1762.
7. Taylor Nelson Healthcare, Epson Survey (1992) England: Copyright Cardiomonitor.
8. Marques-Vidal P, Tuomilehto J (1997) Hypertension awareness, treatment and control in the community: is the 'rule of halves' still valid? *J Hum Hypertens* 11:213–220.
9. Nieto FJ, Alonso J, Chambless LE, et al. (1995) Population awareness and control of hypertension and hypercholesterolemia. The Atherosclerosis Risk in Communities study. *Arch Intern Med* 155:667–684.
10. Flack JM, Neaton J, Grimm R Jr, et al. (1995) Blood pressure and mortality

among men with prior myocardial infarction. Multiple Risk Faction Intervention Trial Research Group. *Circulation* 92:2437–2445.

11. The sixth report of the Joint National Committee on Prevention, Detection, Evaluation and Treatment of High Blood Pressure (1997) *Arch Intern Med* 157:2413–2446.

12. Neutel JM, Rolf CN, Valentine SN, et al. (1996) Low dose combination therapy as first line treatment of mild-to-moderate hypertension: the efficacy and safety of bisoprolol/HCTZ versus amlodipine, enalapril and placebo. *Cardiovasc Rev Rep* 71:1.

13. Kuschnir E, Acuna E, Sevilla D (1996) Treatment of patients with essential hypertension: amlodipine 5mg/benazepril 20mg compared with amlodipine 5mg/benazepril 20mg and placebo. *Clin Ther* 18:6–12.

14. Tatti P, Pahor M, Byington RP, et al. (1998) Outcome results of the Fosinopril Versus Amlodipine Cardiovascular Events Randomized Trial (FACET) in patients with hypertension and NIDDM. *Diabetes Care* 21:597–603.

15. Fogari R, Zoppi A, Malanani GD, Lusardi P, Destro M, Corradi L (1997) Effects of amlodipine vs enalapril on microalbuminuria in hypertensive patients with type II diabetes. *Clin Drug Invest* 13(Suppl. 1):42–49.

16. MacMahon S, Petro R, Cutler J, et al. (1990) Blood pressure, stroke and coronary heart disease. Part I. Prolonged differences in blood pressure: prospective observational studies corrected for the regression dilutional bias. *Lancet* 335:765.

17. Stamler J, Stamler R, Neaton JD (1993) Blood pressure, systolic and diastolic and cardiovascular risks. US Population Data. *Arch Intern Med* 153:598.

21 How to Monitor Progress in Hypertensive Patients

Ehud Grossman, MD

Hypertension is a major risk factor for cardiovascular morbidity and mortality. The risk of cardiovascular morbidity and mortality is remarkably increased by the coexistence of hypertension with other risk factors. These are mainly diabetes mellitus, hypercholesterolemia, smoking, obesity, and positive family history. The existence of target organ damage (TOD) such as left ventricular hypertrophy (LVH), congestive heart failure (CHF), ischemic heart disease, stroke or transient ischemic attack, renal failure or proteinuria, peripheral vascular disease, and retinopathy also increases remarkably the risk of cardiovascular morbidity and mortality *(1,2)*. Lowering blood pressure (BP) reduces the risk of stroke by about 40% and the risk of coronary heart disease by about 20% *(3)*. Controlling additional risk factors may even increase the benefit obtained from lowering BP. Because hypertension is frequently associated with other risk factors, it is therefore important to

From: *Hypertension Medicine*
Edited by: M. A. Weber © Humana Press Inc., Totowa, NJ

identify and control all these risk factors as well. When a patient has elevated BP levels, repeated measurements will determine whether initial elevations persist and require prompt attention or have returned to normal and need only periodic surveillance (1).

CONFIRMATION OF HYPERTENSION AND DETERMINATION OF SEVERITY

Unless BP levels are extremely elevated (above 180/110 mmHg), a 1- to 3-mo period is allowed for confirming the existence and to define the severity of hypertension. During this period BP levels should be measured repeatedly in the clinic in a standardized fashion using equipment that meets certification criteria (4). Alternatively, 24-h ambulatory BP measurements, or self-administered BP measurements at home can be performed. While the patient is in the process of confirmation and determination of the severity of hypertension, lifestyle modifications should be encouraged. These include losing weight if the patient is overweight (body mass index > 25 kg/m^2), cessation of smoking, increasing the level of physical activity such as 30–45 min of brisk walking most days of the week, and moderating alcohol and dietary sodium intake. Additional dietary changes such as increasing potassium and calcium intake and other measures such as relaxation and biofeedback, meditation, and yoga may be tried.

Once the diagnosis of hypertension has been confirmed, an initial evaluation should be performed. The purpose of the evaluation is to exclude secondary hypertension, to assess the presence or absence of TOD, and to identify associated diseases and other cardiovascular risk factors. Important information can be obtained from medical history, physical examination, and laboratory tests. Medical history and physical examination should be directed mainly to answering specific questions (see Tables 21-1 and 21-2). Laboratory work-up should include urinalysis, complete blood cell count, blood chemistry (potassium, sodium, creatinine, fasting glucose, fasting triglycerides, total cholesterol, and high- and low-density lipoprotein cholesterol), and 12-lead electrocardiogram.

Optional tests include urine analysis for microalbumin, blood calcium, uric acid, glycated hemoglobin, limited echocardiography, and renal ultrasound. Additional diagnostic procedures may be indicated when the initial evaluation raises the suspicion of secondary hypertension, or when BP is resistant to treatment. When the diagnosis of

Table 21-1
Taking a Medical History of a Patient with Hypertension

Severity of Hypertension
  Duration and levels of elevated BP (when was the last time normal BP
  was measured)

Symptoms and factors suggesting secondary hypertension
  Muscle weakness (hypokalemia, hyperaldosteronism)
  Tachycardia, tremor, and perspiration (pheochromocytoma)
  Intermittent claudication (peripheral vascular disease, renal artery
    stenosis)
  Use of agents or chemicals that may raise BP or interfere with the
    effectiveness of antihypertensive drugs
  History of weight gain
  Snoring and day somnolence suggesting sleep apnea
  Dietary assessment including intake of sodium, alcohol, saturated fat,
    and caffeine
  Psychosocial and environmental factors

Associated risk factors
  Smoking, lack of physical activity, diabetes mellitus, hyperlipidemia
  Detailed family history (hypertension or premature cardiac disease,
    stroke, diabetes, dyslipidemia, renal disease, or pheochromocytoma)

Evidence of TOD
  History or symptoms of coronary heart disease, heart failure,
    cerebrovascular accident, peripheral vascular disease, renal disease

Data that may guide treatment
  Response and adverse effects of previous antihypertensive therapy
  Sexual function
  Prostatism

essential hypertension is confirmed, a decision should be made whether
to start antihypertensive medication or to continue with lifestyle modification. The decision should be based on BP levels, associated risk
factors, and TOD (Table 21-3). The management of hypertensive
patients should include, in addition to lowering BP, recommendations
to control other risk factors and to treat associated diseases. Close
monitoring to assess BP control, compliance, quality of life, possible
side effects or treatment complications, development of other risk factors, and TOD is mandatory.

Table 21-2
Important Parameters of Physical Examination

- Two or more BP measurements in the sitting and standing position on both arms
- Height, weight, and waist circumference
- Funduscopic examination for hypertensive retinopathy
- Examination of the neck for carotid bruits, distended veins, or an enlarged thyroid gland
- Examination of the heart for abnormalities in rate and rhythm, increased size, precordial heave, clicks, murmurs, and third and fourth heart sounds
- Examination of the lungs for evidence of CHF or bronchospasm
- Examination of the abdomen for bruits, enlarged kidneys, masses, and abnormal aortic pulsation
- Examination of the extremities for peripheral arterial pulsations, bruits, and edema
- Neurologic assessment

Table 21-3
Indications to Start Antihypertensive Drug Therapy

BP level (mmHg)	Associated conditions[a]
≥160/≥100	Regardless of risk factors, or TOD/CVD
140–159/90–99	DM, two risk factors, TOD/CVD
130–139/85–89	DM, CHF, renal failure

[a]TOD, target organ damage; CVD, cardiovascular disease; DM, diabetes mellitus; CHF, congestive heart failure.

FOLLOW-UP

Hypertension is a chronic risk factor that requires long-term treatment, and this should be explained to the patient when antihypertensive treatment is initiated. It is noteworthy that BP increases with age *(5)* and antihypertensive treatment lowers BP but does not prevent the increase over time (Fig. 21-1). Therefore, even if BP is well controlled and stable, it may become uncontrolled over time, and additional treatment may be required.

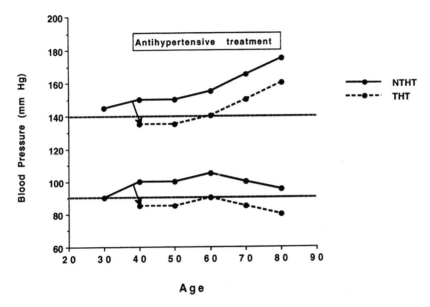

Fig. 21-1. Change in BP with age in nontreated (—•—) and treated (– –•– –) hypertensive patients. In both groups BP increased with age, but in treated patients, it was lower than in nontreated patients. Therefore, patients who are well controlled with a certain treatment may become uncontrolled after a few years.

MONITORING ADEQUACY OF BP CONTROL

Treatment should be targeted to lower BP levels to below 140/90 mmHg in all patients, and below 130/85 mmHg in diabetic patients and those with renal failure or CHF (1). With some agents, such as diuretics, angiotensin-converting enzyme (ACE) inhibitors, angiotensin receptor blockers (ARBs), and β-blockers, a decrease in BP may be expected only after 2–4 wk of treatment. Therefore, the first visit after initiating antihypertensive treatment should be scheduled 4 wk after beginning treatment. If the desired target BP is not achieved, increasing the dose or adding a second agent is recommended. Physicians and patients should understand that achieving BP control may take a few months. The risk of mild hypertension would take years to manifest itself, and therefore a few months of uncontrolled BP does not pose a major risk and should not alarm the patient. If BP is not well controlled with three agents after 3 mo of treatment, further evaluation should be done, or referral to a specialist is recommended, to exclude secondary hypertension.

Follow-up should include measurements of heart rate, BP, and body weight. Heart rate is important to guide antihypertensive treatment. A young patient with relative tachycardia is a good candidate for a β-blocker and a bad candidate for dihydropyridine calcium antagonists. Moreover, dose adjustment of β-blockers should be based on heart rate.

BP should be measured in the sitting position on the arm with the higher BP levels. In some patients, particularly older persons and those with orthostatic symptoms, monitoring should include BP measurement in the seated position and after standing quietly for 2–5 min.

BP control should be based on measurements obtained in the late afternoon or evening to monitor control across the day and in the early morning, at trough effect, to ensure adequate modulation of the surge BP after rising. This may pose a problem for many patients who are unable to come to the clinic early in the morning. To overcome this problem, self-measurements at home can be used. Self-measurements can be done with either validated electronic devices or aneroid sphygmomanometers with appropriate-sized cuffs that have proven to be accurate according to standard testing (6). Two or more readings separated by 2 min should be taken. If the first two readings differ by more than 5 mmHg, additional readings should be obtained. Self-measurements may also identify patients with white coat hypertension (which appears in about 20–25% of hypertensive patients). Indeed, levels reported by patients at home tend to be lower than the actual levels (7), but Sega et al. (8) showed that home measurements are reliable and close to values achieved by 24-h monitoring. To increase reliability of home measurements, one can use an electronic device that stores BP levels, heart rate, date, and hour. The devices should be checked periodically for accuracy against a mercury sphygmomanometer. There is no universally agreed-on upper limit of normal home BP, but readings of 135/85 mmHg or greater should be considered elevated (9). Despite the advantage of self-measurements at home, this method should not be recommended to patients who suffer from panic attacks or anxiety and stress, who may overuse the device and can become addicted to it. This phenomenon may by itself increase the level of panic and stress and thereby increase BP.

Once BP is stabilized at the desirable range, follow-up at 3- to 6-mo intervals with measuring BP once a month is generally appropriate. If an abrupt rise in BP occurs in a medicated patient whose BP was well controlled and stable over a long period, repeated BP measurement should be performed before any decision is made. Usually the increase in BP is transient and related to an underlying cause (Table 21-4).

Table 21-4
Causes of BP Increase in a Stable Medicated Patient

1. Stress or panic attacks
2. Withdrawal of antihypertensive treatment
3. Severe pain (low back pain, abdominal pain, tooth pain)
4. Use of drugs or agents that may increase BP or may blunt the action of antihypertensive agents (typically nonsteroidal anti-inflammatory drugs)
5. The appearance of secondary hypertension (e.g., renal failure)
6. Weight gain or excessive salt intake

Therefore, it is recommended not to change the antihypertensive regimen immediately, but to try to identify the cause and treat it accordingly. Only when no treatable underlying cause is identified should the antihypertensive regimen be modified.

MONITORING LABORATORY PARAMETERS

The frequency of laboratory follow-up depends on baseline laboratory values, associated medical problems and risk factors, and type of drugs used. If a diuretic, ACE inhibitor, or ARB is prescribed, laboratory evaluation, which includes glucose, blood urea nitrogen, creatinine, sodium, and potassium levels, should be recorded within 2 wk. Initiation of a β-blocker, an α-blocker, or a calcium antagonist does not require frequent laboratory evaluation. A slight increase in creatinine levels is expected after administration of an ACE inhibitor or ARB. An increase in serum creatinine of <1 mg/dL allows drug continuation, with close monitoring to confirm stabilization of renal function. A slight decrease in serum potassium and sodium is expected with diuretic use. However, these changes are mild and insignificant when a low dose of diuretic is used. Elderly women are more prone to develop diuretic-induced hyponatremia *(10),* and therefore this subgroup of patients should be closely monitored for serum electrolytes. Note that although most patients develop electrolyte disturbance during the first month of treatment, there are patients who may develop hyponatremia even after long-term use of diuretics especially when a precipitating event such as infection or diarrhea occurs. Any abnormal laboratory results observed in the first work-up, such as low levels of sodium or potassium or elevated creatinine, glucose, or lipid levels, require frequent repeated measurements until they are stabilized in the accepted range. Patients

Table 21-5
Medical History During Follow-up

1. Weakness (hypotension, bradycardia from β-blockers, orthostasis from treatment).
2. Dyspnea (signs of CHF, or exacerbation of asthma in patients using β-blockers)
3. Chest pain—anginal syndrome (signs of ischemic heart disease)
4. Intermittent claudication, Raynaud phenomenon (side effects of β-blockers or development of peripheral vascular disease).
5. Leg edema (side effect of calcium antagonists or signs of CHF)
6. Bowel movements (constipation as a side effect of calcium antagonists)
7. Nutritional status—assessing salt and caloric intake (to understand lack of response to treatment)
8. Headache (related to hypertension or side effect of drugs)
9. Sexual activity (side effect of drugs)
10. Nocturia (side effect of diuretic or calcium antagonists, may guide to change treatment to α-blocker)
11. Hypertrophy of the gums (side effect of calcium antagonists)
12. Cough (side effect of ACE inhibitors, or signs of CHF)
13. Insomnia (a marker of depression or side effect of β-blockers)
14. Snoring (a sign of sleep apnea)

with renal failure require close monitoring of renal function and electrolytes during treatment.

Laboratory work-up should also aim to identify worsening in other risk factors and TOD. Therefore, it is justified to measure fasting glucose, lipid profile, and urinalysis, including urine for microalbumin.

If the first laboratory results are normal, evaluation once a year is recommended. If glucose or lipid levels are slightly elevated, repeated evaluation is recommended.

MONITORING COMPLIANCE, ADVERSE EFFECTS, ASSOCIATED RISK FACTORS, AND TOD

Most patients should be seen within 1 to 2 mo after the initiation of therapy to confirm compliance and identify the presence of adverse effects. A targeted history and physical examination should be done to recognize adverse effects and TOD (Tables 21-5 and 21-6). The frequency of patient follow-up depends on the findings of the last visit.

Table 21-6
Physical Examination and Additional Tests During Follow-up

1. BP—sitting and standing BP on the arm where BP is higher.
2. Heart rate—to adjust the dose of β-blocker and to guide the treatment.
3. Weight—to identify weight gain that may explain uncontrolled BP and to encourage patients to lose weight.
4. Venous engorgement and other signs of CHF.
5. Bruits over the carotid arteries and abdomen.
6. Legs for peripheral pulses and edema.
7. Fundoscopy—once a year if the initial evaluation showed hypertensive retinopathy, or when there is doubt whether the patient is well controlled. If the initial evaluation is normal and the patient is well controlled, less frequent evaluation is required.
8. Electrocardiogram—once a year to detect arrhythmia or signs of LVH and strain.
9. Echocardiogram—should be done when a decision should be made whether or not to start medication, such as in patients with borderline hypertension, or when white coat hypertension is suspected. It should also be done for patients with LVH to observe reduction in ventricular mass (indirect evidence of the efficacy of treatment) and to assess left ventricular function in patients with dyspnea.

A patient whose BP is stable and who has no TOD or associated risk factors can be seen once in 6 mo. Any change in drug regimen requires an additional visit within 1 to 2 mo after the change.

Monitoring and treatment of associated risk factors is part of the management of hypertensive patients. About 10% of the patients with hypertension also have diabetes mellitus. These patients require close monitoring of their diabetes, and therefore frequent measurements of glucose levels, glycated hemoglobin, and microalbumin in the urine should be done. In addition, a more thorough physical examination including fundoscopy should be performed more frequently. Many hypertensive patients also suffer from hyperlipidemia. These patients also should be evaluated frequently until lipid profile is normal.

Encouraging a patient to lose weight, exercise, stop smoking, and avoid alcohol should be emphasized on each visit. The physician should, however, be aware that smoking withdrawal is associated with weight gain and trying to convince patients to do both at the same time will usually fail. Therefore, it may be better to encourage patients first to stop smoking and only after 6 mo to try a weight reduction program.

CONCLUSION

Adequate control of BP and additional risk factors requires prudent and cost-effective monitoring of the patients' progress. Following the recommendations given herein will improve and prolong the patient's life.

REFERENCES

1. The Sixth Report of the Joint National Committee on prevention, detection, evaluation, and treatment of high blood pressure (1997) *Arch Intern Med* 157:2413–2446.
2. Guidelines Subcommittee (1999) World Health Organization—International Society of Hypertension Guidelines for the Management of Hypertension. *J Hypertens* 17:151–183.
3. MacMahon S, Peto R, Cutler J, Collins R, Sorlie P, Neaton J, Abbott R, Godwin J, Dyer A, Stamler J (1990) Blood pressure, stroke, and coronary heart disease. Part 1. Prolonged differences in blood pressure: prospective observational studies corrected for the regression dilution bias. *Lancet* 335:765–774.
4. Perloff D, Grim C, Flack J, Frohlich ED, Hill M, McDonald M, Morgenstern BZ, for the Writing Group (1993) Human blood pressure determination by sphygmomanometry. *Circulation* (1996) 88:2460–2467.
5. Amad S, Rosenthal T, Grossman E (1996) The prevalence and awareness of hypertension among Israeli Arabs. *J Hum Hypertens* 10 (Suppl. 3):S31–S33.
6. White WB, Berson AS, Robbins C, Jamieson MJ, Prisant LM, Roccella E, Sheps SG (1993) National standard for measurement of resting and ambulatory blood pressures with automated sphygmomanometers. *Hypertension* 21:504–509.
7. Mengden T, Hernandez Medina RM, Beltran B, Alvarez E, Kraft K, Vetter H (1998) Reliability of reporting self-measured blood pressure values by hypertensive patients. *Am J Hypertens* 11:1413–1417.
8. Sega R, Cesana G, Milesi C, Grassi G, Zanchetti A, Mancia G (1997) Ambulatory and home blood pressure normality in the elderly: data from the PAMELA population. *Hypertension* 30:1–6.
9. Pickering T, for an American Society of Hypertension ad hoc panel (1995) Recommendations for the use of home (self) and ambulatory blood pressure monitoring. *Am J Hypertens* 9:1–11.
10. Sharabi Y, Ilan R, Cohen H, Kamari Y, Nadler M, Messerli FH, Grossman E (1999) Diuretic induced hyponatremia is a significant side effect mainly in elderly hypertensive women. *J Hypertens* 17(Suppl. 3):S58.

22 Problems of Treatment Compliance and Polypharmacy

Gordon S. Stokes, MD, FRACP
and Philip A. Atkin, BPHARM, PHD

CONTENTS

It is well recognized that it is the physician's responsibility to diagnose when hypertension is present, to rule out remediable causes, and to prescribe appropriate therapy. Less recognized is the physician's duty of care to ensure that therapy is effective in the long term. For this reason, careful instruction and follow-up of the patient is necessary to ensure that the therapy is taken as prescribed and produces a continued antihypertensive effect without troublesome side effects.

Ineffective treatment owing to poor patient compliance has been recognized as an important pharmacotherapeutic problem *(1)*, but little research has been conducted to evaluate the health consequences of noncompliance *(2)*. Several studies have shown that poor patient compliance can be serious enough to cause hospital admission *(3–6)*. Rates of noncompliance as high as 70% of patients omitting 40% of their doses during long-term treatment have been reported *(7–16)*. Observed rates may depend on many factors, including dosing schedules, patients'

From: *Hypertension Medicine*
Edited by: M. A. Weber © Humana Press Inc., Totowa, NJ

enthusiasm for the doctor, the disease being treated, and the patients' perception of the importance of the disease.

The difficulty with ensuring treatment compliance in hypertension is that this condition is usually symptomless. The patient must be made to realize that when hypertension-related symptoms develop, they mostly stem from cardiovascular damage and represent the end result of failure to apply effective antihypertensive therapy.

Even if a patient is sufficiently motivated at the time of initial diagnosis to adhere to the treatment program, compliance may tend to slip away with time. Contributing factors may be forgetfulness, a lack of positive reinforcement by medical attendants and family, a perception that the taking of any drugs is "unhealthy," the impact of side effects, or the expense of medication. All these factors should be taken into account prospectively, from the time of the initial physician visit. A routine to forestall their occurrence should be practiced at that time. At subsequent visits, further steps are needed to diagnose and deal with suspected noncompliance.

PREVENTION OF TREATMENT NONCOMPLIANCE

Motivation

Rational treatment requires a sensible contract of agreement between the prescriber and the patient. Any competent life insurance salesperson knows that he or she must engender a sense of need for the product in a prospective customer. Yet some physicians provide little incentive for patients to follow their medication schedules. It is essential for the hypertensive patient to understand the connection between antihypertensive treatment and prevention of cardiovascular morbidity and mortality. Some basic survey of the history of placebo-controlled antihypertensive treatment trials would be appropriate for many subjects. Others would be better served by simple analogies of cardiovascular disease, e.g., an analogy of excessive pressure in a hose pipe. In either case, the potential benefits of blood pressure (BP) reduction on mortality and morbidity from stroke and other cardiovascular disease should be discussed clearly in language the patient understands. However, it must be recognized that there is little point in prescribing at all for a patient who has impaired cognitive function or memory, unless specific steps are taken to ensure supervision by a third party in whom the prescriber has also engendered the sense of need.

The degree of motivation to access medications is an important determinant of compliance. Motivation may be diminished by various factors ranging from poor manual dexterity in handling medication packaging to lack of education issues or literacy. For example, there is evidence that difficulty with handling medication packaging can cause reduced compliance *(17)*. Also, therapeutic management of "silent" disease processes such as hypertension is prone to high levels of poor compliance among populations with low levels of literacy *(18)*.

Information

In accounting in general for patient noncompliance, there is no doubt that a measure of culpability exists on the part of those doctors and pharmacists who hold the responsibility for imparting appropriate information along with medication prescriptions. Lack of knowledge of drugs is an important reason that 30–50% of patients deviate from their prescribed regimens *(4,5,19)*.

The presentation of the case for therapy should be direct and personal. People are better able to identify with a message if it affects their own personal situation. This is exemplified by the common observation that patients often first seek attention for hypertension when a family member has a stroke. It is important to realize too that there are strong countercurrents against therapy that one must try to overcome.

Case story: A 15-yr-old boy was brought by his mother to a physician for consultation. He had severe hypertension for which no underlying cause had been found. The physician prescribed a regimen of drug therapy. The father, furious that his son had been told to take drugs, telephoned the physician and could not be satisfied that this approach was correct. He said that he himself had hypertension and was healthy although he had never taken any medications. The boy's mother then called to apologize for her husband's attitude and to report that her husband had experienced a heart attack and three strokes over several years.

Both the potential positive and negative effects of family members should always be considered. It is usually helpful to have the spouse or partner present when new therapy is prescribed. With the elderly, particularly those suffering short-term memory loss or having no partner, a younger family member may be willing to come to the office visit if requested. A medication schedule should be written at the time of the interview and given to the patient or consort. Information must be provided about the cost and possible side effects of the medication prescribed. Apart from the issue of medication compliance, it should be remembered that giving specific details of drug toxicity constitutes part of the legal responsibility of duty of care that the physician owes the patient.

Optimizing Therapy

Optimal antihypertensive therapy is that combination of lifestyle and pharmacotherapeutic measures that achieves target BP without side effects and with the minimal number of medication doses. Design factors in reaching this goal are the simplicity of the drug dosage regimen, the specificity of the agent or agents chosen, the careful profiling of patients, and the recognition of drug interactions.

Designing for simplicity of the chosen treatment regimen is an overriding principle in securing good compliance. The most significant factor associated with compliance is the daily dose frequency *(20–23)*. Whereas the level of compliance remains the same regardless of the number of drugs prescribed *(21,24)*, the relationship between compliance and daily dose frequency is a linear one *(23)*. Eisen et al. *(20)* have shown that as the daily prescribed dose frequency decreased from three times to once daily, medication compliance improved by 42% *(20)*. Again, although the demographic attributes of patients *(14,20)* and doctors *(16)* have occasionally been observed to contribute to differences in compliance, they do not abrogate the large effect on compliance of simplicity in the dose regimen *(20)*. Indeed, most investigations have found little consistent relationship among compliance and age, sex, education level, socioeconomic status, occupation, or marital status *(2,21)*.

Specificity in medication (i.e., targeting the pathophysiology) in the particular case of hypertension is often not attainable, because for most cases we do not yet know the precise operative pathogenetic mechanisms. However, for those cases in which we do know, choice of the appropriate medication can secure great benefits.

Case story: A 60-yr-old woman with presumed essential hypertension was receiving combination therapy with an angiotensin-converting enzyme (ACE) inhibitor, a low-dose diuretic, and a calcium antagonist. She developed a troublesome cough. BP was poorly controlled and treatment noncompliance was suspected. Substitution of an α-adrenoceptor antagonist for the ACE inhibitor resulted in disappearance of the cough, but BP control remained poor and the patient objected to the number of medications and their expense. A finding of frequent nocturia prompted aldosterone studies, and primary hyperaldosteronism was diagnosed. Treatment with a single daily dose of spironolactone and cessation of other therapy resulted in satisfactory control of BP without side effects.

Patient profiling utilizes detailed knowledge of the patient to select therapy that will not exaggerate, or may even benefit, any disorder coexisting with his or her hypertension. Thus, a patient with migraine and hypertension may be well suited to β-blocker therapy, but such a choice would be inappropriate for a patient with asthma.

Drug interactions are to be kept in mind particularly when building a stepwise regimen of antihypertensive therapy in patients with hypertension resistant to single-agent treatment. For instance, there is a positive interaction between ACE inhibitors and diuretics, and a potentially negative one between β-blockers and other negative inotropes such as diltiazem or verapamil.

DIAGNOSING AND DEALING WITH SUSPECTED TREATMENT NONCOMPLIANCE

At follow-up visits the patient should be asked to either produce or recite a list of the medications taken. The physician then checks this against his last notation. Discrepancies are often found. These may arise because of a misunderstanding between the physician and patient at the previous visit, or because the patient or another physician has altered the therapy.

If the patient cannot give a clear account of therapy taken, he or she should be asked to bring in all their packages of medication for identification; this tactic is also useful in detecting polypharmacy. Such measures should be routine because under ordinary conditions doctors find it difficult to predict their patients' compliance more accurately than can be arrived at by random chance *(25)*. Both direct measures of compliance (blood levels, urinalysis, tracer identification) and indirect measures (therapeutic or preventative outcome, dispensary data, tablet counts, patient interview) appear to have serious limitations. Establishing the degree of compliance through patients' self-reporting has repeatedly underestimated noncompliance when compared to objective methods *(26)*; patients often underreported but seldom exaggerated their noncompliance *(27)*. Nevertheless, sympathetic questioning of patients is essential. It has been noted that better results are sometimes obtained by interview alone than by the combined use of self-reporting and diagnostic biochemical tests *(13)*.

If noncompliance is detected or suspected, it is essential to determine the cause. The cause may be simply the occurrence of side effects that the patient may or may not have reported to the physician. Either dose reduction of the medication responsible or replacement by an antihypertensive agent of another class is indicated. Reducing the dose is applicable only if the particular side effect is known to be dose related. For example, the dependent edema caused by dihydropyridine calcium antagonists is dose dependent, whereas the cough caused by ACE inhibitors usually is not. Inability to adhere to the dose schedule is a frequent cause of noncompliance. In this case, simplification of the schedule may improve compliance, and this is best achieved by switching to once daily medications. Indeed, because drugs from most antihypertensive drug classes are suitable for once daily administration, there is usually no justification in keeping a patient on multiple-dose regimens. The exception perhaps is during the stage of initiation of therapy, when in some cases it is safer to titrate to the requisite dosage with a short-acting preparation before switching to an equivalent dose of a longer-acting congener.

POLYPHARMACY

Both at initial visits and at follow-up, it is important not to assume that the physician's prescribing role can be limited to the disorder with which the patient has presented. Although most physicians would carefully enquire about concurrent disease and medication, there is reluctance to become involved with "natural remedies," self-prescribed or given by an alternative medicine provider. However, polypharmacy is exponentially associated with an increased likelihood of adverse drug events, independently of the nature of the drugs taken and of the patient's underlying pathology *(28)*. Therefore, it is part of the physician's role to tailor therapy to minimize the number of compounds taken, including natural remedies.

This minimalist goal may seem at odds with comprehensive therapeutic plans developed for those with high cardiovascular risk. In a patient with severe hypertension, hyperlipidemia, diabetes mellitus, and hyperuricemia, it may be difficult to avoid the use of multiple medications. In helping to resolve this dilemma, appropriate application of lifestyle modifications is a key strategy.

Case story: An obese 50-yr-old man with treated but poorly controlled hypertension had his first attack of gouty podagra. He was found to have hyperuricemia, fasting hyperglycemia, and a raised serum total cholesterol concentration. After consultations with several specialists, his therapy included allopurinol, an oral antidiabetic agent, and a lipid-lowering agent, as well as his previous antihypertensive therapy with the diuretic chlorthalidone and a β-blocker. The patient objected to the number and expense of medications. In consultation with a nutritionist, dietary goals were set to reduce his high dietary intake of alcohol, saturated fats, and sugars. A graded exercise program was started. The patient agreed to adhere to these lifestyle modifications provided that his drug burden could be reduced. The diuretic and the β-blocker were stopped, and an α-adrenoceptor antagonist, doxazosin, was substituted. All other drugs were discontinued. Hyperlipidemia and hyperglycemia did not recur, despite only a 4% weight loss. There was mild continuing mild hyperuricemia, but no further attacks of gout occurred. BP control improved.

Comment: The benefits in this case were thought to occur because of withdrawing the adverse metabolic effects of the diuretic (hyperuricemia, hyperglycemia, and hyperlipidemia) and possibly of the β-blocker (hyperlipidemia), substituting a drug (doxazosin) with neutral or possibly beneficial effects on plasma lipids, and applying lifestyle measures.

CONCLUSION

Apart from the complexity of dosing schedules, evidence suggests that inadequate communication about drugs is one of the principal reasons that patients deviate from their prescribed regimens. For most patients with established hypertension, lifelong antihypertensive therapy is indicated and can obtain a vastly improved outcome in terms of cardiovascular morbidity and mortality. Treatment compliance is a key issue in securing this outcome: it greatly depend on the willingness of the physician and others in the health care team to inform and motivate patients so that they continue with their therapy.

REFERENCES

1. Bergman U, Wiholm BE (1981) Drug related problems causing admission to a medical clinic. *Eur J Clin Pharmacol* 20:193–200.

2. Stewart RB (1991) Noncompliance in the elderly: is there a cure? *Drugs Aging* 1:163–167.
3. Atkin PA, Finnegan TP, Ogle SJ, Talmont DM, Shenfield GM (1994) Prevalence of drug related admissions to a hospital geriatric service. *Aust J Ageing* 13:17–21.
4. Davidson F, Haghfelt T, Gram LF, Brosen K (1988) Adverse drug reactions and drug non-compliance as primary causes of admission to a cardiology department. *Eur J Clin Pharmacol* 34:83–86.
5. Levy M, Mermelstein L, Hemo D (1982) Medical admissions due to non-compliance with drug therapy. *Int J Clin Pharmacol Ther Toxicol* 20:600–604.
6. Col N, Fanale JE, Kronholm P (1990) The role of medication noncompliance and adverse drug reactions in hospitalizations of the elderly. *Arch Intern Med* 150:841–845.
7. Stewart RB, Cluff LE (1972) A review of medication errors and compliance in ambulant patients. *Clin Pharmacol Ther* 13:463–468.
8. Griffith S (1990) A review of the factors associated with patient compliance and the taking of prescribed medicines. *Br J Gen Pract* 40:114–116.
9. Pullar T, Birtwell AJ, Wiles PG, Hay A, Feely MP (1988) Use of a pharmacological indicator to compare compliance with tablets prescribed to be taken once, twice, or three times daily. *Clin Pharmacol Ther* 44:540–545.
10. Dirks JF, Kinsman RA (1982) Nondichotomous patterns of medication usage: the yes-no fallacy. *Clin Pharmacol Ther* 31:413–417.
11. Pullar T, Kumar S, Tindall H, Feely M (1989) Time to stop counting the tablets? *Clin Pharmacol Ther* 46:163–168.
12. Cramer JA, Mattson RH, Prevey ML, Scheyer RD, Ouellette VL (1989) How often is medication taken as prescribed? *JAMA* 261:3273–3277.
13. Wright EC (1993) Non-compliance—or how many aunts has Matlida? *Lancet* 342:909–913.
14. Holmberg L, Bottiger LE (1983) The drug consuming patient and his drugs. II. The drugs. *Acta Med Scand* 213:211–216.
15. Darnell JC, Murray MD, Martz BL, Weinberger M (1986) Medication use by ambulatory elderly: an in-home survey. *J Am Geriatr Soc* 34:1–4.
16. Spagnoli A, Ostino G, Borga AD, D'Ambrosio R, Maggiorotti P, Todisco E, Prattichizzo W, Pia L, Commelli M (1989) Drug compliance and unreported drugs in the elderly. *J Am Geriatr Soc* 37:619–624.
17. McIntire MS, Angle CR, Sathees K (1977) Safety packaging: what does the public think? *Am J Public Health* 67:169–171.
18. Branche GCJ, Batts JM, Dowdy VM, Field LS, Francis CK (1991) Improving compliance in an inner-city hypertensive patient population. *Am J Med* 91(1A):37S–41S.
19. Kessler DA (1991) Sounding board: communicating with patients about their medications. *N Engl J Med* 325:1650–1652.
20. Eisen SA, Miller DK, Woodward RS, Spitznagel E, Przybeck TR (1990) The effect of prescribed daily dose frequency on patient medication compliance. *Arch Intern Med* 150:1881–1884.
21. Gilmore JE, Temple DJ, Taggart HM (1989) A study of drug compliance, including the effect of a treatment card, in elderly patients following discharge home from hospital. *Aging Milano* 1:153–158.
22. Black DM, Brand RJ, Greenlick M, Hughes G, Smith J (1987) Compliance to treatment for hypertension in elderly patients: the SHEP pilot study. *J Gerontol* 43:552–557.

23. Bloom BS (1988) Direct medical costs of disease and gastrointestinal side effects during treatment for arthritis. *Am J Med* 84:20–24

24. Seki A (1989) Medication compliance in cardiovascular disease. *Nippon Ronen Igakkai Zashi* 26:115–119.

25. Caron HS, Roth HP (1968) Patients' cooperation with a medical regimen: difficulties in identifying the noncooperator. *JAMA* 203:922–926.

26. Bergman U, Wiholm BE (1981) Patient medication on admission to a medical ward. *Eur J Clin Pharmacol* 20:185–191.

27. Norell SE (1981) Accuracy of patient interviews and estimates by clinical staff in determining medication compliance. *Soc Sci Med* 15:57–61.

28. Smith JW, Seidel LG, Cluff LE (1966) Studies on the epidemiology of adverse drug reactions. *Ann Intern Med* 65:629–634.

23 Should Treatment Differ in African-American and Caucasian Patients?

W. Dallas Hall, MD, MACP

CONTENTS

Should treatment differ in African-Americans and Caucasians? The answer is yes and no. Yes, the choice of initial monotherapy should differ in hypertensive African-Americans and Caucasians. No, the selection and use of antihypertensive drugs should not differ once the patient needs the addition of a second or third drug. No, the compelling clinical indications for specific antihypertensive drug classes do not differ between African-Americans and Caucasians.

INITIAL CHOICE OF MONOTHERAPY

General

Diuretics or calcium channel blockers (CCBs) are the preferred initial therapy in hypertensive African-Americans *(1,2)*. This therapy is preferred because the blood pressure (BP)–lowering effect of monotherapy with β-blockers or angiotensin-converting enzyme (ACE)

From: *Hypertension Medicine*
Edited by: M. A. Weber © Humana Press Inc., Totowa, NJ

inhibitors is blunted, likely related to the lower renin profile of African-Americans. For example, the average BP reduction following monotherapy with ACE inhibitors in hypertensive African-Americans is only about 7.2/6.8 mmHg *(3)*, or a reduction in mean arterial pressure of about 10 mmHg *(4)*. Similar results apply to most of the β-blockers. Limited data on monotherapy with the angiotensin II receptor blockers also suggest blunting of the BP response in hypertensive African-Americans, similar to the ACE inhibitors.

Randomized Clinical Trials

A large randomized double-blind study in 345 hypertensive African-Americans documented a better ($p \leq 0.01$) response to a CCB (sustained-release verapamil, −13.3/−12.9 mmHg) than either a β-blocker (atenolol, −9.8/−10.2 mmHg) or an ACE inhibitor (captopril, −8.2/−9.6 mmHg) *(5)*. In this study, the response rate to captopril improved from 44 to 57% when a higher dose (100 mg daily) was given. The absolute reductions in BP, however, were 151.8/100.7 to 143.6/92.2 mmHg (i.e., −8.2/−8.5) with 50 mg daily of captopril, and 150.2/100.4 to 142/90.8 mmHg (i.e., −8.2/−9.6) with 100 mg daily of captopril. The difference in BP response between the low dose and higher dose was thus 0/1.1 mmHg. The improved response rate with higher doses of captopril was partly because the group began with an average diastolic BP (DBP) of 100.4 mmHg and response rate was defined as a DBP below 90 mmHg. A study of trandolapril (another ACE inhibitor) also reported a larger decrease in BP with the use of higher doses *(6)*. The response of 68 hypertensive African-Americans to 1-, 2-, or 4-mg daily doses of trandolapril was a decrease in sitting DBP by 2.0, 3.8, and 6.5 mmHg, respectively, which was less than in Caucasians (6.1, 8.1, and 8.9 mmHg, respectively) and not significantly different from placebo (3.2 mmHg). The blunted response of hypertensive African-Americans to monotherapy with an ACE inhibitor is improved by a low-salt diet *(7)*, perhaps reflecting both the increased salt sensitivity of African-Americans and the renin stimulation by the low-salt diet.

Diuretics in Elderly vs Young Hypertensive African-Americans

A comparison of six different antihypertensive monotherapies in 621 African-Americans and 654 Caucasian hypertensive patients was reported in a Veterans Affairs study *(8,9)*. Overall, the response rates (DBP <95 mmHg after 1 yr) to diltiazem (72%), clonidine (62%), hydrochlorothiazide (HCTZ) (55%), prazosin (54%), and captopril (50%) were better than placebo (31%). This study is sometimes quoted as showing that elderly African-Americans have a better response to diuretics (i.e., HCTZ, 12.5–50 mg daily) than younger African-Americans. However, the average age of the "elderly" ($\geq$60 yr) African-Americans was 66 yr and the average age of the "younger" (<60 yr) African-Americans was 50 yr. Moreover, BP was reduced from 157/100 to 141/88 (i.e., −16/−12 mmHg) in the older group and from 147/100 to 133/90 (i.e., −14/−10) in the younger group. These differences in response are of borderline clinical significance at best, and should not restrain the use of diuretics in young hypertensive African-Americans.

Initial Therapy with Low-Dose Combination Drugs

Low-dose combination therapy with a diuretic plus an ACE inhibitor or a β-blocker is also appropriate first-line antihypertensive therapy in African-Americans *(1)*. Such combinations can enhance the reduction in BP and also reduce adverse effects. These positive effects might decrease the number of office visits and the time needed to achieve control of BP, although this is unproven. Examples of low-dose combinations that are approved by the Food and Drug Administration for initial therapy include the combination of captopril and HCTZ *(10)* and the combination of bisoprolol and HCTZ *(11)*.

Current Prescribing Patterns

Despite the recommendations of the Sixth Joint National Committee on the Prevention, Detection, Evaluation and Treatment of High Blood Pressure (JNC VI) and the evidence that monotherapy with diuretics or CCBs reduces BP better than β-blockers or ACE inhibitors, a recent national survey of primary care physicians' use of antihypertensive therapy in African-Americans revealed initial selection of diuretics in only 43% of patients, CCBs in 23%, ACE inhibitors in 20%, and β-blockers in 9% *(12)*.

TWO- AND THREE-DRUG THERAPY

General

The issue regarding which drug class to choose as initial monotherapy in hypertensive African-Americans is relatively moot because the

Table 23-1
JNC VI Recommended Goals of Hypertension Therapy[a]

Condition	SBP	DBP
Hypertension (HBP)[b]	<140	<90
Isolated systolic HBP	<140	—
Diabetes mellitus	<130	<85
Renal failure	<130	<85
Proteinuria > 1 g/d	<125	<75

[a]Reprinted with permission from the July 1999 issue of *American Family Physician*. Copyright © American Academy of Family Physicians.
[b]HBP, high blood pressure.

Table 23-2
Number of Drugs Required to Achieve Control of BP

Clinical trial[a]	African-Americans (%)	Target BP (mmHg)	Baseline control (%)	Follow-up control (%)	Number of HBP drugs
AASK (13)	100	<140/<90	24	81	3.23
HOT (14)	<10	DBP <80	0	57	approx 1.6
Diabetics					
UKPDS (15)	8	<150/<85	0	56	≥3.0 (in 29%)
NIDDM (16)	54	<130/<85	0	?	4.2

[a]AASK, African-American Study of Kidney Disease and Hypertension; HBP, high blood pressure; HOT, Hypertension Optimal Treatment study; UKPDS, United Kingdom Prospective Diabetes Study; NIDDM, noninsulin-dependent diabetes mellitus study.

majority of hypertensive African-Americans will require two or more drugs to achieve the new goals for systolic blood pressure (SBP) and DBP. Table 23-1 provides a summary of the BP goals recommended by JNC VI. Table 23-2 shows that the average number of drugs needed to reach goal BP can range from 1.6 to 3.2 in nondiabetic hypertensive patients *(13,14)*. In diabetic hypertensive patients, a recent United Kingdom study (8% African-Americans) reported that 29% required three or more drugs to reduce BP to <150/85 mmHg *(15)*. Bakris *(16)* reported an average use of 4.2 drugs to achieve a BP reduction to <130/85 mmHg in a biracial group of diabetics.

If not chosen initially, low-dose diuretics (e.g., 12.5–25 mg of HCTZ daily) are usually necessary as second-line therapy in hypertensive

Table 23-3
Morisky Scale for Medication Adherence *(20)*

1. Do you ever forget to take your medicine?
2. Are you careless at times about taking your medicine?
3. When you feel better, do you sometimes stop taking your medicine?
4. Sometimes if you feel worse when you take the medicine, do you stop taking it?

African-Americans. Whenever a diuretic is used in combination with an α-blocker, a β-blocker, an ACE inhibitor, or an angiotensin II receptor blocker, there is no difference in the BP-lowering effect in African-Americans and Caucasians *(17,18)*. In other words, racial differences in the BP response to monotherapy are abolished by the use of a diuretic.

Managing the Patient with Uncontrolled BP

BP is very difficult to control in some hypertensive African-Americans *(19)*. The two most common reasons are nonadherence to medications and an often occult, very high dietary salt intake. Nonadherence can be suspected by one or more "yes" answers to the simple four-item Morisky scale (*see* Table 23-3) *(20)*. An extreme dietary salt intake can be suspected if a 24-hr urinary sodium excretion level is 200–400 meq/d. Control of BP will not be achieved if the patient continues not to adhere to medications or consumes a high-salt diet.

In a medication-adherent patient, the most common cause of refractory hypertension is inadequate diuretic therapy *(21)*. Clinical management may require increasing the dose of HCTZ (e.g., from 12.5 to 25–50 mg daily), switching a thiazide-like diuretic to a loop diuretic if the serum creatinine level exceeds 1.5–2 mg/dL (133–177 μmol/L), or switching a once daily dose of furosemide to a twice daily schedule (i.e., 40 mg daily to 40 mg twice daily) or to a longer-acting loop diuretic (e.g., torsemide, 5–10 mg daily).

Compliant hypertensive African-Americans with true resistant hypertension should have screening tests for secondary causes (*see* Chapter 13), especially sleep apnea. In the absence of a secondary cause, additional therapy to block the sympathetic nervous system (e.g., a central α-agonist such as clonidine or a peripheral α-antagonist such as doxazosin) is useful in some patients. Direct vasodilators (hydralazine, then minoxidil) can also improve BP and are useful in those with heart rates below 80–90 beats/min. Referral to a hypertension specialist is indicated for positive screening tests for secondary causes or persistently elevated BP despite these therapies (*see* Chapter 41).

COMPELLING CLINICAL INDICATIONS

General

JNC VI *(1)* identified four compelling clinical indications for the use of specific antihypertensive drug classes (if not contraindicated):

1. Acute myocardial infarction (MI)—Use β-blockers; use ACE inhibitors for an ejection fraction <35–40%.
2. Systolic heart failure—Use ACE inhibitors and diuretics.
3. Type 1 diabetes with proteinuria—Use ACE inhibitors.
4. Isolated systolic hypertension—Use diuretics (preferred) or long-acting dihydropyridine CCBs.

These indications do not differ in African-Americans and Caucasians.

Use of β-Blockers After Acute MI

β-Blockers are underused in patients with acute MI. For example, Soumeral et al. *(22)* reported that during 1987–1991, β-blockers were prescribed for only 21% of 3737 elderly survivors of acute MI in New Jersey. In a large Medicare database, Gottlieb et al. *(23)* found that in 1994–1995, the use of β-blockers at the time of discharge after an acute MI was only 35% in Caucasians and 32% in African-Americans. By 1997, the physician self-reported use of β-blockers post-MI had risen to 66% *(12)*, but self-reported choices can differ considerably from actual prescribing practice. There are still far too many post-MI patients who do not receive the proven benefit of β-blockers in this setting, even without contraindications for their use.

Use of ACE Inhibitors for Systolic Heart Failure

The Studies of Left Ventricular Dysfunction found that the mortality from symptomatic or asymptomatic left ventricular dysfunction was even higher in African-Americans (men or women) than in Caucasians *(24)*. In African-Americans, a 25–36% excess risk of death remained after adjustment for age, severity or cause of the heart failure, coexisting conditions, and use of medications. The benefit of ACE inhibitor therapy for heart failure is proven, yet ACE inhibitors are underprescribed *(25)*. An analysis of 1529 office visits (1989–1994) for congestive heart failure revealed the use of ACE inhibitors by only 27% of Caucasians and 21% of African-Americans *(26)*. In 1997, 82% of primary care physicians self-reported the use of ACE inhibitors in this setting *(12)*. This study, however, did not give these results separately for African-American and Caucasian patients.

There is no scientific reason for the lower use of either β-blockers post-MI or ACE inhibitors for heart failure in African-Americans, especially since the benefits of these drugs on survival derive from many mechanisms in addition to their effects on BP.

GOAL BP

Table 23-1 provides a summary of JNC VI recommendations for the level to which SBP and DBP should be reduced. The 1991–1994 Third National Health and Nutrition Examination Survey data, however, indicate that SBP <140 and DBP <90 mmHg are present in only 27% of all adult hypertensive patients in the United States and in only 49% of those receiving treatment *(1)*. More recent analyses suggest that control of SBP to <140 mmHg is only half as likely as is control of DBP to <90 mmHg *(27)*. How bad these control rates would be if the specific new lower goal BPs for diabetes and so on were used in the analyses is unknown.

There are no large-scale data sets to suggest that the goal BP levels should differ in African-Americans and Caucasians. The broad challenge is to attain successfully the stated goal BP in all ethnic groups. This will often require special attention to medication adherence, compliance to lifestyle modifications, and use of multiple-drug therapy.

REFERENCES

1. Joint National Committee on Prevention, Detection, Evaluation and Treatment of High Blood Pressure (JNC VI) (1997) The Sixth Report of the Joint National Committee on Prevention, Detection, Evaluation, and Treatment of High Blood Pressure. *Arch Intern Med* 27:2413–2446.
2. Hall WD (1999) A rational approach to the treatment of hypertension in special populations. *Am Fam Physician* 60:156–162.
3. Hall WD, Israili ZI (1995) The use of ACE inhibitors in blacks and whites. In

Schacter M, ed. *ACE Inhibitors: Current Use and Future Prospects,* London: Martin Dunitz pp. 123–143.

4. Jamerson K (1998) Calcium antagonists in African-American patients. *Ethn Dis* 8:120–123.

5. Saunders E, Weir MR, Kong BW, et al. (1990) A comparison of the efficacy and safety of a β-blocker, a calcium channel blocker, and a converting enzyme inhibitor in hypertensive blacks. *Arch Intern Med* 150:1707–1713.

6. Weir MR, Gray JM, Paster R, et al. (1995) Differing mechanisms of action of angiotensin-converting enzyme inhibition in black and white hypertensive patients. *Hypertension* 25:124–130.

7. Weir MR, Chrysant SG, McCarron DA, et al. (1998) Influence of race and dietary salt on the antihypertensive efficacy of an angiotensin-converting enzyme inhibitor or a calcium channel antagonist in salt-sensitive hypertensives. *Hypertension* 31:1088–1096.

8. Materson BJ, Reda DJ, Cushman WC, et al. (1993) Single-drug therapy for hypertension in men: a comparison of six antihypertensive agents with placebo. *N Engl J Med* 328:914–921.

9. Materson BJ, Reda DJ, Cushman WC, et al. (1995) Department of Veterans Affairs single-drug therapy of hypertension study: revised figures and new data. *Am J Hypertens* 8:189–192.

10. Katz LA, Cobbol C (1988) Treating black hypertensives with Capozide. *Am J Hypertens* 1(Suppl.): 224S–226S.

11. Prisant LM, Neutel JM, Ferdinand K, et al. (1999) Low-dose combination therapy as first-line antihypertensive treatment for blacks and nonblacks. *J Natl Med Assoc* 91:40–48.

12. Mehta SS, Wilcox CS, Schulman KA (1999) Treatment of hypertension in patients with comorbidities. *Am J Hypertens* 12:333–340.

13. Wright JT Jr (1999) VA First Annual Hypertension Conference. *Improvement in the Management of Hypertension in 2000 and Beyond: Challenges and Opportunities.* Washington, DC.

14. Hansson L, Zanchetti A (1997) The Hypertension Optimal Treatment (HOT) study: 24-month data on blood pressure and tolerability. *Blood Press* 6:313–317.

15. UK Prospective Diabetes Study Group (1998) Tight blood pressure control and risk of macrovascular and microvascular complications in type 2 diabetes. *BMJ* 317:703–713.

16. Bakris GL (1999) Renal disease progression. *Semin Hypertens Management* 2(1):12–15.

17. Veterans Administration Cooperative Study Group on Antihypertensive Agents (1982) Comparison of propranolol and hydrochlorothiazide for the treatment of hypertension. I. Results on short-term titration with emphasis on racial differences in response. *JAMA* 248:1996–2003.

18. Veterans Administration Cooperative Study Group on Antihypertensive Agents (1982) Racial differences in response to low-dose captopril are abolished by the addition of hydrochlorothiazide. *Br J Clin Pharmacol* 14(Suppl. 2):97S–101S.

19. Oparil S, Calhoun DA (1998) Managing the patient with hard-to-control hypertension. *Am Fam Physician* 57:1007–1013.

20. Morisky DE, Green LW, Levine DM (1986) Concurrent and predictive validity of a self-reported measure of medication adherence. *Med Care* 24:67–74.

21. Graves JW, Bloomfield RL, Buckalew VM Jr (1989) Plasma volume in resistant hypertension: guide to pathophysiology and therapy. *Am J Med Sci* 298:361–365.

22. Soumeral SB, McLaughlin TJ, Spiegelman D, et al. (1997) Adverse outcomes of underuse of β-blockers in elderly survivors of acute myocardial infarction. *JAMA* 277:115–121.

23. Gottlieb SS, McCarter RJ, Vogel RA (1998) Effect of beta-blockade on mortality among high-risk and low-risk patients after myocardial infarction. *N Engl J Med* 339:489–497.

24. Dries DL, Exner DV, Gersh BJ, et al. (1999) Racial differences in the outcome of left ventricular dysfunction. *N Engl J Med* 340:609–616.

25. Smith NL, Psaty BM, Pitt B, et al. (1998) Temporal patterns in the medical treatment of congestive heart failure with angiotensin-converting enzyme inhibitors in older adults, 1989 through 1995. *Arch Intern Med* 158:1074–1080.

26. Stafford RS, Saglam D, Blumenthal D (1997) National patterns of angiotensin-converting enzyme inhibitor use in congestive heart failure. *Arch Intern Med* 157:2460–2464.

27. Lapuerta P, L'Italien GJ (1999) Awareness, treatment, and control of systolic blood pressure in the United States. *Am J Hypertens* 12(4, pt. 2):92A (abstract).

24 Measuring the Benefits of Antihypertensive Treatment

Michael A. Weber, MD

Not only physicians and scientists, but also governmental agencies and health insurers are finding it important to use objective measurements of the benefits and cost-effectiveness of antihypertensive treatment. These outcomes can be classified as short-, intermediate-, and long-term. The short-term outcomes are most relevant to the practitioner and include such measures as BP control, laboratory changes, and quality of life. By contrast, the long-term outcomes, typically measured in randomized clinical trials, are of particular interest to policy makers and guidelines writers and focus on whether treatments affect survival and the incidence of major cardiovascular events. Intermediate outcomes, usually measurable within months of starting treatment, deal with such clinical surrogates as treatment-induced changes in left ventricular structure, arterial compliance, and renal function. No longer are the traditional short-term outcomes adequate to describe a new drug; hypertension specialists, formulary committees, health care economists, and even regulatory agencies now expect sponsors to plan studies that define a drug's full range of outcomes. This chapter discusses some of the criteria for these outcome measures.

From: *Hypertension Medicine*
Edited by: M. A. Weber © Humana Press Inc., Totowa, NJ

Although awareness of hypertension is greater than it was 20 yr ago, national surveys, such as the National Health and Nutrition Examination Survey, indicate that hypertension is still not adequately controlled (1). It is estimated that less than one quarter of hypertensive patients are controlled at a target blood pressure (BP) of 140/90 mmHg. Although intensive management of hypertension reduces the incidence of stroke and heart failure, coronary events are still the most common result of hypertension. Hypertension-related morbidity and mortality will not decrease until changes are made in treatment protocols, and these changes must be based on quantifiable outcome measures.

The Sixth Joint National Committee on the Prevention, Detection, Evaluation and Treatment of High Blood Pressure (JNC VI) identifies short-, intermediate-, and long-term outcomes for the evaluation of antihypertensive therapy (2). Short-term outcomes, such as BP levels, are commonly measured at the initiation of antihypertensive therapy. Both short- and intermediate-term outcomes are used to assess how successfully hypertension therapy controls BP and prevents end-organ damage. Long-term outcomes assess the success of hypertension treatment in the prevention of coronary disease, heart failure, stroke, renal failure, and mortality over many years.

Because the ultimate goal of treating hypertension is prevention of long-term effects, one can make a strong argument for including long-term outcomes in hypertension management protocols. However, long-term outcomes generally take several years and huge expenditure to document, and therefore the cost-effectiveness of gathering these data vs their potential health benefits becomes a separate, measurable outcome.

SHORT-TERM OUTCOMES

Short-term outcomes, e.g., BP levels, treatment compliance, clinical chemistries, and side effects, assess the initial effects of therapy. Table 24-1 provides a complete list of short-term outcomes and how they are measured.

Short-term outcomes are generally quantified in numerical values. Recent data from studies such as the Hypertension Optimum Treatment (HOT) trial have shown that clinical events occur less frequently in patients whose diastolic blood pressure (DBP) levels are in the low 80s, compared with patients whose DBP levels are in the upper 80s (3). In addition, reducing BP levels to <125/75 mmHg appears to

Table 24-1
Short-Term Outcome Measures

Outcome	How outcome was measured

Blood pressure
  Office
  Indices of 24-h efficacy
	Numerical values (direct measure)

Symptomatic side effects	Present/absent Mild/moderate/severe on analog scale

Quality of life
  Patients
  Perception of spouses or others
	Numerical values

Compliance with treatment
  Drug utilization, self-reported
  Timely prescription refills
  Adherence to clinical appointments
	Yes/no
	Percentage achievement of optimal performance

Lifestyle modifications
  Weight control
  Weekly aerobic exercise
  Alcohol reduction
  Smoking cessation
	Numerical values (direct measure or self-reported)
	Yes/no

Routine clinical chemistries
  Electrolytes
  Renal function
  Glucose
	Numerical value (measured variables)

Number of drugs taken	Numerical value (measured variables)
Frequency of physician visits Complexity of treatment	Numerical value (measured variables)
Frequency of clinical tests	Numerical value (measured variables)
Total direct medical costs of treatment[a]	Numerical value (calculated)

Indirect costs of treatment
  Travel expenses
  Loss of productivity
  Increased insurance costs
	Numerical value (calculated cost and direct measure)

Global evaluation: patient Subjective perception of satisfaction	Analog scale
Global evaluation: physician Subjective perception of satisfaction	Analog scale

[a]Costs = drug cost + monitoring cost + side effects cost − savings in management of underlying disease.

preserve renal function most effectively *(4)*. The JNC VI also advocates a lower target BP level of <130/85 mmHg for patients with concomitant disease or evidence of end-organ damage *(2)*. Addressing these short-term outcomes may reduce the incidence of long-term morbidity.

Many antihypertensive therapies have side effects that diminish patients' quality of life and thus lead to poor compliance. Instruments to validate quality of life were introduced to allow for more quantifiable measures of how hypertension and hypertension treatment affect patients' lifestyles. These instruments allow physicians to select drugs, or adjust drug doses, on the basis of improving a patient's quality of life (i.e., diminishing the side effects that discourage a patient from continuing with treatment). Other quantifiable, short-term measures include routine laboratory tests, the number of drugs used, the frequency of physician visits, and the cost of treatment.

Some short-term outcomes are more difficult to measure because they rely on self-reporting by patients. These include lifestyle modifications and patient global evaluations. Despite the subjective nature of self-evaluation, a patient's perception of the success of therapy is an important variable of long-term compliance.

INTERMEDIATE-TERM OUTCOMES

Table 24-2 presents intermediate-term outcomes, which are measured approx 6 mo after the start of antihypertensive therapy. At this point, presumably, dose adjustments have been made and the patient's treatment regimen and short-term measurements are fairly stable. The purpose of intermediate-term outcomes is to monitor signs indicating end-organ damage, such as impaired renal function, echocardiography changes, or altered left ventricular function. There is no clearly established causal link between intermediate-term outcomes and long-term clinical events. However, the relationship between chronic hypertension and clinical events suggests that monitoring of intermediate-term outcomes may aid in the early identification of end-organ damage.

Intermediate-term outcomes include all short- and intermediate-term clinical and economic outcomes, such as lost workdays and health resources utilization (Table 24-2). Lost workdays during initiation of treatment may be attributed to visits to the clinic for BP monitoring and general assessment, whereas days missed in the intermediate phase

Table 24-2
Intermediate-Term Outcome Measures

Outcome[a]	How outcome was measured
All short-term clinical and economic outcomes	See Table 24-1

Concomitant metabolic risk factors
    Lipid profile
    Glucose tolerance, HbA$_{1c}$
	Numerical values (direct measure)

Renal outcome measures
    Renal function
    Proteinuria/microalbuminuria
	Numerical value (direct measure)

Cardiac outcomes: ischemia ECG changes	Present/absent: yes/no New findings: yes/no

Cardiac outcomes: left ventricular structure and function
    ECHO left ventricular mass
    Doppler diastolic function
    ECG left ventricular hypertrophy
	Numerical values (direct measure): yes/no

Cardiac outcomes: arrhythmias
    Symptoms
    ECG/ambulatory monitoring
	Present/absent
	Numerical values

Arterial compliance Noninvasive estimates of arterial stiffness	Numerical value (direct measure)

Clinical evidence of atherosclerosis
    New-onset angina pectoris
    Findings of carotid stenosis
    Renovascular findings
    Changes in optic fundi
	Present/absent: yes/no (or measure of severity of vascular changes)

Patient days lost from work	Numerical value (measured variable)

Health resources utilization
    Related hospitalizations
    Clinical visits
    Advanced imaging or other tests
	Numerical value

[a]ECHO, echocardiography; ECG, electrocardiography.

might result from hypertension-related complications. Physicians must consult with patients during this phase in order to determine whether missed workdays or health care utilization are clearly related to hypertension symptoms or treatment. The economic impact of these outcomes is quantifiable.

Table 24-3
Long-Term Outcome Measures

Outcome	How outcome was measured
All short-term and intermediate-term clinical and economic outcomes	*See* Tables 24-1 and 24-2
Mortality	Yes/no
Cardiovascular	
Noncardiovascular	
Cardiac events	Yes/no
Sudden death	
Myocardial infarction	
Angina pectoris	
Coronary artery bypass surgery	
Precutaneous transluminal coronary angioplasty	
Congestive heart failure	
Clinically significant arrhythmias	
Cerebrovascular events	Yes/no
Strokes, hemorrhagic or thrombotic	
Transient ischemic attacks	
Renal events	Yes/no
Renal insufficiency	Numerical value
Renovascular disease	
Aortic and peripheral vascular disease	Yes/no
Cost-effectiveness	Numerical values
Cost per year of life saved	(calculated)
Cost of health resources	
Patient and indirect costs	
Costs of lost productivity	

LONG-TERM OUTCOMES

The events of cardiac, cerebrovascular, renal, and vascular diseases are associated with long-term hypertension. Prevention of morbidity and mortality owing to clinical events is the ultimate goal of antihypertensive therapy. However, it generally takes years, even decades, for the long-term outcomes of hypertension and antihypertensive therapy to become apparent.

Long-term outcomes include all short- and intermediate-term outcomes, as well as the incidence of hypertension-related clinical events and mortality (Table 24-3). Mortality resulting from cardiovascular disease can be attributed, at least in part, to hypertension, whereas mortality resulting from causes other than cardiovascular disease may indicate that antihypertensive therapy was effective during the patient's lifetime.

Long-term outcomes may aid assessments of the costs of antihypertensive treatment and the value of antihypertensive therapy in the context of reducing morbidity and mortality. By using large population studies, one can evaluate the cost per year of each life saved, as well as quality-adjusted life years. In addition, long-term evaluation of antihypertensive agents may identify the drugs of optimal benefit to patients, e.g., those with antiproliferative properties that can inhibit vascular changes.

CONCLUSION

Most clinical studies use only short-term outcome measures to determine the efficacy of a particular drug because they can be assessed immediately and economically. The causal connection between short- and intermediate-term outcomes and long-term morbidity and mortality is still under investigation. However, all three ranges of outcomes should be considered in assessments of how effectively antihypertensive therapies prolong life and reduce clinical events. Short-term measures are easily attainable. However, intermediate- and long-term measures are obtained over many years of patient monitoring, and the process is costly.

If clinical trials are expanded to include short-, intermediate-, and long-term outcomes, they may lead to hypertension-management regimens that reduce morbidity and mortality, improve quality of life, and provide economic justification for prescribing newer, promising drugs.

REFERENCES

1. Burt VL, Culter JA, Higgins M, Horan MJ, Labarthe D, Whelton P, Brown C, Roccella EJ (1995) Trends in the prevalence, awareness, treatment, and control of hypertension in the adult US population: data from the health examination surveys, 1960 to 1991. *Hypertension* 26:60–69.
2. The sixth report of the Joint National Committee on prevention, detection, evaluation, and treatment of high blood pressure (1997) *Arch Intern Med* 157:2413–2466.
3. Hansson L, Zanchetti A, Carruthers SG, Dahlof B, Elmfeldt D, Julius S, Menard J, Rahn KH, Wedel H, Westerling S (1998) Effects of intensive blood-pressure lowering and low-dose aspirin in patients with hypertension: principal results of

the Hypertension Optimal Treatment (HOT) randomised trial. HOT Study Group. *Lancet* 351:1755–1762.

4. Lazarus JM, Bourgoignie JJ, Buckalew VM, Greene T, Levey AS, Milas NC, Paranandi L, Peterson JC, Porush JG, Rauch S, Soucie JM, Stollar C (1997) Achievement and safety of a low blood pressure goal in chronic renal disease. The Modification of Diet in Renal Disease Study Group. *Hypertension* 29:641–650.

IV MAJOR HYPERTENSIVE DRUG CLASSES

25 Diuretics in Hypertension Therapy

James Sowers, MD, Joel Neutel, MD and Matthew Weir, MD

CONTENTS

REFERENCES

Diuretics have been and remain an important class of antihypertensive agents. They are a critical component of the hypertension therapeutic regimen, particularly for patients with systolic hypertension, the elderly, African Americans and diabetic patients. In large controlled clinical trials, diuretic therapy has consistently lowered morbidity and mortality for cardiovascular disease as well as stroke. For this reason, diuretic therapy is an important component of the overall antihypertensive regimen.

The first availability of the thiazide diuretics in the late 1950s greatly improved the therapeutic outlook for patients with hypertension and simplified its management. Over the past 40 yr there has been an evolution in the understanding of diuretics that has resulted in a change in the use of these drugs from high dose monotherapy of 50–200 mg of hydrochlorothiazide (HCTZ) to lower doses (6.25, 12.5 mg) used either as monotherapy or in combination therapy with other drugs. There are several reasons for this change in diuretic dosing: (1) it was realized that diuretics effectively reduce blood pressure (BP) at doses much lower than initially recommended; (2) they have far fewer side effects and are better tolerated at lower doses; and (3) many of the metabolic and electrolyte abnormalities associated with high dose diuretic therapy are rare at low doses.

It has also now become clear that diuretics have antihypertensive actions beyond that of natriuresis. A number of studies have

From: *Hypertension Medicine*
Edited by: M. A. Weber © Humana Press Inc., Totowa, NJ

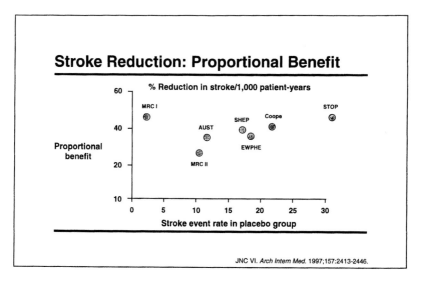

Fig. 25-1. Effects of diuretic-based treatment on stroke rates in several antihypertensive trials. MRC, Medical Research Council; SHEP, Systolic Hypertension in the Elderly Program; AUST, Australian Trial in Mild Hypertension; EWPHE, European Working Party on Hypertension in the Elderly; and STOP, Systolic Trial in Old People.

demonstrated that the predominant long-term antihypertensive action of diuretics is vasodilation. The mechanism of this effect is not well understood. It is possible that it is related to shifts in cellular concentrations of electrolytes such as sodium, calcium, or even magnesium. Volume reduction is a modest effect and volume usually returns to baseline, or near baseline levels, within 3 d.

The JNC VI recommendation *(1)* that diuretics should be used as first line therapy for the treatment of patients with essential hypertension is based on numerous clinical trials demonstrating consistent reduction in cardiovascular morbidity and mortality. This benefit is especially evident in elderly patients, primarily manifesting elevations in systolic blood pressure, where diuretics have exhibited substantial ability to reduce morbidity and mortality related to stroke, myocardial infarction, and congestive heart failure. Many of these trials utilized diuretics as the initial therapy but allowed addition of other agents, usually β-blockers, in order to achieve goal BP. Summary data from diuretic-based trials are given in Fig. 25-1 and Table 25-1.

Thiazide diuretics are also beneficial in hypertensive diabetics. In the Systolic Hypertension in the Elderly Program trial (SHEP), the

Table 25-1
Effects of diuretic-based treatment on rates of major cardiovascular
endpoints in several antihypertensive trials. MRC, Medical Research
Council, SHEP, Systolic Hypertension in the Elderly Program; AUST,
Australian Trial in Mild Hypertension; EWPHE, European Working Party
on Hypertension in the Elderly; and STOP, Systolic Trial in Old People.

Mild Hypertension Trials: Percent
Change in Fatal and Nonfatal Event Rates

	Australian	EWPHE	SHEP	STOP	MRC
Stroke	-34	-36*	-36*	-47*	-25*
All cardiac	-19	-20	-27*	-13‡	-19†
All CV	-24	-34*	-32*	-40*	-17*

NR = not reported.
*P<0.05; †IHD; ‡MI.

Adapted from Beard L et al. *BMJ.* 1992;304:412-416.

diabetic cohort of patients with isolated systolic hypertension had reductions in cardiovascular events that equaled or exceeded the reductions in the overall patient population studied. This indicates that diuretics can be effectively used as first line therapy in the diabetic population, especially when used in low doses to minimize adverse metabolic effects. The JNC VI consensus report suggests that diuretics in low dosages may be used as first line therapy in diabetic patients with hypertension, alone or in combination with other drugs. In the diabetic hypertensive, a combination of low-dose diuretic with either an ACE inhibitor or an angiotensin receptor blocker is an ideal way to facilitate the more intensive BP reduction (<130/85 mmHg) that these patients require. Thiazide diuretics can be considered as "blood vessel conditioning" agents in that they can facilitate blood pressure reduction with other classes of medication, particularly those that block the renin angiotensin system. This is very helpful in patients who are more resistant to antihypertensive therapy due to different response pattern such as the elderly, diabetics, African Americans, or those who are more salt sensitive.

Older clinical data with high doses of diuretics raised concern about potential adverse metabolic effects of these drugs. This was of particular concern in patients with impaired glucose tolerance or those with clinical diabetes mellitus. However, carefully conducted trials with low-dose thiazide (6.25–12.5 mg) diuretics have demonstrated no association with adverse effects on lipids, glucose and insulin metabolism, or electrolyte balance. These results are in direct contrast to what has been reported for hydrochlorothiazide at doses >25 mg. Since the majority of hypertensive patients require combination therapy to achieve lower BP goals, low-dose combination drugs are becoming an alternative first line therapy in an effort to obtain better BP control with diminished adverse events and metabolic side effects.

In summary, thiazide diuretics have undergone a resurgence in use. Our appreciation of how best to use them in lower doses and in conjunction with other medications has improved their therapeutic index. Moreover, they are cost-effective and have been demonstrated to be especially effective in the treatment of systolic hypertension and in enhancing BP responsiveness in combination therapy. In addition, diuretics also have a consistent track record for reducing hypertensive morbidity and mortality.

REFERENCES

1. The Sixth Report of the Joint National Committee on Prevention, Detection, Evaluation and Treatment of High Blood Pressure (1997) *Arch Intern Med* 157:2413–2446.
2. SHEP Cooperative Research Group (1991) Prevention of stroke by antihypertensive drug treatment in older persons with isolated systolic hypertension: final results of the Systolic Hypertension in the Elderly Program (SHEP). *JAMA* 265(24):3255–3264.
3. MRC Working Party (1992) Medical Research Council trial of treatment of hypertension in older adults: principal results. *BMJ* 304(6824):405–412.
4. Mac Mahanon S, Rodgers A (1993) The effects of blood pressure reduction in older patients: an overview of five randomized controlled trials in elderly hypertensives. *Clin Exp Hypertens* 15(6):967–978.
5. Neutel JM, Weir M, Sowers J (1996) Metabolic manifestations of low-dose diuretics. *Am J Med* 101(Suppl.):715–825.
6. Bakris GL, Weir MR, Sowers JR (1996) Therapeutic challenges in the obese diabetic patient with hypertension. *Am J Med* 101(Suppl 3A):33S–46S.
7. Neutel JM, Black HR, Weber MW (1996) Combination therapy with diuretics: An evolution of understanding. *Am J Med* 101(suppl 3A):61S–70S.
8. Jamerson K, DeQuattro V (1996) The impact of ethnicity on response to antihypertensive therapy. *Am J Med* 101(Suppl 3A):22S–32S.
9. Weir MR, Flack JM, Applegate WB (1996) Tolerability, safety, and quality of life and hypertensive therapy: The case for low-dose diuretics. *Am J Med* 101(Suppl 3A):83S–92S.

26 β-Adrenergic Blocker Treatment of Hypertension

Pharmacodynamics and Guide to Patient Selection

Jon D. Blumenfeld, MD

β-Adrenergic receptor blockade is a principal treatment for cardiovascular disease, including ischemic heart disease and heart failure *(1,2)*. Hypertension is a leading risk factor for these major causes of death in modern society. Although β-blockers lower blood pressure (BP) in many patients *(3,4)*, their antihypertensive efficacy varies widely among individuals, indicating the pathophysiologic heterogeneity of hypertension *(5,6)*. In fact, of all the hypertensive patients in the United States who are treated with an antihypertensive medication, fewer than half achieve a target pressure of ≤140/90 mmHg *(7)*. This chapter reviews some of the mechanisms by which β-blockers lower BP and

From: *Hypertension Medicine*
Edited by: M. A. Weber © Humana Press Inc., Totowa, NJ

provides a rational approach for identifying the hypertensive patient
who is most likely to have a favorable response to this treatment.

PHARMACOLOGY

β-Adrenergic receptor blockers are competitive antagonists characterized as β_1-selective or β_1-nonselective *(4)*. Cardiac tissue contains
both β_1- and β_2-receptors; therefore, cardioselectivity is an inaccurate
term when describing β-blocker actions.

β-Blockers can be classified further depending on the presence of
partial β-agonist activity, referred to as intrinsic sympathomimetic
activity, and also by other features including lipid solubility. Highly
lipid soluble drugs (e.g., propranolol) are excreted by hepatic metabolism, whereas the kidneys eliminate more hydrophilic drugs (e.g., atenolol) *(8)*. β-Blockers that are extensively metabolized by the liver are
cleared at a rate approaching hepatic blood flow (~1.5 L/min), whereas
renal clearance is much slower, approximating the glomerular filtration
rate (120 mL/min). It is therefore reasonable to select the drug that is
cleared independently of the diseased organ.

OVERVIEW OF HEMODYNAMIC EFECTS OF β-BLOCKADE

Poiseuille's law states that, in a cylindrical tube, the ratio of the
pressure gradient (ΔP) to flow (Q) is a function of the dimensions of
the tube (length L and radius r) and the viscosity (η) of the fluid. The
ratio of the mean pressure gradient to mean flow is indicative of the
resistance (R) to flow through the system. Accordingly,

$$R = \Delta P/Q$$
in which $R = (8\eta l/\pi r^4)$

Assuming that Poiseuille's law can be applied to the vasculature,
then BP is directly related to cardiac output (CO), a primary determinant
of blood flow, and to peripheral vascular resistance (TPR) (Fig. 26-1):

$$BP = CO \times TPR$$

When propranolol, a nonselective β-blocker, is infused intravenously, heart rate and CO fall acutely *(4)* (Fig. 26-2). The reduction
in CO is correlated to the decline in heart rate. As CO falls, TPR
increases by a baroreceptor mechanism, and, hence, BP is not reduced
acutely during β-blockade *(9)*. This rapid rise in peripheral resistance

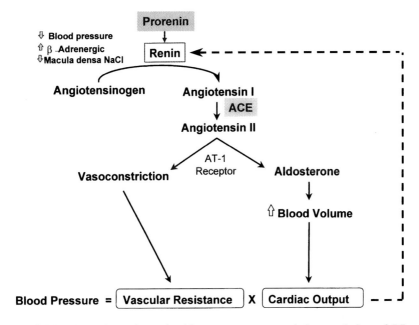

Fig. 26-1. The renin-angiotensin-aldosterone system and the regulation of BP. Solid lines indicate stimulation, and dotted line indicates inhibition.

can be prevented by pretreatment with a σ-adrenergic receptor blocker (e.g., phentolamine). However, within hours to days after initiation of β-blockade, TPR declines, and, consequently, BP falls in those patients who are responders to treatment. Thus, a characteristic feature of antihypertensive efficacy during chronic therapy with β-blockers is the fall in vascular resistance at any given CO.

Vasodilation by epinephrine is mediated by β_2-adrenergic receptors. Nonselective β-blocking agents attenuate this effect, and, thus, epinephrine binds preferentially to the σ-adrenergic receptor. As a consequence of the unopposed σ_1-mediated vasoconstriction by epinephrine and norepinephrine, BP can rise paradoxically during nonselective β-blockade *(4,10)*. This increase in BP can be striking in patients with pheochromocytoma.

As with most other antihypertensive agents, fewer than half of all hypertensive patients have a satisfactory reduction in BP during treatment with β-blockers. However, Buhler et al. *(11,12)* reported that the plasma renin activity (PRA) level was useful for predicting the antihypertensive efficacy of these agents. BP was controlled by β-blocker monotherapy in 75% of hypertensive patients with a high

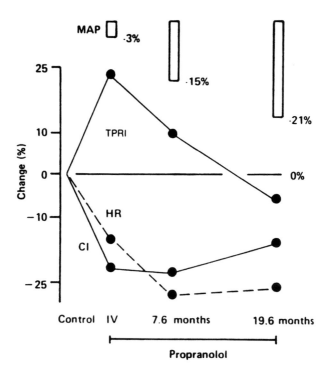

Fig. 26-2. Hemodynamic response to acute and chronic β-blockade. Immediately after propranolol infusion, BP does not fall because the reduction in cardiac index (CI) and heart rate (HR) are offset by the rise in peripheral resistance (TPRI). Chronically, TPRI and BP fall in patients with an antihypertensive response. (Reproduced from ref. *4.*)

PRA level, 65% with a medium renin level, and only 10% with a low renin level (Fig. 26-3). Moreover, the fall in PRA during treatment with propranolol was directly related to the reduction in BP (Fig. 26-4). This was the first demonstration that the efficacy of an antihypertensive agent could be predicted by a blood test—in this case the PRA level.

RENIN-ANGIOTENSIN SYSTEM AND BP HOMEOSTASIS

To understand the relationship between the renin system and the antihypertensive efficacy of β-blockers, a brief review of the renin-angiotensin system is warranted (Fig. 26-1).

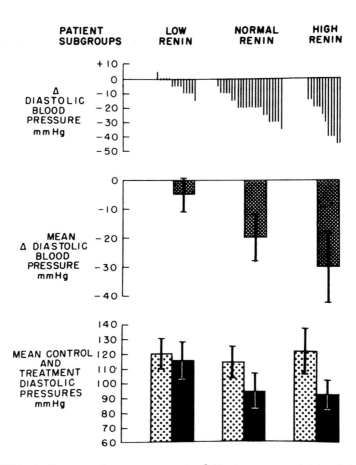

Fig. 26-3. Antihypertensive response to the β-blocker propranolol is related to the pretreatment PRA level. Patients in the high-renin subgroup had the greatest magnitude of reduction in diastolic BP compared to the normal and low-renin subgroups (top, individual values; middle, mean values for each subgroup). **(Bottom)** Mean BP values during pretreatment control (▨) and during treatment with propranolol (■) in the renin subgroups. (Reproduced from ref. *11*.)

The renin-angiotensin-aldosterone system regulates peripheral vascular resistance and renal reabsorption of sodium and water *(13)*. Renin is normally secreted by renal juxtaglomerular cells into the systemic circulation in situations in which BP is reduced, such as during upright posture and during sodium depletion. Specific renal stimuli include reduced renal perfusion pressure, increased $β_1$-adrenergic stimulation, and reduced chloride delivery to the macula densa located at the distal

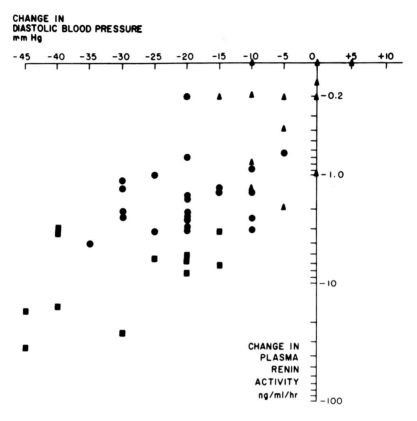

Fig. 26-4. Propranolol-induced changes in diastolic BP in relation to decrements in PRA in patients with low- (▲), normal (●), and (■) high-renin subgroups. (Reproduced from ref. *11*.)

nephron. Renin cleaves the decapeptide angiotensin I from angiotensinogen. Angiotensin II, an octapeptide, is then formed from angiotensin I by angiotensin-converting enzyme (ACE). Angiotensin II (Ang II), the main effector substance of this system, raises BP toward normal by stimulating vascular smooth muscle contraction and, hence, increasing vascular resistance. It increases blood volume by stimulating renal sodium and water reabsorption directly at the proximal tubule and indirectly by increasing adrenal cortical production and release of aldosterone. These actions are transduced by the type 1 Ang II receptor *(14)*. The consequent rise in BP to normal exerts negative feedback inhibition of renin secretion. These coordinated renal and adrenal responses maintain BP within the normal range.

Disruption of these mechanisms provides a pathophysiologic basis for hypertension *(15)*. High renal perfusion pressure should suppress renin secretion. However, approx 70% of hypertensive patients do not have a low PRA level despite high BPs *(16)*. That excess renin-angiotensin activity maintains high BP is supported by the fact that drugs that interrupt the renin system lower BP *(17)* (e.g., ACE inhibitors, Ang II receptor antagonists, and β-blockers).

β-BLOCKADE AND RENIN SYSTEM ACTIVITY: RELATIONSHIP TO ANTIHYPERTENSIVE EFFICACY

In the 1960s and early 1970s, the nonselective β-blocker propranolol was found to significantly reduce PRA levels in normotensive subjects and hypertensive patients in a dose-dependent manner, whereas diuretics stimulated PRA and did not lower BP when renin was elevated. Buhler et al. *(11)* reported a significant correlation between the pretreatment PRA level and the fall in BP during β-blocker monotherapy (Fig. 26-4). Furthermore, D-propranolol, which has the quinidine-like effect but not the β-blocking properties of DL-propranolol, the clinically used racemate, does not suppress renin secretion and does not lower BP *(9)*. Subsequent studies found that this renin response was transduced by renal β_1-adrenergic receptors and that all β-blockers reduce the PRA level, although this effect may be attenuated in agents with intrinsic sympathomimetic activity.

We have evaluated mechanisms whereby β-blockers lower renin secretion. Campbell et al. *(18)* have shown that the plasma total renin level, defined as the sum of plasma prorenin + PRA, is directly related to (pro)renin gene expression. This indicates that that the product of (pro)renin gene expression (i.e., prorenin) circulates in proportion to its production rate either as prorenin or as renin *(18)*. In both normotensive subjects and hypertensive patients, PRA decreases significantly during β-blockade. This occurs without affecting plasma total renin because there is a reciprocal increment in plasma prorenin *(19,20)* (Fig. 26-5). Therefore, β-blockers appear to suppress renin secretion by reducing the proportion of prorenin that is processed to renin within the kidney, without affecting (pro)renin gene expression.

Although renin secretion is the regulated step in the formation of Ang II, it is Ang II that stimulates vasoconstriction and aldosterone production. Plasma Ang II levels, like PRA levels, also decline during β-blockade in normotensive subjects and hypertensive patients and are

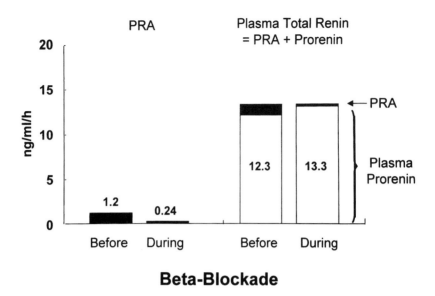

Beta-Blockade

Fig. 26-5. Effect of β-blockade on PRA (■), prorenin (□), and plasma total renin (PRA + prorenin; combined white and black bars. PRA is significantly reduced during β-blockade. Plasma prorenin increases modestly, so that total renin is unchanged. (Reproduced from ref. *20.*)

highly correlated with PRA levels *(20,21)* (Fig. 26-6). As predicted by the reduction in PRA and Ang II, aldosterone excretion also falls during treatment with β-blockers, although to a lesser extent than PRA and Ang II because potassium excretion decreases when aldosterone production falls. Taken together, these findings indicate that β-blockade suppresses the major components of the renin system, and this relates to the antihypertensive efficacy of β-blockers.

In contrast to β-blockers, which reduce Ang II levels by suppressing PRA, ACE inhibitors decrease the rate of Ang II formation from angiotensin I. In view of the different mechanisms by which β-blockers and ACE inhibitors reduce Ang II formation, the addition of an ACE inhibitor during β-blockade might be expected to reduce BP further if the Ang II level was not already maximally suppressed. Indeed, acute captopril administration enhances the antihypertensive effect of β-blockade, consistent with the further acute reduction in Ang II. In essential hypertension, Pickering et al. *(22)* demonstrated that propranolol lowered BP and suppressed PRA, whereas captopril monotherapy caused a comparable reduction in BP, but PRA rose. When these agents were administered together, their antihypertensive effect was enhanced.

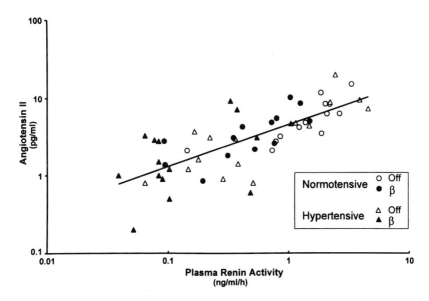

Fig. 26-6. Direct relationship between PRA and plasma Ang II level before and during β-blockade in normotensive and hypertensive subjects. $R^2 = 0.55$; $p < 0.0001$.

This amplified response was attributed to their complementary antirenin system actions, since the PRA rise that occurred during the administration of captopril was blunted by propranolol. Furthermore, aldosterone decreased further during combined treatment, indicating reduced Ang II levels.

Several studies have suggested that elderly patients are less responsive to antihypertensive treatment with a β-blocker (5,23). Some studies have found PRA levels to decline with advancing age, and thus provide one mechanism for the higher rate of failure to respond to β-blocker monotherapy in the elderly (9).

β-BLOCKADE AND PREVENTION AND TREATMENT OF ACUTE MYOCARDIAL INFARCTION

β-Blocker treatment during the earliest phase of an acute myocardial infarction (MI) prolongs survival and reduces the risk of recurrent MI (1). This salutary response has been attributed to several factors, including reduction in myocardial oxygen utilization and attenuation of the proarrhythmic and prothrombotic effects of excess adrenergic activity that occur during acute MI *(24)*.

Several lines of evidence suggest that excess renin system activity is associated with an increased risk of MI and that the risk of reinfarction can be reduced by treatment strategies that interrupt the renin system. First, Ang II infusion causes acute MI in experimental animal models *(25)*. Second, prospective and retrospective studies have demonstrated that ambulatory hypertensive patients with high PRA levels are at threefold greater risk for suffering an MI compared with those with low- and medium-renin levels *(16,26)*. Third, ACE inhibitor treatment during acute MI reduces the risk of reinfarction *(27)*. Fourth, patients who present to an emergency room with chest pain and an acute MI have PRA levels that are more than twofold higher than those in whom the diagnosis of acute MI is ruled out *(28)*. These findings form the basis for the hypothesis that the therapeutic effects of β-blockade during acute MI are, in part, owing to the drug-induced suppression of renin system activity.

SUMMARY

The importance of renin system suppression in the antihypertensive efficacy of β-adrenergic receptor blockade is supported by the direct relationship between the antihypertensive efficacy and the pretreatment renin level, the suppression of renin by all types of β-blockers, the correlation between the reduction in renin and the long-term fall in BP and peripheral vascular resistance, and the comparable antihypertensive efficacy of β-blockers and other antirenin system drugs (i.e., ACE inhibitors, Ang II receptor blockers) *(17)*. Lack of antihypertensive responsiveness to β-blockade in an individual patient indicates that other nonrenin mechanisms are predominant, including σ-adrenergic vasoconstriction or sodium-volume–sensitive hypertension. Although a subset of hypertensive patients can be identified by excess adrenergic activity, plasma catecholamine levels are not reliable predictors of the antihypertensive efficacy of β-blockers.

In the antihypertensive response to β-blockade, cardiac output is depressed initially, thereby promoting baroreceptor activation and σ-adrenergic-mediated vasoconstriction. Although the PRA level falls promptly during treatment, the vasodilating effect is offset by brisk σ-adrenergic-mediated vasoconstriction. Within days to weeks, σ-adrenergic activity decreases, vasodilation then occurs because renin system activity is suppressed, and BP falls.

REFERENCES

1. Gottlieb SS, McCarter RJ, Vogel RA (1998) Effect of beta-blockade on mortality among high-risk and low risk patients after myocardial infarction. *N Engl J Med* 339:489–497.
2. Packer M, Bristow MR, Cohn JN, et al. (1996) The effect of Carvedilol on morbidity and mortality in patients with chronic heart failure. *N Engl J Med* 334:1349–1355.
3. Kannel WB (1996) Blood pressure as a cardiovascular risk factor: prevention and treatment. *JAMA* 275:1571–1576.
4. Prichard BNC, Cruickshank JM (1995) Beta-blockade in hypertension: past, present, and future. In: Laragh JH, Brenner BM, eds. *Hypertension: Pathophysiology, Diagnosis, and Management,* vol. 2, New York: Raven, pp. 2827–2859.
5. Preston RA, Materson BJ, Reda DJ, et al. (1998) Age-race subgroup compared with renin profile as predictors of blood pressure response to antihypertensive therapy. Department of Veterans Affairs Cooperative Study Group on Antihypertensive Agents. *JAMA* 280:1168–1172.
6. Blumenfeld JD, Laragh JH (1998) Renin system analysis: a rational method for the diagnosis and treatment of the individual patient with hypertension. *Am J Hypertens* 11:894–896.
7. Burt VL, Whelton P, Roccella EJ, et al. (1995) Prevalence of hypertension in the U.S. population: results from the Third National Health and Nutrition Examination Survey, 1988–1991. *Hypertension* 25:305–314.
8. McDevitt DG (1981) Differential features of beta-adrenoceptor blocking drugs for therapy. In: Laragh JH, Buhler FR, eds. Selding, D.W., vol. 1, Frontiers in Hypertension Research, New York: Springer-Verlag, pp. 473–481.
9. Buhler FR. Antihypertensive actions of beta-blockers. In: Laragh JH, Buhler FR, Seldin DW, eds. *Frontiers in Hypertension Research,* vol. 1, New York: Springer-Verlag, pp. 424–435.
10. Blumenfeld JD, Vaughan ED Jr (1999) Hypertensive adrenal disorders. In: Brady HR, Wilcox CS, eds. *Therapy in Nephrology and Hypertension,* vol. 1, Philadelphia: W. B. Saunders, pp. 451–462.
11. Buhler FR, Laragh JH, Baer L, Vaughan ED Jr, Brunner HR (1972) Propranolol inhibition of renin secretion: a specific approach to diagnosis and treatment of renin-dependent hypertensive diseases. *N Engl J Med* 287:1209–1214.
12. Buhler FR, Laragh JH, Vaughan ED Jr, Brunner HR, Gavras H, Baer L (1973) Antihypertensive action of propranolol: specific antirenin responses in high and normal renin forms of essential, renal, renovascular and malignant hypertension. *Am J Cardiol* 32:511–522.
13. Laragh JH, Sealey JE (1992) Renin-angiotensin-aldosterone system and the renal regulation of sodium, potassium, and blood pressure homeostasis. In: Windhager

EE, ed. *Handbook of Physiology, Renal Physiology,* vol. 2, New York: Oxford University Press, pp. 1409–1541.

14. Goodfriend TL, Elliott ME, Catt KJ (1996) Angiotensin receptors and their antagonists. *N Engl J Med* 334:1649–1654.

15. Sealey JE, Blumenfeld JD, Bell GM, Pecker MS, Sommers SC, Laragh JH (1988) On the renal basis for essential hypertension: nephron heterogeneity with discordant renin secretion and sodium excretion causing a hypertensive vasoconstriction-volume relationship. *J Hypertens* 6:763–777.

16. Brunner HR, Laragh JH, Baer L, et al. (1972) Essential hypertension: renin and aldosterone, heart attack and stroke. *N Engl J Med* 286:441–449.

17. Laragh JH (1995) Renin system understanding for analysis and treatment of hypertensive patients: a means to quantify the vasoconstrictor elements, diagnose curable renal and adrenal causes, assess risk of cardiovascular morbidity, and find the best fit drug regimen. In: Laragh JH, Brenner BM, eds. *Hypertension: Pathophysiology, Diagnosis, and Management,* vol. 2, New York: Raven, pp. 1813–1836.

18. Campbell WG Jr, Gahnem F, Catanzaro DF, et al. (1996) Plasma and renal prorenin/renin, renin mRNA, and blood pressure in Dahl salt-sensitive and salt-resistant rats. *Hypertension* 27:1121–1133.

19. Atlas SA, Sealey JE, Laragh JH, Moon C (1977) Plasma renin and "prorenin" in essential hypertension during sodium depletion, beta-blockade, and reduced arterial pressure. *Lancet* 2:785–789.

20. Blumenfeld JD, Sealey JE, Mann SA, et al. (1999) Beta-adrenergic receptor blockade as a therapeutic approach for suppressing the renin-angiotensin-aldosterone system in normotensive and hypertensive subjects. *Am J Hypertens* 12:451–459.

21. Bragat AC, Blumenfeld J, Sealey JE (1997) Effect of high-performance liquid chromatography on plasma angiotensin II measurements in treated and untreated normotensive and hypertensive patients. *J Hypertens* 15:459–465.

22. Pickering TG, Case DB, Sullivan PA, Laragh JH (1982) Comparison of antihypertensive and hormonal effects of captopril and propranolol at rest and during exercise. *Am J Cardiol* 49:1566–1588.

23. Messerli FH, Grossman E, Goldbourt U (1998) Are beta-blockers efficacious as first-line therapy for hypertension in the elderly? A systematic review. *JAMA* 279:1903–1907.

24. McAlpine HM, Mortin JJ, Leckie B, Rumley A, Gillen G, Dargie HJ (1988) Neuroendocrine activation after acute myocardial infarction. *Br Heart J* 60:117–124.

25. Gavras H, Brown JJ, Lever AF, et al. (1971) Acute renal failure, tubular necrosis, and myocardial infarction induced in the rabbit by intravenous angiotensin II. *Lancet* 2:19–22.

26. Alderman MH, Madhavan S, Ooi WL, Cohen H, Sealey JE, Laragh JH (1991) Association of the renin-sodium profile with the risk of myocardial infarction in patients with hypertension. *N Engl J Med* 324:1098–1104.

27. ACE Inhibitor Myocardial Infarction Collaborative Group (1998) Indications for ACE inhibitors in the early treatment of acute myocardial infarction: systematic overview of the individual data from 100,000 patients in randomized trials. *Circulation* 97:2202–2212.

28. Blumenfeld JD, Sealey JE, Alderman MH, Cohen H, Lappin R, Laragh JH Association between plasma renin activity and acute myocardial infarction in normotensive and hypertensive patients. *Am J Hypertens,* to be published.

27 Calcium Antagonists

Franz H. Messerli, MD,
Jayant Dey, MBBS, MD,
and Zhanbin Feng, MD

CONTENTS

Calcium antagonists have been available for study and clinical use since the 1960s. As a class of antihypertensive agents, they are the most heterogeneous in their chemical structure, modes of action, and clinical indications. However, they all share a common physiologic action: decreasing the intracellular availability of calcium ions in cardiac and vascular smooth muscle cells, thereby directly inhibiting their contractility. At least four different receptors, with varying affinities to calcium antagonists, regulate calcium ion movement across the cell membrane *(1)*. In addition, some of the diversity of this class of drugs may be explained by the difference in intracellular calcium ion release

From: *Hypertension Medicine*
Edited by: M. A. Weber © Humana Press Inc., Totowa, NJ

Table 27-1
Calcium Antagonists Approved for Treatment of
Hypertension in the United States[a]

Drug	Form	PO dose for SR
Amlodipine (Norvasc)	Tablet	2.5–10 mg QD
Diltiazem (Cardizem CD, Dilacor XR, etc.)	IV, IR, SR	180–480 mg QD (CD)
Felodipine (Plendil)	SR	2.5–10 mg QD
Isradipine (Dynacirc)	Tablet	2.5–10 mg QD
Nicardipine (Cardene SR)	IV, IR, SR	30–60 mg BID (SR)
Nifedipine (Procardia XL, Adalat CC)	IR, SR	30–120 mg QD
Nisoldipine (Sular)	SR	20–40 mg QD
Verapamil (Isoptin SR, Calan SR, etc.)	IV, IR, SR	120–480 mg QD

[a]PO, oral; IV, intravenous preparation available; IR, immediate release tablet; SR, sustained release tablet; QD, once a day; BID, twice a day.

from the sarcoplasmic reticulum and the mitochondria as well as binding to specific intracellular proteins (e.g., calmodulin).

CLINICAL PHARMACOLOGY

Eight calcium antagonists are currently approved in the United States for use in the treatment of hypertension (*see* Table 27-1). Other than verapamil and diltiazem, all other calcium antagonists have a dihydropyridine core structure. Most are metabolized in the liver via CYP3A, a subset of the cytochrome P450 family of oxidative enzymes, to less active metabolites. Verapamil and diltiazem can inhibit the clearance of other CYP3A substrates (e.g., carbamazepine, cyclosporine, lovastatin, simvastatin, midazolam). Most often this interaction is of little clinical significance. Inducers and inhibitors of CYP3A-mediated drug biotransformation can affect the metabolism of the calcium antagonists *(2)*.

Of all the calcium antagonists, verapamil consistently increases digoxin blood levels. Combining amiodarone, digoxin, or β-blockers with verapamil or diltiazem can cause synergistic inhibition of sinus node and atrioventricular node conduction. Intravenous verapamil coadministration with β-blockers is contraindicated owing to the risk of asystole *(3)*. Lithium-induced neurotoxicity has been reported to be

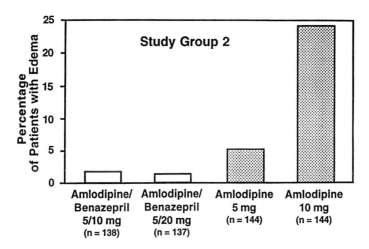

Fig. 27-1. Percentage of patients presenting with edema of all forms on various treatment strategies *(4)*.

predisposed by concurrent use of verapamil. Interestingly, concurrent intake of grapefruit juice with certain dihydropyridine calcium antagonists enhances their bioavailability, and patients should be warned not to drink grapefruit juice with calcium antagonists.

Vasodilatory edema has been reported for all calcium antagonists. It seems to be more common with the dihydropyridines than the nondihydropyridines, and more common in women than in men. Vasodilatory edema is dose dependent and does not respond to diuretic therapy. It often limits high doses of monotherapy of dihydropyridine calcium antagonists. However, vasodilatory edema has been shown to respond quite well to the addition of either an angiotensin-converting enzyme (ACE) inhibitor or an angiotensin receptor blocker (Fig. 27-1). *(4)*.

Constipation occurs as a direct extension of the pharmacologic effect from vascular to gastrointestinal smooth muscle relaxation. Constipation is more common with the nondihydropyridine calcium antagonists than with the dihydropyridines. Headache is frequently reported with the use of rapid-acting calcium antagonists, but less commonly noted with the slow onset and sustained release preparations. In fact, some calcium antagonists, particularly verapamil, have been used for the treatment of migraine. Gingival hyperplasia can occur with prolonged use of all calcium antagonists and, again, seems to be counteracted by the addition of an ACE inhibitor or an angiotension receptor antagonist.

HEART RATE AND CARDIAC CONDUCTION

Calcium antagonists lower arterial pressure by decreasing total peripheral resistance. Consequently, reflexive tachycardia and an increase in activity of the sympathetic nervous system are commonly seen, particularly with the first dose. It has been shown that with sustained therapy, heart rate and norepinephrine levels remained unchanged or only slightly elevated with long-acting dihydropyridines; both heart rate and norepinephrine levels decreased with long-acting nondihydropyridines *(5)*. Sympathetic activity has been well identified as a powerful independent risk factor for cardiovascular morbidity and mortality *(6)*. Conceivably, the increased mortality reported in some studies in which short-acting calcium antagonists were inappropriately used could have been related to increased sympathetic activity. Alderman et al. *(7)* have shown a five- to eightfold difference in morbidity and mortality between short- and long-acting calcium antagonists.

In pharmacologic doses, most calcium antagonists diminish automaticity of the sinus node, slow conduction in the atrioventricular node, and have little if any effect on the automaticity of the myocytes. These effects are considerably more pronounced with the nondihydropyridine calcium antagonists than with the dihydropyridine derivatives. The combination of the nondihydropyridine calcium antagonists with β-blockers is therefore relatively contraindicated. The dihydropyridine calcium antagonists generally have little if any effect on cardiac conduction and can be combined with β-blockers *(8)*.

CARDIAC CONTRACTILITY AND HYPERTROPHY

In general, calcium antagonists are negative inotropic agents and therefore are likely to impair cardiac pump function to some extent. The most profound negative inotropic effect is seen with verapamil and diltiazem. This direct effect is partially overridden by afterload reduction and reflexive sympathetic drive elicited by most of the dihydropyridine derivatives.

Left ventricular hypertrophy (LVH) has been identified as a significant pressure-independent risk factor and a harbinger of sudden death, myocardial infarction (MI), congestive heart failure, and other events leading to cardiovascular morbidity and mortality *(9)*. Not all antihypertensive agents are equally effective in regressing LVH. In a recent meta-analysis of 50 randomized, double-blind trials, calcium antagonists

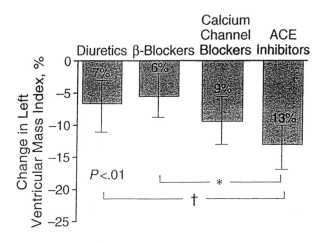

Fig. 27-2. Percentage of change in left ventricular mass index with the four antihypertensive drug classes. Mean values and 95% confidence intervals adjusted for duration are given. $p < 0.01$ between drug classes; † $p < 0.10$ between drug classes (Bonferroni correction) (Reprinted with permission from ref. *10.*)

decreased left ventricular mass by 9% compared with a 7% decrease with diuretics, 6% decrease with β-blockers, and 13% decrease with ACE inhibitors (Fig. 27-2) *(10,11)*.

It seems that the dihydropyridine calcium antagonists have a somewhat less powerful effect on left ventricular mass than the nondihydropyridines when the antihypertensive efficacy is taken into account *(12)*. Thus, for any given decrease in arterial pressure, verapamil and diltiazem may reduce left ventricular mass more than dihydropyridine derivatives. This difference, at least to some extent, may be related to the effects of the respective calcium antagonists on sympathetic activity.

CORONARY BLOOD FLOW AND MYOCARDIAL ISCHEMIA

All calcium antagonists are vasodilators and therefore increase coronary blood flow. In addition to coronary blood flow, determinants of myocardial ischemia such as heart rate, contractility, and arterial pressure are also profoundly and variably affected by calcium antagonists. Their overall effects on myocardial oxygenation depend on an interplay of these mechanisms, either directly or through reflex sympathetic stimulation. It should therefore not be surprising that, in certain clinical situations, some calcium antagonists may even have a detrimental effect on myocardial oxygenation.

Acute exacerbation of angina and even acute MI have been observed when arterial pressure was excessively lowered by short-acting nifedipine *(13)*. Short-acting nifedipine has never been approved for the treatment of any form of hypertension, emergent or not. Messerli and Grossman recently documented that the use of this drug can lead to serious, even fatal, adverse events *(14)*. Based on that study, the Sixth Joint National Committee on the Prevention, Detection, Evaluation and Treatment of High Blood Pressure JNC VI has now labeled short-acting calcium antagonists as unacceptable for use in hypertension *(15)*.

Clearly, the situation is different with long-acting calcium antagonists, particularly with the nondihydropyridines *(16)*. In the post-MI patient, nondihydropyridine calcium antagonists, such as verapamil, should be considered as an alternative if β-blockers are contraindicated or not well tolerated. Several studies now attest to the benefits of the nondihydropyridine calcium antagonists in the post-MI patient *(17–20)*. The benefits may be particularly pronounced in post-MI patients who are hypertensive.

CLINICAL USE OF CALCIUM ANTAGONISTS
IN HYPERTENSION

All calcium antagonists lower arterial pressure when given acutely and with prolonged administration. Tachyphylaxis of the antihypertensive effect has not been reported. In general, there is little, if any, difference in blood pressure (BP)-lowering potency among the various agents, provided that an adequate dose is given. The effect on arterial pressure seems to be somewhat more powerful in the elderly or African American patients who are characterized by a low activity of the renin-angiotensin system than in the younger or Caucasian patients *(21)*. In general, calcium antagonists are well tolerated and metabolically inert and have been documented to reduce or prevent target organ disease in the heart, brain, kidneys, and vascular tree. Recent data from the Systolic Hypertension in Europe (Syst-EUR) study (Fig. 27-3) have shown that calcium antagonists diminish morbidity and mortality in the elderly patient with isolated systolic hypertension *(22)*. Based on

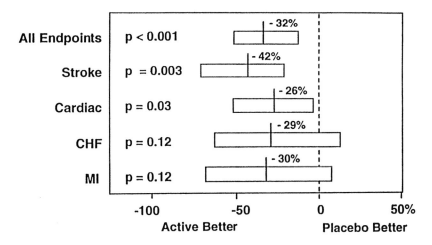

Fig. 27-3. Syst-EUR: fatal and nonfatal stroke in 4695 randomized patients.

the Syst-EUR study, JNC VI has labeled long-acting dihydropyridine calcium antagonists as an appropriate alternative in older patients. Similarly, in the Systolic Hypertension in China (Syst-CHINA) study, a reduction in morbidity and mortality was seen with a dihydropyridine calcium antagonist when compared with placebo *(23)*. Thus, apart from the diuretics, calcium antagonists are the only drug class for which two independent, prospective, randomized studies documented a significant reduction in morbidity and mortality. A recent substudy of the Syst-EUR showing a 50% reduction in dementia of all causes, mostly of the Alzheimer type, with calcium antagonists in the elderly makes these drugs even more attractive. Recent large prospective randomized trials such as STOP II, NORDIL, and INSIGHT, attest to the safety and efficacy of this drug class.

CLINICAL USE OF CALCIUM ANTAGONISTS IN HYPERTENSIVE PATIENTS WITH DIABETES

Both the Syst-EUR and the Syst-CHINA studies document a greater reduction in morbid events in the diabetic than in the nondiabetic

Table 27-2
Syst-EUR: Benefits in Diabetic Patients *(22)*

End point	Diabetics (n = 446)	Nondiabetics (n = 4250)	p value
Total mortality	0.46	0.93	<0.06
Cardiovascular mortality	0.24	0.86	<0.03
All cardiovascular events	0.32	0.73	<0.03
All cardiac end points	0.29	0.80	<0.06
Fatal/nonfatal stroke	0.38	0.59	<0.44

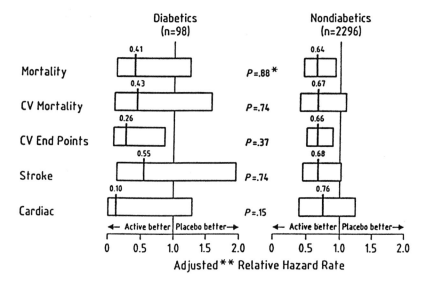

Fig. 27-4. Relative hazard rates of active treatment compared with placebo in diabetic and nondiabetic patients with adjustments for the covariates. *P for interaction; ** for sex, cardiovascular complications, age, entry SBP and DBP, smoking, and residence in Northern China. (Reprinted with permission from ref. *23.*)

subpopulation (Table 27-2; Fig. 27-4) *(24,25)*. Thus, by itself, is not surprising because hypertension is a powerful risk factor for cardiovascular morbidity and mortality in the diabetic patient, and any reduction of arterial pressure can be expected to confer some benefits. However, of interest is the comparison of the Syst-EUR with the Systolic Hypertension in the Elderly Program (SHEP) *(24)* study. In the SHEP study, chlorthalidone was used as step 1 therapy, whereas in the Syst-EUR

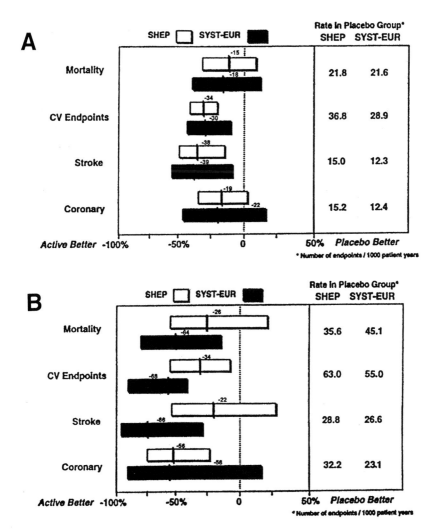

Fig. 27-5. Comparison of Syst-EUR and SHEP studies. Mortality and morbidity in **(A)** nondiabetic and **(B)** diabetic patients. (Reprinted with permission from ref. *24*.)

nitrendipine was the initial therapy. In the nondiabetic population, there was not much difference between the two treatment strategies. Both reduced stroke or cardiovascular events (Fig. 27-5). However, in the diabetic subpopulation, nitrendipine had a significantly greater effect than chlorthalidone. Interestingly, in the Hypertension Optimal Treatment study in which felodipine was used as initial therapy, there was a distinctly greater trend of reduction in cardiovascular events with BP lowering in the diabetic when compared with the nondiabetic population. In diabetic patients, the use of felodipine in the treatment group with a target of diastolic pressure <80 mmHg led to more than a 50% reduction in cardiovascular events than in the one with a target of 90 mmHg *(26)*. Recent data from the Appropriate Blood Pressure Control in Diabetes study have shown that there was no difference in renal outcome (proteinuria, glomerular filtration rate) between ACE inhibitors and dihydropyridine calcium antagonists after 5 yr of therapy in the diabetic hypertensive patient.

Lack of adverse effects on glucose metabolism, lipid metabolism, and renal perfusion make the calcium antagonists an attractive therapeutic choice for use in diabetic patients *(27)*.

CONCLUSION

By definition, all antihypertensive drugs, including calcium antagonists, lower arterial pressure. However, calcium antagonists, in addition to lowering arterial pressure, have a variety of beneficial effects in patients with hypertensive heart disease. They reduce LVH and improve its sequelae, such as ventricular dysrhythmias, impaired filling, and contractility, and the heart rate–lowering calcium antagonists reduce the risk of postinfarct reinfarction. Although the efficacy with regard to some of these properties clearly varies from one calcium antagonist to another, these drugs remain a cornerstone for therapy in patients with essential hypertension, particularly in African American, elderly, and diabetic patients.

The short-acting calcium antagonists should no longer be used in hypertensive patients. In fact, most of the short-acting calcium antagonists have not been approved for the treatment of hypertension. The practice of using oral or sublingual nifedipine in a hypertensive emergency or pseudoemergency should be abandoned because it can lead to serious side effects such as syncope, MI, stroke, and even death. By contrast, as shown by several studies, the use of the long-acting formulations seems to be safe and promising in patients with essential hypertension.

It should be emphasized that hypertension remains a surrogate end point and that not all drugs that reduce BP will *paribus passu* reduce morbidity and mortality. A prime example of failure of the so-called surrogate end point concept is provided by a recent meta-analysis in hypertension in the elderly: although β-blockers did lower BP, they consistently failed to reduce heart attacks and mortality from cardiovascular and all causes *(28)*. This means that numerous elderly hypertensive patients are exposed to the side effects, inconvenience, and cost of β-blockers without harvesting any benefits.

Many large, prospective randomized trials against placebo, such as the Shanghai Trial of Nifedipine in the Elderly (STONE) *(29)*, Syst-EUR, and Syst-CHINA, and against active therapy, such as the Swedish Trial in Old Patients with Hypertension-2 (STOP II) *(30)*, the Nordic Diltiazem (NORDIL) study *(31)*, and the International Nifedipine GITS Study Intervention as a Goal in Hypertension Treatment (INSIGHT) *(32)*, have recently attested to the safety and efficacy of calcium antagonist in the treatment of essential hypertension. With the exception of the diuretics, calcium antagonists, within a very short period of time, have emerged as the best documented drug class in the antihypertensive arsenal.

REFERENCES

1. Catterall WA, Stiessnig J (1992) Receptor sites for Ca++ channel antagonists. *Trends Pharmacol Sci* 13:256–262.
2. Guengerich FP, Brian WR, Iwasaki M, Sari M-A, Baarnhielm C, Bretsson P (1991) Oxidation of dihydropyridine calcium channel blockers and analogues by human liver cytochrome P-450 IIIA4. *J Med Chem* 34:1838–1844.
3. Albernethy DR (1997) Pharmacological properties of combination therapies for hypertension. *Am J Hypertens* 10:13S–16S.
4. Messerli FH, Oparil S, Feng Z (2000) Comparison of effectiveness and side effects of combined calcium antagonist (nifedipine or amlodipine) and angiotensin-converting enzyme inhibitor (benazepril) versus high-dose calcium antagonist monotherapy for systemic hypertension. *Am J Cardiol*, in press.
5. Grossman E, Messerli FH (1997) Effect of calcium antagonists on plasma norepinephrine levels, heart rate, and blood pressure. *Am J Cardiol* 80:1453–1458.
6. Zuanetti G, Mantini L, Hernandez-Bernal F, Barlera S, di Gregorio D, Latini R, Maggioni AP (1998) Relevance of heart rate as a prognostic factor in patients with acute myocardial infarction: insights from the GISSI-2 study. *Eur Heart J* 19:F19–F26.
7. Alderman MH, Cohen H, Roqué R, Madhavan S (1997) Effect of long-acting and short-acting calcium antagonists on cardiovascular outcomes in hypertensive patients. *Lancet* 349(9052):594–598.
8. Singh BN, Nademanee K (1987) Use of calcium antagonists for cardiac arrhythmias. *Am J Cardiol* 59:153B–162B.
9. Messerli FH, Ventura HO, Elizardi DJ, Dunn FG, Frohlich ED (1984) Hypertension and sudden death: increased ventricular ectopy activity in left ventricular hypertrophy. *Am J Med* 77:18–22.

10. Schmieder RE, Martus P, Klingbeil A (1996) Reversal of left ventricular hypertrophy in essential hypertension: a meta-analysis of randomized double-blind studies. *JAMA* 275:1507–1513.

11. Schmieder RE, Schlaich MP, Klingbeil AU, Martus P (1998) Update on reversal of left ventricular hypertrophy in essential hypertension (a meta-analysis of all randomized double-blind studies until December 1996). *Nephrol Dial Transplant* 13:564–569.

12. Cruickshank JM, Lewis J, Moore V, Dodd C (1992) Reversibility of left ventricular hypertrophy by differing types of antihypertensive therapy. *J Hum Hypertens* 6:85–90.

13. Wilson DJ, Schwarts GL, Textor SC, Zachariah PK, Sheps SG (1991) Precipitous fall in blood pressure in the treatment of chronic hypertension. Paper presented at the 5th International Symposium on Calcium Antagonists: Pharmacology and Clinical Research, Houston, TX.

14. Messerli FH, Grossman E (1998) Antihypertensive agents and the risk of cancer. *JAMA* 280:600.

15. The Sixth Report of the Joint National Committee on Prevention, Detection, Evaluation, and Treatment of High Blood Pressure (1997) *Arch Intern Med* 157:2413–2446.

16. Laragh JH, Held C, Messerli F, Pepine C, Sleight P (1996) Calcium antagonists and cardiovascular prognosis: a homogenous group? *Am J Hypertens* 9:99–109.

17. Messerli FH, Boden WE, Fischer Hansen J, Schechtman KB (1996) Heart rate lowering calcium antagonists (HRL-CA) in hypertensive post MI patients. *Am Coll Cardiol* 27:178A (abstract).

18. Messerli FH (1996) What, if anything, is controversial about calcium antagonists? *Am J Hypertens* (12 pt. 2):177S–181S.

19. Rehnqvist N, Hjemdahl P, Björkander I, et al. (1985) Primary prevention in patients with coronary heart disease: the APSIS study. *Cardiovasc Drugs Ther* 9(Suppl. 3):493.

20. Parker JD (1998) Clinical outcome studies of anti-anginal drug therapy for patients with stable coronary disease: an indication for clinical trials. *Eur Heart J* 19(Suppl. I):I15–I19.

21. Erne P, Bolli P, Bertel O, et al. (1983) Factors influencing the hypertensive effects of calcium antagonists. *Hypertension* 5:II97–II102.

22. Staessen JA, Fagard R, Thijs L, et al. (1997) Randomised double-blind comparison of placebo and active treatment for older patients with isolated systolic hypertension. The Systolic Hypertension in Europe (Syst-Eur) Trial Investigators. *Lancet* 350:757–764.

23. Liu L, Wang JG, Gong L, Liu G, Staessen JA (1998) Comparison of active treatment and placebo in older Chinese patients with isolated systolic hypertension. Systolic Hypertension in China (Syst-China) Collaborative Group. *J Hypertens* 16(12, Pt. 1):1823–1829.

24. Tuomilehto J, Rastenyte D, Birkenhager WH, et al. (1999) Effects of calcium-channel blockade in older patients with diabetes and systolic hypertension: Systolic Hypertension in Europe Trial Investigators. *N Engl J Med* 340:677–684.

25. Wang JG, Staessen JA, Gong L, Liu L (2000) Chinese trial on isolated systolic hypertension in the elderly. Systolic Hypertension in China (Syst-China) Collaborative Group. *Arch Intern Med* 160:211–220.

26. Hansson L, Zanchetti A, Carruthers SG et al. (1998) Effects of intensive blood-pressure lowering and low-dose aspirin in patients with hypertension: principal

results of the Hypertension Optimal Treatment (HOT) randomised trial. *Lancet* 351:1755–1762.

27. National High Blood Pressure Education Program Working Group report on hypertension in diabetes (1994) *Hypertension* 23:145–158.

28. Messerli FH, Grossman E, Goldbourt U (1998) Are β-blockers efficacious as first-line therapy for hypertension in the elderly? A systematic review. *JAMA* 279:1903–1907.

29. Gong L, Zhang W, Zhu Y, Zhu J, 11 collaborating centres in the Shanghai area, Kong D, Pagé V, Ghadirian P, LeLorier J, Hamet P (1996): Shanghai trial of nifedipine in the elderly (STONE). *J Hypertens* 14:1237–1245.

30. Hansson L, Lindholm LH, Ekbom T, Dahlöf B, Lanke J, Scherstén B, Wester P-O, Hedner T, de Faire U, for the STOP-Hypertension-2 study group (1999). Randomised trial of old and new antihypertensive drugs in elderly patients: cardiovascular mortality and morbidity the Swedish Trial in Old Patients with Hypertension-2 study. *Lancet* 354:1751–1756.

31. The Nordic Diltiazem Study (NORDIL) (2000). *Lancet,* to be published.

32. International Nifedipine GITS Study Intervention as a goal in Hypertension Treatment (INSIGHT) (2000). *Lancet,* to be published.

28 Angiotensin-Converting Enzyme Inhibitors

Irene Gavras, MD
and Haralambos Gavras, MD

CONTENTS

ANGIOTENSIN- AND BRADYKININ-MEDIATED
ACTIONS
CLINICAL EXPERIENCE WITH ACE INHIBITORS
REFERENCES

The introduction of angiotensin-converting enzyme (ACE) inhibitors for the treatment of hypertension and heart failure is probably the most important advance in cardiovascular pharmacotherapy in the last few decades. Although the role of the renin-angiotensin system (RAS) in cardiovascular diseases had been investigated extensively for more than 70 yr, the therapeutic application of this knowledge became possible only after the introduction of a practical way to block this system. It is now well established that activation of the RAS has a detrimental effect on the cardiovascular system and promotes arterial, myocardial, and renal damage. ACE inhibition was shown to diminish morbidity and mortality in patients with ischemic cardiomyopathy after myocardial infarction (MI), in patients with left ventricular impairment ranging from subclinical diastolic dysfunction to advanced systolic dysfunction with decompensated congestive heart failure (CHF), and in patients with diabetic nephropathy. Accordingly, these conditions are now compelling indications for treatment with ACE inhibitors *(1)*, even in non-hypertensive patients.

From: *Hypertension Medicine*
Edited by: M. A. Weber © Humana Press Inc., Totowa, NJ

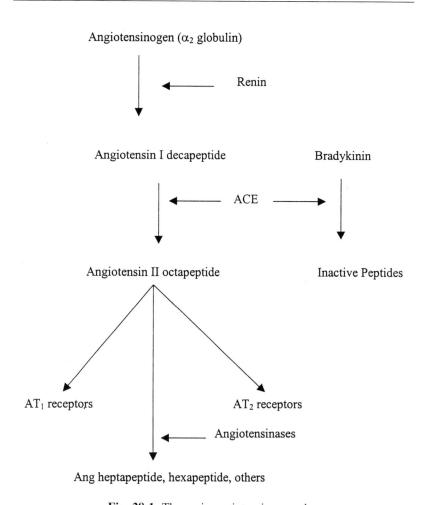

Fig. 28-1. The renin-angiotensin cascade.

ANGIOTENSIN- AND BRADYKININ-MEDIATED ACTIONS

When ACE inhibitors were first introduced in the treatment of human hypertension *(2),* their effects were attributed solely to blockade of the generation of angiotensin II (Ang II). It is now known that ACE inhibition has a dual effect in vivo: it interrupts partially the formation of the vasoconstrictor Ang II and it interrupts the degradation of the vasodilator bradykinin *(3).* Figure 28-1 is a simplified representation of the renin-angiotensin cascade. Accordingly, the results of ACE inhibition are attributable in part to Ang II withdrawal and in part to

Table 28-1
Angiotensin- and Bradykinin-Mediated Effects That Are Attenuated and
Potentiated, Respectively, During ACE Inhibition

Angiotensin-mediated effects	Bradykinin-mediated effects
Systemic vascular resistance	Protection from injury of ischemia/ reperfusion
Preload and afterload	Perfusion of vulnerable areas (regional)
Myocardial contractility	Rheology of blood (antithrombotic)
Myocardial oxygen consumption	Glucose supply and metabolism
Perfusion of heart and other vital organs	Antiarrhythmogenic effects
	Antimitotic-antiproliferative effects
Cellular growth and proliferation	Proinflammatory effect
	Nociception

bradykinin potentiation (Table 28-1). In general, the systemic hemodynamic changes (e.g., decrease in peripheral arterial resistance, fall in
blood pressure (BP), reduction of preload and afterload) are attributable
mainly to Ang II withdrawal, whereas bradykinin tends to redistribute
regional blood flows within organs (e.g., increase flow to subendocardial
rather than subepicardial regions in the heart, or to papillary rather
than medullary regions in the kidney). Notably, because of different
sensitivity of the vasculature of various organs to the vasoconstricting
effect of Ang II, ACE inhibition causes general redistribution of blood
flow favoring perfusion of vital organs; that is, it enhances the coronary,
renal, adrenal, and cerebral circulation at the expense of the musculo-
skeletal and cutaneous circulation *(4)*. This is of particular importance
in patients who benefit from very low systemic BPs (such as patients
with chronic CHF or diabetic nephropathy), which might otherwise
compromise the perfusion of vital tissues *(5)*. Under normal conditions,
ACE inhibition does not alter cardiac output or heart rate. However,
in patients with decompensated heart failure, characterized by neurohormonal activation (including activated RAS and catecholamines),
ACE inhibition increases cardiac output and decreases heart rate while
diminishing myocardial oxygen demands.

Two distinct types of Ang II receptors have been identified on
cell membranes and are designated as AT_1 and AT_2. Under normal
conditions, all of the currently known effects of Ang II are exerted via
activation of the AT_1 type of receptors. The AT_2 type of receptors are
believed to play a role mostly in fetal development, because their

Table 28-2
Actions of Ang II via AT_1 Receptor Stimulation

Systemic (endocrine) effects of circulating Ang II
  Vasoconstrictive (preferentially coronary, renal, cerebral)
  Steroidogenic (aldosterone)
  Dipsogenic (central nervous system effect)
  Renin-suppressing (negative feedback)

Tissue-specific effects of Ang II as local hormone
  Trophic/mitogenic (cardiac and vascular myocytes)
  Inotropic/contractile (cardiomyocytes)
  Chronotropic/arrythmogenic (cardiomyocytes)
  Thrombogenic (plasminogen activator inhibitor)
  Oxidative (generation of reactive oxygen species)
  Ion transport channels (myocytes, renal cells)
  Neuroexcitation (sympathetic nerve terminals)
  Endothelin stimulation (endothelial cells)

numbers decline sharply in the postnatal period. However, they increase again under pathologic conditions, such as the failing myocardium, in which they may be involved in apoptosis (i.e., cell death). In recent years it has become apparent that Ang II acts both as a circulating "endocrine" substance and as a locally generated autacoid exerting paracrine, autocrine, and intracrine effects (Table 28-2). The local effects are tissue specific; that is, they depend on the cell type responding to the Ang II stimulation. Thus, activation of AT_1 receptors in cardiomyocytes and vascular smooth muscle cells elicits changes in the electrophysiologic milieu (enhancing contractility and electric current conduction), as well as changes in the production of intracellular proteins, including protooncogenes and growth factors, leading to cell hypertrophy and proliferation (6). Endothelial cells respond by producing various autacoids (e.g., endothelin), neural cells by modulating release of neurotransmitters, fibroblasts and platelets by releasing growth factors, and so on.

Bradykinin also exerts its effects via specific receptors. The B_1 type of receptors are generated de novo under conditions of tissue inflammation or injury and mediate endotoxic shock. The physiologically important local hemodynamic and metabolic effects of bradykinin are mediated via the B_2 type of receptor. Stimulation of B_2 receptors results in the local release of autacoids, including nitric oxide and products of activation of the arachidonic acid cascade (e.g., protacyclin), which mediate the local vasodilatory, metabolic, and tissue-protective effects of bradykinin *(7)*. An important metabolic effect is the facilitation of insulin-dependent glucose transport across cell membranes. Essential hypertension is almost always associated with some degree of insulin resistance, which frequently progresses to overt type 2 diabetes mellitus. (The constellation of hyperinsulinemia, hyperglycemia, hyperlipidemia, hypertension, and abdominal adiposity—each trait being an independent coronary risk factor in its own right—is known as metabolic syndrome X and is encountered in 40–50% of patients with essential hypertension.) ACE inhibition tends to decrease insulin resistance, whereas other antihypertensive agents, such as thiazides and, to a lesser extent, β-adrenergic blockers, tend to accentuate it further. Experimental studies using specific antagonists to the B_2 bradykinin receptor and to various autacoid intermediaries, have determined that the effect on glucose transport is a direct effect of bradykinin itself *(8)*.

Bradykinin is also believed to be responsible for some of the adverse reactions to ACE inhibition, namely, cough and angioedema *(9)*. Both are attributed to the nociceptive and proinflammatory properties of bradykinin. The incidence of cough varies between 3% and 39% *(10)*, depending on the demographic characteristics of the population (more frequent in females vs males, in older vs younger patients, and in Caucasians vs African Americans with Orientals being the most sensitive). It is also aggravated by coexisting conditions, such as chronic CHF causing pulmonary congestion, or atmospheric pollutants causing heightened tracheobronchial irritability. Angioedema is extremely rare (about 1 in 2000 or less) but can be fatal if not recognized. It can occur at any time, even years after initiation of ACE inhibition, possibly triggered by allergens, which might have otherwise produced a minor reaction, that gets exaggerated by ACE inhibition. Both of these adverse effects are "class effects" encountered with all ACE inhibitors. Adverse reactions to withdrawal of Ang II are also "class effects" and will recur with every other ACE inhibitor as they are part of the drugs' pharmacologic profile (see Table 28-3). In contrast, adverse reactions due to idiosyncrasy of the patient against a particular compound are attributed to a drug's specific chemical structure. Such reactions are more common with captopril, especially at higher doses, but are rare with the "second generation" ACE inhibitors. Captopril is the only ACE inhibitor available in the U.S. that contains a sulfhydryl group in its molecule, which makes it likely to cause adverse reactions similar to those of other –SH– containing drugs with unrelated pharmacologic effects (e.g., penicillamine or thiureas). Idiosyncratic reactions will resolve upon changing to another drug of the same class, whereas

Table 28-3
Adverse Effects of ACE Inhibitors

Class effects
  Cough
  Angioedema
  Hyperkalemia
  Renal insufficiency (in bilateral renal artery disease)
  Hypotension (in hypovolemia)
  Teratogenesis (in pregnancy)

Idiosyncratic effects
  Allergic reactions (rash, fever)
  Interstitial nephritis
  Bone marrow suppression
  Taste alterations

Table 28-4
ACE Inhibitors Available in the United States

Generic name	Trade name	Daily dose range (mg)
Captopril	Capoten	50–200 (divided)
Enalapril	Vasotec, Renitec	2.5–40
Lisinopril	Zestril, Prinivil	5–80
Quinapril	Accupril	20–80
Benazepril	Lotensin	10–40
Fosinopril	Monopril	10–40
Ramipril	Altace	2.5–10
Trandolapril	Mavik	4–16
Moexipril	Univasc	7.5–15
Perindopril	Aceon	4–16

adverse reactions owing to the drug's pharmacologic properties require change to an agent from a different class.

CLINICAL EXPERIENCE WITH ACE INHIBITORS

The first orally active ACE inhibitor, captopril, was released in 1981 and was soon followed by a dozen second-generation ACE inhibitors. Table 28-4 lists those currently available in the United States along with the recommended daily doses for hypertension. In the treatment of CHF the starting doses should be the lowest. In fact, in patients with decompensated heart failure treated with diuretics, it is often recommended to start with low-dose captopril until it can be determined that the patient tolerates ACE inhibition without developing hypotension or functional renal insufficiency. Once tolerability has been ensured, the patient can be switched to one of the long-acting agents for convenience. In stable patients initiation of treatment with any ACE inhibitor is appropriate. All except captopril are long-acting once-a-day drugs, whose absorption is unaffected by the presence of food. They are effective as monotherapy in about 60% of unselected hypertensive patients, with no gender predilection. Preexisting levels of plasma renin activity do not predict the BP response of an individual—indeed, elderly patients who usually tend to have suppressed renin levels have nonetheless excellent response to ACE inhibition at lower doses than young or middle-aged patients *(11)*. African-American hypertensive patients tend to respond less well to monotherapy than Caucasians. However, the addition of a diuretic, which makes the BP more renin dependent, enhances the response of all patients to ACE inhibition and dissipates any racial differences. In addition to raising the response rate to >80%, this combination is also particularly effective in maintaining metabolic stability, because ACE inhibition attenuates the common side effects of diuretics (e.g., hypokalemia, hyperglycemia, hyperuricemia). A fixed combination of an ACE inhibitor with a thiazide can be used for convenience after an effective dose has been established.

Advantages of ACE inhibitors include the lack of side effects common to other antihypertensive classes (e.g., fatigue, drowsiness, impotence, forgetfulness) and the absence of adverse effects on coexisting conditions or concurrent treatments (e.g., chronic obstructive pulmonary disease, diabetes mellitus, ischemic heart diseases, heart failure, renal failure). Far from being contraindicated, for most of these conditions, the hemodynamic and metabolic consequences of ACE inhibition present distinct benefits: the enhanced insulin sensitivity is helpful in type 2 diabetes; the decrease in systemic vascular resistance and afterload is helpful in CHF; and the preferentially enhanced coronary blood flow and renal flow and the diminished intraglomerular pressures are beneficial for ischemic heart disease, renal insufficiency, and diabetic nephropathy, respectively. Because of its effect on intrarenal hemodynamics *(12)* (i.e., preferential vasodilation of efferent vs afferent arterioles with decreased intraglomerular pressure), ACE inhibition decreases proteinuria and protects the patient from developing glomerulosclerosis and renal failure. Chronic renal failure is no contraindication to the use of ACE inhibitors, provided the doses are adjusted to the level of creatinine clearance. Bilateral renal artery stenosis or stenosis of the artery to a single kidney is a contraindication, because ACE inhibition will precipitate functional renal insufficiency that can be reversed only by switching to a different class of drug.

Within tissues of target organs, the inhibition of locally generated Ang II and potentiation of local effects of bradykinin exert additional vasculoprotective, renoprotective, and cardioprotective actions in terms of prevention or reversal of vascular wall hypertrophy, nephrosclerotic lesions, left ventricular hypertrophy, and remodeling. In particular, ACE inhibition has been shown to protect the myocardium from acute ischemic and reperfusion injury, such as occurs after MI and reperfusion postthrombolysis.

The cardioprotective and renoprotective properties of ACE inhibition, first demonstrated in small clinical studies, have now been confirmed by a number of large, controlled, longitudinal multicenter trials in CHF *(13–15)* post MI *(16–19)*, diabetic nephropathy *(20)*, and chronic renal insufficiency *(21)*. All these trials, even those in which cardioprotection was not the primary objective, have established that ACE inhibitors protect the already injured myocardium from further damage. Indeed, they diminish the rate of recurrence of new events *(22)* and attenuate the rate of progression of heart failure *(13–19);* that is, they confer secondary cardioprotection. What has not yet been established is whether they can also confer primary cardioprotection, i.e., prevent or retard the onset of coronary disease in otherwise healthy hypertensive patients. Evidence from studies designed for other purposes, such as the Appropriate Blood Pressure Control in Diabetes (ABCD) trial *(23)*, the Fosinopril Amlodipine Cardiovascular Events Trial *(24)*, and Multicenter Isradipine Diuretic Atherosclerosis Study (MIDAS) *(25)*, as well as evidence from studies of chronic heart failure *(13–15)*, suggest that treatment with ACE inhibitors may indeed diminish the incidence of first heart attacks by about 25% *(22,26)*.

As many classes of safe and effective antihypertensive agents have become available over the past few decades, the goals of treatment have shifted from immediate BP lowering—which is taken for granted—to quality of life and long-term protection from cardiovascular complications. A favorable side effect profile is one of the most important factors in enhancing patient compliance and maintenance of good BP control, especially in otherwise healthy and asymptomatic patients. Effective BP lowering by any drug can successfully decrease the incidence of malignant hypertension, renal failure, stroke, and heart failure; however, the incidence of heart attacks has remained disproportionately elevated *(27)*, even with optimal BP control. A large, ongoing, long-term trial funded by the National Institutes of Health, the Antihypertensive Lipid Lowering Trial to Prevent Heart Attack *(28)*, is designed to compare the capacity of various classes of antihypertensives drugs to confer primary cardioprotection. Meanwhile, ACE inhibitors (and probably Ang II antagonists, as well), on the basis of their excellent tolerability and tissue-protective properties, seem to best fulfill both of the afore-mentioned goals.

REFERENCES

1. The Sixth Report of the joint National Committee on Prevention, Detection, Evaluation and Treatment of High Blood Pressure (1997) *Arch Intern Med* 157:2413–2446.
2. Gavras H, Brunner HR, Laragh JH, Sealey JE, Gavras I, Vukovich RA (1974) An angiotensin converting enzyme inhibitor to identify and treat vasoconstrictor and volume factors in hypertensive patients. *N Engl J Med* 291:817–821.
3. Erdos EG (1975) Angiotensin I converting enzyme. *Circ Res* 36:247–255.
4. Gavras H, Liang C, Brunner HR (1978) Redistribution of regional blood flow after inhibition of the angiotensin converting enzyme. *Circ Res* 43(Suppl. 1):59–63.
5. Faxon DP, Creager MA, Halperin JL, Gavras H, Coffman JD, Ryan TJ (1980) Central and peripheral hemodynamic effects of angiotensin inhibition in patients with refractory congestive heart failure. *Circulation* 61:925–931.
6. Dostal DE, Baker KM (1995) Biochemistry, molecular biology, and potential roles of the cardiac renin—angiotensin system. In Dhalla NS, Takeda N, Nagano M, eds. *The Failing Heart,* Philadelphia: Lippincott-Raven, pp. 275–294.
7. Regoli D, Rhaleb NE, Drapeau G, et al. (1989) Basic pharmacology of kinin: pharmacologic receptors and other mechanisms. In: Abe K, Moriya F, Fuji S, eds. *Kinins V,* Plenum NY, pp. 398–407.
8. Kohlman O Jr, De Assis Rocha Neves F, Ginoza M, Tavares A, Cezaretti ML, Zanella MT, Ribeiro AB, Gavras I, Gavras H (1995) Role of bradykinin in insulin sensitivity and blood pressure regulation during hyperinsulinemia. *Hypertension* 25:1003–1007.
9. Gavras I (1992) Bradykinin-mediated effects of ACE inhibition. *Kidney Int* 42:1020–1029.
10. Israili ZH, Hall WD (1992) Cough and angioneurotic edema associated with angiotensin-converting enzyme inhibitor therapy. *Ann Intern Med* 117:234–342.
11. Mulinari R, Gavras I, Gavras H (1987) Efficacy and tolerability of enalapril monotherapy in mild-to-moderate hypertension in older patients compared to younger patients. *Clin Ther* 9(6):678–692.
12. Anderson S, Rennke HG, Brenner BM (1986) Therapeutic advantage of converting enzyme inhibitors in arresting progressive renal disease associated with systemic hypertension in the rat. *J Clin Invest* 77:1993–2000.
13. The CONSENSUS Trial Study Group (1987) Effects of enalapril on mortality in

severe congestive heart failure: result of the Cooperative North Scandinavian Enalapril Survival Study (CONSENSUS). *N Engl J Med* 316:1429–1435.

14. The SOLVD Investigators. (1992) Effect of enalapril on mortality and the development of heart failure in asymptomatic patients with reduced left ventricular ejection fractions. *N Engl J Med* 327:685–691.

15. Cohn JN, Johnson G, Ziesche S, et al. (1991) A comparison of enalapril with hydralazine-isosorbide dinitrate in the treatment of chronic congestive heart failure. *N Engl J Med* 325:303–310.

16. Sharpe N, Murphy J, Smith H, Hannan S (1988) Treatment of patients with symptomless left ventricular dysfunction after myocardial infarction. *Lancet* 1:255–259.

17. Pfeffer MA, Lamas GA, Vaughan DE, Paris AF, Braunwald E (1988) Effect of captopril on progressive ventricular dilation after anterior myocardial infarction. *N Engl J Med* 319:80–86.

18. Pfeffer MA, Braunwald E, Moye LA, et al. (1992) Effect of captopril on mortality and morbidity in patients with left ventricular dysfunction after myocardial infarction: results of the Survival and Ventricular Enlargement trial. *N Engl J Med* 327:669–677.

19. The AIRE Study Investigators (1993) Effect of ramipril on mortality and morbidity of survivors of acute myocardial infarction with clinical evidence of heart failure. *Lancet* 342:821–828.

20. Clark CM Jr, Lee DA (1995) Prevention and treatment of the complications of diabetes mellitus. *N Engl J Med* 332:1210–1217.

21. The GISEN Group (1997) Randomized placebo-controlled trial of effect of ramipril on decline in glomerular filtration rate and risk of terminal renal failure in proteinuric, non-diabetic nephropathy. *Lancet* 349:1857–1863.

22. Yusuf S, Pepine CJ, Garces C, et al. (1992) Effect of enalapril on myocardial infarction and unstable angina in patients with low ejection fractions. *Lancet* 340:1173–1178.

23. Estacio RO, Jeffers BW, Hiatt WR, Biggi SL, Gifford N, Schrier RW (1998) The effect of nisoldipine as compared with enalapril on cardiovascular events in patients with non-insulin-dependent diabetes and hypertension. *N Engl J Med* 338:645–652.

24. Tatti P, Pahor M, Byington RP, DiMauro P, Guarisco R, Strollo F (1997) Results of the Fosinopril Amlodipine Cardiovascular Events Trial (FACET) in hypertensive patients with non-insulin dependent diabetes mellitus (NIDDM). *Circulation* 96(Suppl. I):I-764 (abstract).

25. Byington RP, Craven T, Furberg CD, Pahor M (1997) Isradipine, raised glycosylated haemoglobin, and risk of cardiovascular events. *Lancet* 350:1075, 1076.

26. Kostis JB (1995) The effect of enalapril on mortal and morbid events in patients with hypertension and left ventricular dysfunction. *Am J Hypertens* 8:909–914.

27. MacMahon SW, Cutler JA, Furberg CD, et al. (1986) The effects of drug treatment for hypertension morbidity and mortality from cardiovascular disease: a review of randomized controlled trials. *Progr Cardiovasc Dis* 29(Suppl. I):99–118.

28. Cavis BR, Cutler JA, Gordon DJ, et al. (1996) Rationale and design for the antihypertensive and lipid lowering treatment to prevent heart attack trial (ALLHAT). *Am J Hypertens* 9:342–360.

29 Angiotensin II Receptor Blockers

Michael A. Weber, MD

The angiotensin II (Ang II) receptor antagonists are the most selective blockers of the renin-angiotensin system (RAS) currently available. The efficacy of these drugs is similar to that of the other major antihypertensive drug classes, but they appear to exhibit fewer side effects. Angiotensin receptor blockers (ARBs) selectively block the angiotensin AT_1 receptors, leaving AT_2 receptors exposed to increased circulating concentrations of Ang II. It is not yet known whether the AT_2 receptor is expressed or mediates meaningful hemodynamic or vascular effects in clinical hypertension. ARB and angiotensin-converting enzyme (ACE) inhibitors differ in their interactions with the RAS, bradykinin, and other neurohormonal mediators; the two drug classes have similar hemodynamic effects, but it is not yet known whether they might have differential impacts on clinical outcomes. Although ARBs are still relatively new, several rigorous clinical trials with morbidity and mortality end points are already in progress.

From: *Hypertension Medicine*
Edited by: M. A. Weber © Humana Press Inc., Totowa, NJ

RATIONALE FOR THE USE OF ARBs IN TREATING HYPERTENSION

Blocking the RAS is a rational approach to treating hypertension. Ang II contributes in two major ways to the clinical picture of hypertension: it raises blood pressure (BP) through its vasoconstrictor actions, and it has trophic actions on the heart and circulation that might contribute directly to cardiovascular and renal events. The RAS can be interrupted by β-blockers, which decrease renal renin secretion, and by ACE inhibitors, which limit conversion of angiotensin I (Ang I) to Ang II. ARBs, however, provide the most direct means for antagonizing this system.

PHARMACOLOGY

The ARBs bind selectively to the AT_1 receptor, thereby blocking the vasoconstrictor and other actions typically exhibited by Ang II. The binding of these nonpeptidic orally administered agents to the AT_1 receptors can be either competitive or nonsurmountable. Some ARBs are prodrugs that require conversion to an active metabolite. To date, there is no evidence of clinical differences between drugs that work in their parent form or those that are prodrugs.

All the available ARBs are effective when dosed once daily, although there may be pharmacokinetic differences among them that could produce differences in BP effects during a 24-h period. Comparisons using ambulatory BP monitoring will be required to determine whether these differences are clinically meaningful. The effects of these agents on renal function, natriuresis, and metabolic factors have not been fully defined, and it is not possible to determine whether some agents might have advantages over others.

Ang II RECEPTORS

At least four Ang II receptors have been described: AT_1, AT_2, AT_3, and AT_4. Only the first two of these have been well defined. The AT_1 receptor mediates most of the known physiologic actions of Ang II. Recently genetic polymorphisms of this receptor have been described, but it is not known whether these variations are important. The AT_2

Table 29-1
Ang II Receptors and Effects of Blockade

Vascular AT_1 receptors
    Constantly expressed
    Mediate vasoconstriction
    Mediate Ang II arterial wall growth effects

Vascular AT_2 receptors
    Expressed only after injury (sustained hypertension might provoke
        expression)
    Mediate vasodilation
    Mediate antiproliferative actions
    Activate other factors (e.g., nitric oxide)

Potential double action of selective AT_1 blockers
    Directly block vasoconstrictor and growth actions of Ang II at AT_1
        receptors
    Increase circulating Ang II levels
    Unblocked AT_2 receptors (if expressed) stimulated by increased Ang II
        activity, mediate vasodilation and growth inhibition
    Net effects: AT_1 blockade plus AT_2 stimulation

---

receptor is found primarily during fetal development and appears to
mediate programmed cell death or apoptosis. The AT_2 receptor can be
expressed in normal adults in response to trauma or other injuries. It
is possible that such stimuli as aging and high BP could sufficiently
affect the vasculature to evoke the expression of these receptors. When
stimulated by Ang II, these receptors mediate vasodilation and inhibi-
tory effects on cell growth. Recently, stimulation of these receptors
has been shown to increase nitric oxide production. Because administration of ARBs increases circulating Ang II levels, it is possible that they
work through a dual mechanism: first, direct blockade of the AT_1
receptor; and, second, stimulation of the AT_2 receptor. Tissue culture
studies have confirmed that AT_1 blockade reduces cell growth and
that AT_2 blockade (with experimental agents) increases cell growth;
simultaneous blockade of the AT_1 receptor and stimulation of the AT_2
receptor (the putative situation when an ARB is used) results in an
enhanced antiproliferative effect. These interesting possibilities, which
have yet to be documented in the clinical setting, are summarized in
Table 29-1.

USE OF ARBs IN HYPERTENSION

The efficacy of ARBs is similar to that found with other widely used antihypertensive drugs. More interesting, though, is the question of whether ARBs exhibit dose-response relationships. The lowest effective dose of losartan, the first of this class to be available, is 50 mg. The efficacy achieved with 100 mg, however, is not greater; moreover, doubling the dose of losartan in patients not responding adequately to 50 mg does not provide substantive further benefit. On the other hand, such agents as valsartan, irbesartan, telmisartan, eprosartan, or candasartan appear to have greater efficacy at higher doses, although even with these agents the dose-response curves tend to be rather shallow. This poses an interesting but still unanswered question: When patients fail to respond fully to an initial dose, should a higher dose be given or should a second drug be added?

ARBs work equally well in older and younger patients as well as in men and women. Preliminary data suggest that African-American patients might also respond to these agents. In particular, with agents such as valsartan and tasosartan there is a shift in the dose-response curves such that higher doses can produce antihypertensive efficacies similar to those observed in Caucasians. It is not clear whether this phenomenon reflects pharmacokinetic differences between the two population groups or whether it reflects lower levels of renin activity in African-American patients. Additional studies are important, particularly because African-American patients are especially vulnerable to the renal and other consequences of hypertension that might be addressed by this new drug class. There have been relatively few studies of ARBs in combination with other antihypertensive agents. As with ACE inhibitors, diuretics appear to be a logical addition to ARBs. Experiences with combinations with other drug classes such as calcium channel blockers have not yet been published.

SIDE EFFECTS

The absence of symptomatic and metabolic adverse events with ARBs is one of their strong attributes. The incidence of side effects is not different from that in placebo-treated patients. Cough is less common than with ACE inhibitors and is probably similar in incidence to other drug classes. Note, however, that there have been rare case reports of angioedema with ARBs. Like ACE inhibitors, they should be avoided during pregnancy and in patients with bilateral renovascular disease.

CLINICAL END POINTS

It is too early for definitive data. Studies of heart effects have been inconsistent: left ventricular hypertrophy has been shown to be regressed or unchanged by ARBs in different trials, though recent studies indicate benefit. Studies in congestive heart failure (CHF) have shown that ARBs have effects on hemodynamics and symptoms similar to those with ACE inhibitors. There have been no studies of the effects of ARBs on arteries in humans, but these drugs have reversed arterial wall hypertrophy in such animal models as the spontaneously hypertensive rat. ARBs have significantly reduced proteinuria in nephrotic patients as well as in hypertensive patients with or without diabetes mellitus. Some early studies indicate that candasartan and losartan might improve insulin sensitivity in hypertension.

Arbs VS ACE INHIBITORS

Beyond their comparable efficacies, there are potentially important differences between ARBs and ACE inhibitors. ACE inhibitors do not fully interrupt the RAS; during chronic treatment, enzymes such as chymase might substitute for ACE and convert Ang I to Ang II. On the other hand, ACE inhibitors reduce bradykinin breakdown, thus increasing bradykinin availability and secondarily increasing vasodilatory prostaglandins and nitric oxide. These substances may contribute to both the hemodynamic and cardioprotective effects of ACE inhibitors. The differential effects of ARBs on the Ang II receptors (discussed earlier) may provide similar but qualitatively different benefits. Because of their differences, combinations of ACE inhibitors and ARBs have been studied both in congestive heart failure (no end point data yet available) and in hypertension. Early evidence suggests that the BP effects of these two classes may indeed be additive, although such study design issues as choosing optimal dosing have limited the conclusions. ACE inhibitors have clear clinical benefits when used in heart failure, following myocardial infarction, and in diabetic nephropathy. No such data are yet available with ARBs. In one small study, losartan was associated with a lower mortality rate than the ACE inhibitor captopril in patients with CHF, but this could not be confirmed in a follow-up study.

CLINICAL TRIALS

It is encouraging that the manufacturers of ARBs are already supporting major clinical outcome studies in hypertension. For example, losartan is being compared with atenolol, and valsartan with amlodipine, in older high-risk hypertensive patients. The end points for these studies are fatal and nonfatal cardiovascular events and strokes. Other ARBs, including irbesartan and candasartan, are being studied for their renoprotective and cardioprotective effects.

SUGGESTED READINGS

Bermann MA, Walsh MF, Sowers JR (1997) Angiotensin-II biochemistry and physiology: update on angiotensin-II receptor blockers. *Cardiovasc Rev* 15(1):75–100.

Messerli FH, Weber MA, Brunner HR (1996) Angiotensin II receptor inhibition: a new therapeutic principle. *Arch Intern Med* 156:1957–1965.

DeGasparo M, Bottari S, Leven NR (1995) Characteristics of angiotensin II receptors and their role in cell and organ physiology. In: Laragh JH, Brenner BM, eds. *Hypertension: Pathophysiology, Diagnosis, and Management,* 2nd ed., New York: Raven, pp. 1695–1720.

Azizi M, Guyene TT, Chatellier G, Wargon M, Monard J (1997) Additive effects of losartan and enalapril on blood pressure and plasma active renin. *Hypertension* (2):634–640.

Benz J, Oshrain C, Henry D, Avery C, Chiang YT, Gatlin M (1997) Valsartan, a new angiotensin II receptor antagonist: a double-blind study comparing the incidence of cough with lisinopril and hydrochlorothiazide. *J Clin Pharmacol* 37(2):101–107.

Almazov VA, Shlyakhto EV, Conrady AO, Brodskaya IS, Zaharov DV (1997) Effects of losartan on left ventricular mass and heart rate variability in hypertensive patients. *Cardiovasc Drugs Ther* 11(Suppl. 2):406.

Chan JNC, Critchley JAJH, Tomlinson B, Chan TYK, Cockram CS (1997) Antihypertensive and anti-albuminuric effects of losartan potassium and felodipine in Chinese elderly hypertensive patients with or without non-insulin-dependent diabetes mellitus. *Am J Nephrol* 17(1):72–80.

Paolisso G, Tagliamonte MR, Gambardella A, Manzella D, Gualdiero P, Varricchio G, Verza M, Varricchio M (1997) Losartan mediated improvement in insulin action is mainly due to an increase in non-oxidative glucose metabolism and blood flow in insulin-resistant hypertensive patients. *J Hum Hypertens* 11(5):307–312.

Pitt B, Segal R, Martinez FA, Meurers G, Cowley AC, Thomas I, Deedwania PC, Ney DE, Snavely DB, Chang PI (1997) Randomised trial of losartan versus captopril in patients over 65 with heart failure (Evaluation of Losartan in the Elderly Study ELITE). *Lancet* 349(9054:747–752.

Weber MA (1997) Angiotensin II receptor antagonists in the treatment of hypertension. *Cardiol Rev* 5(2):72–80.

30 Selective α_1-Blockers

Joseph L. Izzo Jr., MD

α_1 Adrenergic blockers (prazosin/Minipress, terazosin/Hytrin, and doxazosin/Cardura) are approved antihypertensive drugs with a generally favorable profile of safety and tolerability. They have not gained widespread sustained use in hypertension because of their relatively limited monotherapeutic efficacy and their tendency to cause significant first-dose hypotension and sustained postural hypotension, both of which are magnified by salt depletion and interactions with diuretics and other antihypertensive medications. Opportunities remain for use in essential hypertension, especially with concomitant hypercholesterolemia or symptoms of prostatism. Other possible areas of use include Raynaud syndrome and cardiac failure, especially in combination with other agents.

α-RECEPTOR PHYSIOLOGY AND BLOCKADE

α-Adrenergic receptors are divided into two major types: α_1 and α_2. Although additional minor subtypes can be defined pharmacologically, their clinical significance is currently unclear. α_1 Receptors, which are

From: *Hypertension Medicine*
Edited by: M. A. Weber © Humana Press Inc., Totowa, NJ

usually located on postganglionic synaptic membranes in cardiac and vascular smooth muscle, cause vasoconstriction through stimulation of inositol triphosphate and phospholipase-C, with subsequent release of intracellular calcium. α_2 Receptors, which are located on both presynaptic and postsynaptic membranes in the central and peripheral nervous systems and on blood vessels, platelets, and white blood cells, are linked to G-proteins and inhibit adenylate cyclase. In general, stimulation of α_2-receptors (with agents such as clonidine, guanfacine, or methyldopa) causes a weak direct peripheral vasoconstriction, which is subsequently overcome by the powerful ability of α_2-agonists to inhibit central sympathetic nervous outflow and neuronal norepinephrine release. As a result, α_2-agonists decrease pressure (BP) in all types of hypertension. By contrast, blockers of α_2-receptors (such as yohimbine) cause weak peripheral vasodilation and marked central nervous sympathetic stimulation, thereby increasing BP.

Blockade of α_1-receptors with prazosin (Minipress), terazosin (Hytrin), or doxazosin (Cardura) effectively displaces norepinephrine and epinephrine from vascular smooth muscle and interrupts peripheral sympathetic neurotransmission. There are negligible effects of α_1-blockers on the central nervous system owing to their inability to effectively penetrate the blood-brain barrier. Hemodynamically, α_1-blockers cause both venous and arterial dilation and thus do not tend to cause a reflex increase in cardiac output. Selective α_1-blockers have greater antihypertensive potency than nonselective α-blockers such as phentolamine or phenoxybenzamine, which today are used primarily in the management of pheochromocytoma.

EFFECTS ON POSTURAL HOMEOSTASIS

Normal assumption of upright posture requires instantaneous reflex activation of the sympathetic nervous system (SNS), which maintains upright BP via instantaneous venous and arterial constriction and a concomitant increase in heart rate. During α_1-blockade, blunted reflex venous and arterial constriction during upright posture results in a tendency for greater pooling of blood in the lower extremities and greater BP reduction in the upright than supine position. In extreme cases, especially during periods of extracellular volume depletion or in individuals with impaired baroreflex sensitivity, symptomatic orthostatic hypotension or dizziness can occur. Orthostatic increases in cardiac sympathetic nerve traffic are not affected by α_1-blockers and postural tachycardia or palpitations are sometimes seen as a result of exaggerated postural sympathetic activation during chronic α₁-blockade.

OTHER CLINICAL EFFECTS

In addition to their effects on BP, α₁-blockers have other potentially favorable effects.

Lipid Lowering

A small decrease in low-density lipoprotein, cholesterol has been reported in short-term studies of α₁-blockers, with little change in high-density lipoprotein cholesterol. Effects on triglycerides are modestly negative, probably owing to the tendency for these drugs to activate the SNS. The true clinical significance of this effect has not been studied, however.

Bladder Emptying

Bladder sphincters are richly innervated by sympathetic neurons, and bladder emptying can be impaired by excessive sympathetic activation. A modest positive effect of moderate doses of α₁-blockers has been observed in men suffering from decreased force of urinary stream, urinary retention, and other symptoms of early prostatism. This effect has caused the widespread use of α₁-blockers by urologists and a clinical indication exists for such symptoms.

Raynaud Syndrome

Raynaud syndrome, a painful manifestation of excessive digital cutaneous vasoconstriction often found in healthy young women and in people with scleroderma, may respond to low doses of α₁-blockers (1 to 2 mg daily in some cases).

Heart Failure

Prazosin in combinaton with diuretics or hydralazine has been used on occasion in patients with chronic heart failure. Although this combined regimen achieves a degree of venous and arterial dilation, the efficacy of α_1-blockers in heart failure appears to be far less than that of angiotensin-converting enzyme (ACE) inhibitors.

PHARMACODYNAMIC INTERACTIONS

The addition of various cardiovascular drugs can affect BP and orthostatic homeostasis when combined with α_1-blockers.

Thiazide Diuretics

Thiazides generally potentiate the antihypertensive effects of α-blockers. Because thiazides are direct-acting arterial vasodilators, they complement the indirect vasodilation of α_1-blockers. As arterial dilators, however, they further activate the SNS and tend to potentiate both favorable BP-lowering effects and unfavorable postural hypotension and tachycardia. The antihypertensive effects of α_1-blockers are dependent on extracellular fluid volume status. To the extent that thiazides affect extracellular fluid volume status (usually minimally), they further enhance the effects of α_1-blockers.

β-Blockers

Postural adaptation is often impaired by the addition of β-blockade to α_1-blockade because the greater heart rate response to upright posture seen during α-blockade is blunted. This pattern is also seen with α-β-blockers such as labetalol.

Nitrates

As strong venodilators, nitrates have their own tendency to favor postural BP decreases, particularly in elderly individuals with impaired cardiac systolic or diastolic function who are dependent on high venous pressure (preload) to drive cardiac output. Particular care must be taken if α-blockers (or nitrates) are to be considered in older individuals, with gradual dose titration and careful monitoring of orthostatic BP changes.

RATIONAL CLINICAL USE

The astute clinician can identify several clinical situations in which α-blockers may be useful. Several points can enhance routine use, which are discussed next.

Monitoring of Orthostasis

It is important to measure postural changes in BP in all patients being considered for drug therapy. With α-blockers in particular, I recommend monitoring upright BPs along with sitting or preferably supine BPs. It is my experience that the symptomatic patients have the greatest differences between upright and supine BPs on therapy.

Dose Times

I do not concur with manufacturers' recommendations that bedtime administration is preferred over morning dosing initially and chronically because of potential problems of orthostatic hypotension. Many older individuals experience chronic nocturia. Given that BP usually decreases during the hours of sleep and that orthostatic tolerance is often impaired in elderly individuals, there is greater potential for orthostatic symptoms to occur overnight. It therefore seems more prudent to administer the first dose in the morning along with the admonition to the patient that initial orthostatic symptoms can be alleviated by recumbency with the legs elevated if necessary.

First-Dose Effects and Chronic Underdosing

A strong first-dose effect is common with α_1-blockers. Manufacturers have therefore recommended that the initial doses be low (usually 1 mg) to minimize the chance of hypotensive symptoms with the first dose. Fortunately, subsequent doses are usually much better tolerated. For the purposes of chronic BP lowering, daily doses of 10–20 mg of any α_1-blocker (prazosin, terazosin, or doxazosin) are often required. Unfortunately, many clinicians fail to titrate to these higher doses, leaving patients with inadequate BP control.

Urologic Use and Unrecognized
Pharmacodynamic Interactions

I have seen several cases in which information that an α_1-blocker was prescribed by a urologist for urinary hesitancy was not relayed to the primary care physician. Subsequent use of other cardiovascular agents, especially thiazide diuretics, β-blockers, nitrates, or ACE inhibitors then caused orthostatic symptoms, which were attributed to the later drug rather than to the pharmacodynamic interaction of the later drug with the α_1-blocker. Good communication between physicians and periodic review of all current medications is essential for prevention of these untoward effects.

REFERENCES

1. Izzo JL Jr (1999) The sympathetic nervous system in human hypertension. In Izzo JL, Black HR, eds. *Hypertension Primer,* Lippincott Williams & Wilkins, pp. 109–112.
2. Berecek KH, Carey RM (1999) Adrenergic and dopaminergic receptors and actions. In Izzo JL, Black HR, eds. *Hypertension Primer,* Baltimore: Lippincott Williams & Wilkins, pp. 3–6.
3. Grimm RH (1999) Alpha adrenergic blockers. In Izzo JL, Black HR, eds. *Hypertension Primer,* Baltimore: Lippincott Williams & Wilkins, pp. 366–367.

31 Centrally Acting Antihypertensive Drugs

Mark Houston, MD, FACP

CONTENTS

The centrally acting antihypertensive drugs are one of the oldest classes still in use for the treatment of hypertension. As a group, their common and unique mechanism of action is to stimulate receptors in the brain that reduce sympathetic nervous system (SNS) activity, and lower blood pressure (BP), heart rate, and systemic vascular resistance while preserving cardiac output *(1)*. The overall hemodynamic and metabolic profiles are quite favorable for these drugs, but their clinical use has been limited owing to side effects of sedation, dry mouth, or mild depression. Recently, newer centrally acting drugs have been developed that are more specific for the imidazoline receptor, which results in excellent antihypertensive effects but minimal to no adverse

From: *Hypertension Medicine*
Edited by: M. A. Weber © Humana Press Inc., Totowa, NJ

effects *(2)*. These newer agents will assume an important role in the future management of hypertension as monotherapy or in combination with other antihypertensive drugs.

CENTRALLY ACTING DRUGS

The centrally acting drugs all stimulate the central postsynaptic α_2-receptor or the imidazoline receptor in the brain stem, which reduces the SNS activity to the periphery *(1–3)*. Methyldopa (Aldomet), clonidine (Catapres), guanabenz (Wytensin), and guanfacine (Tenex) stimulate the α_2-receptor more than the I_1-imidazoline receptor *(2)*. Reserpine depletes catecholamine stores in both the central and peripheral nervous systems and differs significantly from the other centrally acting drugs in virtually all respects. Its use is quite limited owing to side effects and therefore is not discussed in this chapter.

MECHANISM OF ACTION

Stimulation of α-adrenergic or imidazoline receptors in the nucleus reticularis lateralis of the rostroventrolateral part of the medulla is the primary mechanism of action of the centrally acting drugs *(1–3)*. The α-adrenergic-binding sites are of two types: presynaptic and postsynaptic. Stimulation of the postsynaptic α_2-receptor centrally lowers BP slightly, but is mostly responsible for the side effects of sedation and dry mouth *(1,3)*.

The imidazoline-binding sites are also of two types: I_1, which is sensitive to clonidine and idazoxan; and I_2, which is sensitive to idazoxan and largely insensitive to clonidine *(2)*. Stimulation of the I_2-imidazoline receptors lowers BP without the side effects of sedation and dry mouth *(2)*. Stimulation of both receptors may be necessary to trigger the central hypotensive response *(2)*. The relative selectivity for the receptors determines the efficacy and the effects of the centrally acting agents.

HEMODYNAMIC EFFECTS

In general, the centrally acting agents lower BP, reduce SNS activity, reduce heart rate, lower systemic vascular resistance, and preserve cardiac output at rest and during exercise *(1,3,4)*. In addition, norepinephrine, aldosterone, angiotensin II (Ang II) levels, and plasma renin activity (PRA) are decreased; renal blood flow, renal plasma flow, and glomerular filtration rate do not change or increase; renal vascular resistance is reduced; and there is a sodium-water diuresis in some patients *(3,4)*. The sodium-water diuresis is especially prominent with rilmenidine and mononidine and, to a lesser extent, with clonidine, guanabenz, and guanfacine, owing to selective binding to renal I_1-imidazoline receptors *(1–4)*. Table 31-1 compares the hemodynamic effects.

PHARMACODYNAMICS, DOSES, AND METABOLIC EFFECTS

Table 31-2 lists the onset of action, peak effects, plasma half-life, metabolism, excretion, and recommended doses *(5)*. Clonidine, guanabenz, and guanfacine all have a neutral or favorable effect on serum lipids and glucose compared with methyldopa, which has an unfavorable effect. Methyldopa reduces high-density lipoprotein cholesterol and increases triglycerides. There is little reason to use methyldopa now because the side effects are greater than and the efficacy is inferior to those of the other centrally acting drugs *(4,5)*.

EFFECTS OF CENTRALLY ACTING DRUGS ON CORONARY HEART DISEASE RISK FACTORS

Centrally acting drugs have an overall favorable effect on coronary heart disease (CHD) risk factors. Of the 18 modifiable CHD risk factors, clonidine, guanabenz, and guanfacine have no adverse effects, giving them a 0:18 CHD relative risk ratio *(see* Table 31-3) *(4,5)*. Methyldopa has a 2:18 CHD relative risk ratio. The newer agents rilmenidine and mononidine are less well studied in this regard.

CLINICAL USE

Antihypertensive efficacy is excellent and similar with all of the centrally acting drugs. Selection of therapy depends more on some of the unique side effects, metabolic and pharmacologic effects, duration

Table 31-1
Hemodynamics of Centrally Acting Drugs[a]

Clonidine	Guanabenz	Guanfacine	Methyldopa	Rilmenidine and Mononidine
MAP reduced	MAP reduced	MAP reduced	MAP reduced	MAP reduced
CO unchanged	CO unchanged	CO unchanged	CO unchanged or some decrease	CO unchanged
HR reduced (10%)	HR reduced (minimal)	HR reduced (10%)	HR slightly decreased	HR reduced
SVR reduced	SVR reduced	SVR reduced	SVR decreased	SVR reduced
RBF, RPF, GFR: no change or increase	RBF, RPF, GFR: no change	RBF, RPF, GFR: no change or increase	RBF, RPR, GFR: no change	RBF, RPF, GFR: no change or increase
RVR reduced	RVR reduced	RVR reduced	RVR reduced	RVR reduced
Plasma and urinary NE and EPI reduced	Plasma and urinary NE and EPI reduced	Plasma and urinary NE and EPI reduced	Ang II reduced	Plasma and urinary NE and EPI reduced
Ang II reduced	Aldosterone reduced	Ang II reduced	PRA reduced	Ang II reduced
PRA reduced	PRA reduced	PRA reduced	Aldosterone reduced	PRA reduced
Aldosterone reduced	Ang II reduced	Aldosterone reduced	Exercise response preserved	Aldosterone reduced
Exercise response preserved	Exercise response preserved	Exercise response preserved	Plasma volume increased	Exercise response preserved
PWP reduced	Plasma volume unchanged	PWP reduced		PWP reduced
Fluid retention: minimal to none	Diuresis in some patients	Fluid retention: minimal to none		Diuresis
Diuresis in some patients		Diuresis in some patients		Natriuresis

[a]CO, cardiac output; EPI, epinephrine; GFR, glomerular filtration rate; HR, heart rate; MAP, mean arterial pressure; NE, norepinephrine; PRA, plasma renin activity; PWP, pulmonary wedge pressure; RBF, renal blood flow; RPF, renal plasma flow; RVR, renal vascular resistance; SVR, systemic vascular resistance.

Table 31-2
Pharmacodynamics[a]

Drug	Preparation	Mechanism of action	Pharmacodynamics	Adverse effects	Contraindications	Daily dosage
Clonidine (Catapres)	0.1 mg (oral) 0.2 mg (oral) 0.3 mg (oral) TTS 1–3	Selective stimulation of postsynaptic α_2-adrenergic receptors in depressor site of vasomotor center of medulla, nucleus tractus solitari, and hypothalamus; reduces efferent sympathetic tone and increases vagal tone to heart, peripheral vasculature, and kidney; reduces SVR, causing vasodilation and lowering BP; spares peripheral reflexes; reduces PRA.	Onset: 1/2–1 h Peak: 3–5 h Plasma half-life: 12–16 h Metabolism: liver (minimal) Excretion: renal TTS—duration of antihypertensive effect: 1 wk	Sedation and drowsiness; dry mouth; dizziness; withdrawal syndrome and rebound hypertension (uncommon with doses <1.2 mg qd); weakness; headache; bradycardia; constipation; impotence (uncommon—4%)	Sick sinus syndrome; second or third-degree AV block	Initial: 0.1 mg hs and increase by 0.1 mg q 3–4 d, giving larger bid doses at bedtime. Some qd. Usually bid Average: 0.4–0.6 mg Maximum: 1.2 mg Range: 0.2–1.2 mg TTS: once per week TTS: 1, 2, or 3
Guanabenz (Wytensin)	4 mg 8 mg	Stimulation of postsynaptic α_2 receptors in medulla reduces sympathetic activity and reduces SVR and PRA.	Onset: 1 h Peak: 4 h Plasma and half-life: 6 h Metabolism: 75% (site undetermined) Excretion: renal, 80%	Dry mouth; sedation and drowsiness; fatigue; impotence; withdrawal syndrome; rebound and overshoot hypertension; dizziness; headache; constipation	Pregnancy	Average dose: 16 mg Range: 8–48 mg Maximum: 48 mg

continued

343

Table 31-2
Continued

Drug	Preparation	Mechanism of action	Pharmacodynamics	Adverse effects	Contraindications	Daily dosage
Guanfacine (Tenex)	1 mg 2 mg	Reduces sympathetic tone, SVR, and HR.	Onset: 1 h Peak: 4 h Plasma half-life: 12 h Excretion: renal	See Clonidine	Allergy to guanfacine	1 mg hs Maximum: 3 mg hs
Methyldopa (Aldomet)	125 mg 250 mg 500 mg Also available in elixir (250 mg/mL)	α-Methylnorepinephrine stimulates a postsynaptic α_2-adrenergic receptor in the medulla and decreases sympathetic outflow, which reduces SVR and PRA. Also has some peripheral action.	Onset: 2–3 h Peak: 5 h Plasma half-life: 12 h Metabolism: hepatic Excretion: renal	Lassitude; drowsiness and sedation; dry mouth; mild orthostasis; positive Coombs Test and anemia; positive rheumatoid factor and lupus erythematosus preparation; impotence; hepatitis withdrawal syndrome; rebound and overshoot hypertension; altered mental acuity; depression	Active hepatic disease	Average: 250–300 mg bid schedule Maximum: 3000 mg
Rilmenidine	1 mg	Stimulates I_1 imidazoline receptor	—	Minimal	—	1–2 mg

[a]AV, atric ventricular; TTS, transdermal therapy; SVR, systonic vascular resistance; PRA, plasma renin activity; HR, heart rate.

Table 31-3
CHD Risk Factors and Centrally Acting Drugs[a]

	Central	Methyldopa
Hypertension	↓	↓
Dyslipidemia	↓	↑
Glucose intolerance	↓	→
Insulin resistance	↓	→
LVH	↓	↓
Exercise	→	→
Potassium	→	→
Magnesium	→	→
Uric acid	→/↓	→/↓
Blood viscosity	→	→
Blood velocity	↓	↑
Catecholamines	↓	↓
Ang II	↓	↓
Arrhythmia potential	↓	↓
Fibrinogen	?	?
Platelet function	↓	→
Thrombogenic potential	?	?
Antiatherogenic	?	?
CHD relative risk ratio	0:18	2:18

[a]↓, Reduced; ↑, increased; →, no change; ?, unknown. LVH, left ventricular hypertrophy; CHD, coronary heart disease.

of action, mode of administration, and cost. All are effective as monotherapy.

Combination therapy with diuretics, calcium channel blockers (CCBs), angiotension-converting enzyme (ACE) inhibitors, and angiotension receptor blockers (ARBs) have added or synergistic activity with reduced side effects, particularly if low-dose combination therapy is used (4,5). Using a centrally acting agent with an α-blocker may result in antagonism in a majority of patients through competing effects at the receptor binding site. Concomitant use with a β-blocker may be effective in most patients but may result in central antagonism in a minority. In addition, there is a higher risk for bradycardia or heart block and a more frequent or more severe withdrawal syndrome if both drugs are discontinued simultaneously or the centrally acting drug is stopped abruptly and the β-blocker is continued (3–6).

Combination therapy may also reduce left ventricular hypertrophy better than with monotherapy especially when CCBs, ACE inhibitors and ARBs *(2–5)* are used with centrally acting drugs. Reduction in SNS activity with centrally acting drugs may reduce cardiac ischemic events and supraventricular and ventricular arrhythmias when used as monotherapy or in combination *(2–5)*. Two centrally acting drugs should never be used together. These drugs should be initiated in low doses with the predominant dose at night to allow the patient to become tolerant to sedative side effects. The dose should be increased gradually every 2–4 wk until the maximum doses are attained or goal BP is achieved.

Clonidine may be administered orally or transdermally. Oral therapy is appropriate for chronic hypertension and in hypertensive urgencies in carefully selected patients *(7)*. Transdermal therapy (TTS) given once a week, has fewer side effects owing to lower steady-state plasma levels, but the efficacy is equal to oral therapy *(4,5)*. In general, the equivalent TTS therapy is three fourths the oral dose (i.e., clonidine at 0.4 mg orally/d = Catapres TTS – 3 once per wk) *(4,5)*. It takes 24–48 h for TTS to achieve adequate plasma levels, but some of the antihypertensive effects persist 48 h after the TTS is discontinued. The other drugs are available only in oral form except methyldopa, which can be administered intravenously or orally. The dose equivalency is as follows: 0.1 mg of clonidine = 4 mg of guanabenz = 0.25 mg of guanfacine = 250–500 mg of methyldopa *(5)*. Oral clonidine and methyldopa must be given twice daily unless renal impairment is present that would reduce excretion. Guanabenz, guanfacine, rilmenidine, and mononidine may be given once daily. The centrally acting drugs have very few contraindications and can be given to patients with many concomitant diseases such as hyperlipidemia, diabetes mellitus, angina, congestive heart failure, renal insufficiency, obstructive lung disease, peripheral vascular disease, and to patients with a history of cerebro-vascular accidents *(4,5)*. Clonidine may be particularly useful in patients with concomitant addictive syndromes (opiates, alcohol, tobacco), anxiety, supraventricular tachycardia, diabetic diarrhea, essential tremor, menopausal symptoms, migraine headache, and mitral valve prolapse *(4,5)*.

ADVERSE EFFECTS

Common side effects of the centrally acting drugs are sedation and dry mouth, which are minimal with low-dose long-term therapy. Concern about a withdrawal syndrome has been overemphasized with all these drugs, particularly clonidine. When low doses are used, the frequency of withdrawal syndrome is minimal and probably less than that with β-blockers. Other adverse effects are given in Table 31-2 *(4,5)*.

DRUG INTERACTIONS

Tricyclic antidepressants, monoamine oxidase inhibitors, and phenothiazines may frequently interfere with the antihypertensive effects. Central nervous system depressant or sedative drugs may be potentiated. β-Blockers may interfere with the antihypertensive effects in a minority of patients. Oral contraceptives may reduce methyldopa's antihypertensive effect, and iron salts may reduce its absorption. Methyldopa may increase lithium levels *(4,5)*.

CONCLUSION

Centrally acting antihypertensive agents are extremely effective antihypertensive drugs with a favorable hemodynamic, metabolic, and CHD risk factor profile. They can be used in many concomitant diseases with excellent effects and are relatively cost-effective. Adverse effects have limited their use, but new agents with selectivity for imidazoline receptors will result in good BP control and a marked reduction in side effects. These agents will add to our growing armamentarium of antihypertensive drugs that can be used as monotherapy or in combination with other agents.

REFERENCES

1. Buhler FR, Krakoff LR, Brunner HR, Buckalew VM, Weber MA (1984) Centrally acting agents in antihypertensive therapy. *J Cardiovasc Pharmacol* 6(Suppl. 5): S725–S858.
2. Bousquet P, Esler MI (1998) Agents in high blood pressure and cardioprotection management: the contribution of rilmenidine. *J Hypertens* 16(Suppl. 3):SI–S62.
3. Houston MC (1981) Clonidine hydrochloride: review of pharmacologic and clinical aspects. *Prog Cardiovasc Dis* 23:337–350.
4. Houston MC (1992) New insights and approaches to reduce end organ damage in the treatment of hypertension: subsets of hypertension approach. *Am Heart J* 123:1337–1367.

5. Houston MC, Meador BP, Schipani LM (1998) *Handbook of Anti-Hypertensive Therapy,* 8th ed., Philadelphia: Hanley and Belfus.
6. Houston MC (1981) Abrupt cessation of treatment in hypertension: consideration of the clinical features, mechanisms, prevention and management of the discontinuation syndrome. *Am Heart J* 102:415–430.
7. Houston MC (1987) Treatment of hypertensive emergencies and urgencies with oral clonidine loading and titration: a review. In: Rogers DE, Des Prez RM, Cline MJ, et al., eds. *The 1987 Year Book of Medicine.* Chicago: Year Book Medical Publishers, pp. 698–700.

V SOLVING PROBLEMS IN HYPERTENSION MANAGEMENT

32 The National Health and Nutrition Examination Survey III

How Are We Doing with Blood Pressure Control?

David A. Calhoun, MD
and Suzanne Oparil, MD

CONTENTS

Untreated and uncontrolled hypertension is a major health problem in the United States. Findings from the Third National Health and Nutrition Examination Survey (NHANES III, phase 2), conducted from 1991 to 1994, indicate that this problem may be worsening (Fig. 32-1) *(1)*. Major decreases in awareness, treatment, and control rates for hypertension have been recorded in the past decade despite extensive educational programs directed toward patients and health care providers, the widespread availability of facilities for diagnosis and treatment, and the development of effective management strategies *(2–4)*. Because of the high prevalence of hypertension in the United States, the observed decline in control rates is estimated to put more than 1 million hypertensive patients at increased risk for target organ damage (TOD) and

From: *Hypertension Medicine*
Edited by: M. A. Weber © Humana Press Inc., Totowa, NJ

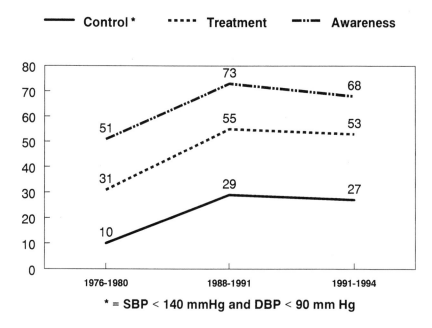

Fig. 32-1. Trends in awareness, treatment, and control of high BP in noninstitution-alized adults in the United States expressed as percentage of the hypertensive population sampled in the NHANES II (1976–1980); NHANES III, Phase 1 (1988–1991); and NHANES III, Phase 2 (1991–1994). (Adapted from ref. 2.)

cardiovascular disease–related morbidity and mortality. Although a causal relationship has not been established, the decline in hypertension detection, treatment, and control rates has coincided with an increase in morbidity and mortality owing to cardiovascular disease (Fig. 32-2) *(5)*. Since 1993, age-adjusted stroke rates have risen, the slope of the age-adjusted rate of decline in coronary heart disease has leveled off, and the incidence of end-stage renal disease and the prevalence of heart failure have increased. These trends support an urgent need for greater emphasis on public awareness of the problem of high blood pressure (BP) and on more aggressive approaches to antihypertensive treatment and BP control by caregivers.

STRATEGIES FOR ENHANCING AWARENESS OF HYPERTENSION

Hypertension can be detected only by measuring BP. This procedure should be carried out at each encounter between a patient and a health

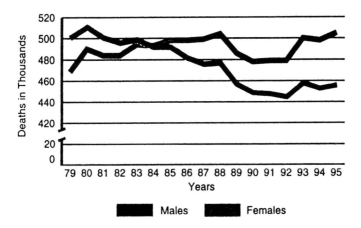

Fig. 32-2. (Reproduced with permission from Heart and Stroke Facts 1998 Statistical Supplement, 1997, American Heart Association.)

Table 32-1
BP Measurement[a]

Patients should be seated with back supported and arm bared and supported.
Patients should refrain from smoking or ingesting caffeine for 30 min prior to measurement.
Measurement should begin after at least 5 min of rest.
Appropriate cuff size and calibrated equipment should be used.
Both SBP and DBP should be recorded.
Two or more readings should be averaged.

[a]SBP, systolic blood pressure; DBP, diastolic blood pressure. (Reproduced from ref. 2.)

care provider. In addition, community screening at health fairs, schools, churches, sporting events, and other gathering places for persons who may not be engaged in the health care system may be useful in identifying previously undiagnosed hypertensive patients. BP should be measured in a standardized fashion using equipment that meets certification criteria (Table 32-1) (6,7). Repeated BP measurements made at intervals are needed to determine whether initial elevations persist and require prompt attention or whether only periodic surveillance is needed (Table 32-2). It is critical that persons in whom a diagnosis of hypertension has been considered not be lost to follow-up, since labile or intermittent hypertension in some people, particularly the young, may lead to fixed

Table 32-2
Recommendations for Follow-up Based on Initial BP
Measurements for Adults[a]

Initial BP (mmHg)		
Systolic	Diastolic	Follow-up recommended
<130	<85	Recheck in 2 yr
130–139	85–59	Recheck in 1 yr
140–159	90–99	Confirm within 2 mo
160–179	100–109	Evaluate or refer to source of care within 1 mo
≥180	≥110	Evaluate or refer to source of care immediately or within 1 wk depending on clinical situation

[a]If systolic and diastolic categories are different, the higher pressure should be used in planning follow-up (e.g., 160/86 mmHg should be evaluated or referred to source of care within 1 mo). The scheduling of follow-up may be modified according to past BP measurements, other cardiovascular risk factors, and/or target disease. All patients should be given information about lifestyle modifications. (Reproduced from ref. 2.)

hypertension later in life. Furthermore, people with high normal BP (130–139/85–89 mmHg) are at greater risk of developing definite hypertension and of experiencing cardiovascular events than the general population. These increased risks should be clearly explained to patients in order to reinforce the need for periodic remeasurement of BP.

Measurement of BP outside of the health care setting by the patient or a friend, relative, or coworker is useful in making or ruling out a diagnosis of hypertension and in following the course of the BP, whether or not antihypertensive treatment is administered. Self-measurement of BP has the particular advantages of distinguishing sustained hypertension from "white coat" hypertension and of enhancing the active role of the patient in his or her own care, thus fostering adherence to treatment. The upper limit of normal for home BP is generally set at 135/85 mmHg.

STRATEGIES FOR ENHANCING ADHERENCE TO ANTIHYPERTENSIVE TREATMENT

Despite its obvious benefits, antihypertensive treatment, whether by lifestyle modification and/or drug administration, is frequently not embraced with enthusiasm by the patient. The reasons for nonadherence to antihypertensive treatment are many, and include the asymptomatic and chronic nature of high BP; the adverse effects of many antihypertensive drugs; the sense of deprivation engendered by lifestyle modification, particularly when dietary restrictions are involved; the cost of medication and other aspects of care, e.g., clinic visits and special diet and exercise programs; and failure of the provider to communicate the benefits of successful treatment and the risks of nonadherence to prescribed therapy. Other barriers to care, such as changes in provider, long waiting times, and restrictions in reimbursement for diagnostic procedures, also contribute to the problem of nonadherence.

In usual medical practice, low patient adherence seriously undermines the effectiveness of antihypertensive therapy. At each step, from detection through long-term follow-up, large numbers of patients drop out of care: up to 50% fail to follow through with referral advice, more than 50% of those who begin treatment drop out of care within 1 yr, and 50–70% of new treatments are changed or discontinued within the first 6 mo in most practices *(8,9)*. The initial choice of antihypertensive drug is an important determinant of adherence to therapy, independent of the cost of the medication. For example, examination of all outpatient prescriptions (more than 3 million) for antihypertensive drugs filled in the Canadian province of Saskatchewan over the period 1989–1994 revealed that 41% of 27,364 newly diagnosed hypertensive patients stopped treatment during the study period *(10)*. The likelihood of stopping was significantly related to the class of the initial agent—greatest for diuretics and smallest for ACE inhibitors. Even for those who remained compliant, fewer than half remained on the initial agent throughout the period of the study (4+ yr). Because Saskatchewan Health funds the prescription drug plan for the province, the cost of medications did not appear to play a role in either the physician's choice of drug or the patient's decision about whether or not to continue therapy. What was important was the number of changes in the drug regimen and the class of initial agent chosen. Patients whose prescriptions were changed frequently were less likely to adhere to the regimens prescribed. Further, angiotensin-converting enzyme (ACE) inhibitors performed better than diuretics, β-blockers, or calcium channel blockers (CCBs), presumably because they were better tolerated. The angiotensin receptor blockers (ARBs), which appear to have an even better tolerability profile, were not available at the time of this study.

The Losartan Effectiveness and Tolerability (LET) study was a 16-wk prospective, open label, randomized study that compared a three-step losartan/hydrochlorothiazide (HCTZ) regimen (50 mg of losartan

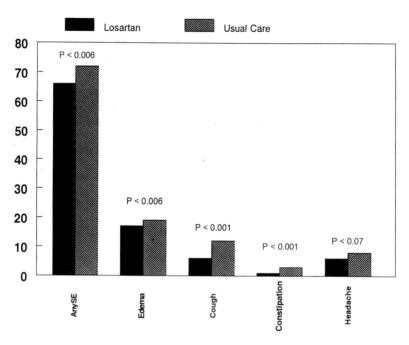

Fig. 32-3. The common side effects (SE5) of antihypertensive treatment were significantly less frequent in subjects randomized to losartan-based treatment (■) than in those randomized to usual care (■), which did not include an ARB, in the community-based LET study. (Adapted from ref. *11*.)

titrated to 50 mg of losartan + 12.5 mg of HCTZ and to 50 mg of losartan + 25 mg of HCTZ) plus additional medications, as needed, to a usual care regimen *(11)*. Enrollees included 2616 outpatients in community care sites who required a switch in antihypertensive therapy owing to either uncontrolled BP (82%) or intolerable adverse effects (18%). Primary end points included the percentage of patients reaching goal BP (<140/90 mmHg) and the frequency of medication switches. Secondary end points were the percentage of patients reaching goal BP without a switch and the frequency of adverse effects for each treatment group. BP control rates were identical (66%) in both groups, but medication switches were significantly less frequent in the losartan group (113/1303, 9%) than in the usual care group (303/1313, 23%) ($p < 0.001$). Figure 32-3 summarizes the adverse effects of medications for the two treatment groups. Note that the antihypertensive drugs used by the usual care group after the initial switch included CCBs (35%), ACE inhibitors (25%), β-blockers (9%), diuretics (±another agent)

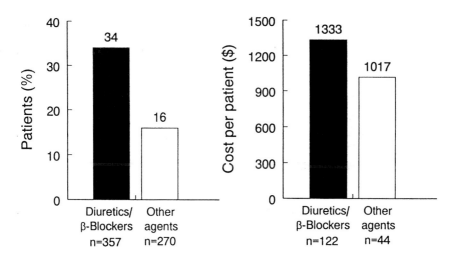

Fig. 32-4. Annual cost of changing antihypertensive drug monotherapy in a tertiary care hypertension clinic was greater with traditional "preferred" diuretic/β-blocker therapy than with other agents because a greater percentage of patients in the former group required a change, and the cost per patient was greater in the former group, offsetting the lower initial acquisition costs of the traditional drugs. (Adapted from ref. *12.*)

(8%), and other classes (22%); twenty-six percent of patients taking losartan received other medications, and only 9% were switched to another class. The investigators concluded that the losartan regimen was as effective as usual care in controlling BP, required fewer switches, and had fewer adverse effects. They hypothesized that if better tolerability translates into better compliance and persistency, a losartan regimen may result in better long-term hypertension control than usual care with the older classes of drugs. Further study is needed to determine whether the hypothesis is correct and whether the benefits seen with the losartan regimens are also seen with other members of the ARB class.

When selecting antihypertensive drug therapy, it is extremely important to consider tolerability and the likelihood that the patient will adhere to the prescribed regimen over time. The cost of poorly tolerated therapy, which often involves changes in the drug program, includes payments for additional clinic visits and laboratory tests, supplemental/ alternative drugs, and treatment of adverse effects. These costs tend to be higher for patients treated with diuretics and β-blockers than with the newer classes of antihypertensive drugs (Fig. 32-4 *(12)*. In one study conducted in a tertiary care hypertension clinic, charges generated

Table 32-3
Suggestions for Increasing Patient Compliance
with Antihypertensive Therapy

Educate patient about hypertension and the importance of following prescribed drug regimen.
Schedule follow-up appointment during office visit and reconfirm by telephone.
Prescribe the drug regimen least likely to result in adverse effects.
Choose the least costly regimen likely to be effective.
Prescribe a once-a-day regimen, if feasible.
Simplify drug regimen by using a fixed-dose combination product.
Track attendance.
Monitor for achievement of BP goal.
Reward/acknowledge progress toward goal.
Inquire about compliance obstacles.
Collaborate with patient in devising new treatment strategies.

[a]Adapted from ref. 13.

for 1 yr after an antihypertensive drug was changed were recorded. Diuretic or β-blocker therapy was changed in 122 of 357 patients, compared with 44 of the 270 given the newer classes of drugs during 4+ yr of follow-up. Per-patient charges generated in switching from diuretic or β-blocker therapy were $1333 ± 130 (mean ± SEM) over the next year, compared with $1017 ± 126 for patients switching from other antihypertensive drugs ($p < 0.001$). Most of the charges were the result of additional clinic visits to monitor BP and laboratory parameters. Additional expenses such as the cost of time off from work and transportation were not included in the analysis. Thus, the cost of antihypertensive therapy includes much more than that of drug acquisition alone. The economic burden of poor BP control, with attendant TOD and cardiovascular events, may ultimately involve disability payments, hospital costs, and payments to physicians and other health care providers for the treatment of advanced cardiovascular disease.

Strategies that enhance adherence and improve patient outcomes must involve both patient education and behavioral modification (Table 32-3) (13,14). Evidence-based approaches that have been shown to be helpful in maximizing long-term adherence to antihypertensive regimens include educating the patient and his or her family about high BP and its treatment, individualizing the regimen, providing feedback to the patient, and promoting social support. With respect to medications, it is reasonable to individualize antihypertensive treatment based on each patient's personal needs with respect to tolerability, convenience, and quality of life. Initiation of treatment with a drug that is expected to be well tolerated and therefore likely to be effective in lowering BP over time is prudent. Long-acting agents are preferable because adherence to therapy and consistency of BP control are superior with once daily dosing. Low-dose, fixed-dose combination therapy can be used in place of monotherapy as initial treatment or as an alternative to adding a second agent of a different therapeutic class to unsuccessful monotherapy. The advantage of this approach is that low doses of drugs that act by different mechanisms may have additive or synergistic effects on BP with minimal dose-dependent adverse effects. Single-tablet dosing provides an additional benefit. The pairing of pill taking with daily habits, such as brushing teeth or shaving, helps minimize missed medication. Furthermore, compliance packaging such as blister packaging helps patients remember when to take their medication and to note errors in pill taking. Self-monitoring of BP at home and/or at work increases patient involvement and ties adherence to a successful treatment outcome—BP lowering.

Whenever possible, multidisciplinary teams that address patients' specific needs and concerns and provide follow-up and feedback should be utilized. This multilevel approach, in which patients, providers, and health care organizations/systems take part, is needed to optimize adherence. Provision of reminders, outreach, and follow-up services is useful. Many of these functions can be carried out by nurses and/or office assistants and by the pharmacists who dispense the patients' medications. Vigilant counseling and surveillance by an interested pharmacist concerning timeliness of prescription refills and possible drug-drug interactions can greatly enhance the quality of antihypertensive treatment.

STRATEGIES FOR IMPROVING BP CONTROL

Data from NHANES III indicate that approx 50% of patients under treatment for hypertension are uncontrolled (BP > 140/90 mmHg). When the more stringent BP goals recommended for diabetics (<130/85 mmHg) and patients with renal dysfunction and proteinuria (125/75 mmHg) are taken into account, control rates are even lower. The reasons are complex, but are most commonly related to patient nonadherence to therapy (previously discussed), and inadequate and inappropriate therapy (Table 32-4) *(15,16)*. Secondary hypertension is a less

Table 32-4

Reasons for Lack of Responsiveness to Hypertension Therapy[a]

Nonadherence to therapy	Drug-related causes	Associated conditions	Volume overload
Cost of medication and related care	Doses too low	Increasing obesity	Inadequate diuretic therapy
Instructions not clear and/or not given to the patient in writing	Inappropriate combinations (e.g., two centrally acting adrenergic inhibitors)	Alcohol intake >1 oz of ethanol/d	Excess sodium intake
Failure of physician to increase or change therapy to achieve BP goals	Rapid inactivation (e.g., hydralazine, oral clonidine [Catapres], captopril [Capoten], short-acting CCBs	Sedentary lifestyle	Fluid retention from reduction of BP
Inadequate or no patient education	Drug interactions: glucocorticoids,	Sleep apnea	Progressive renal damage
Lack of involvement of the patient in the treatment plan	mineralocorticoids, NSAIDS, tyramine and MAO inhibitors, appetite		Secondary hypertension
Side effects of medication	suppressants, phenothiazines,		
Organic brain syndrome (e.g., memory deficit)	oral contraceptives, sympathomimetics,		
Inconvenient dosing schedule	antidepressants, adrenal steroids, nasal decongestants, cocaine, cyclosporine (Sandimmune, neoral), erythropoietin		

[a]NSAIDs, nonsteroidal anti-inflammatory drugs; MAO, monoamine oxidase. (Adapted from ref. 17.)

360

At Enrollment										Final Visit

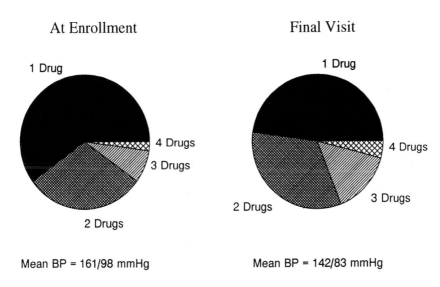

Mean BP = 161/98 mmHg							Mean BP = 142/83 mmHg

Fig. 32-5. Main reduction in BP and high rates of BP control were achieved in the HOT study by increasing the intensity of treatment from one drug to two to four drugs in the majority of patients. (Adapted from ref. *15.*)

common (<5% of cases overall) but nevertheless important cause of uncontrolled hypertension, and it is potentially curable. (*See* Chapter 13 for a discussion of screening procedures for secondary hypertension.) Because definitive diagnosis and treatment of these conditions can be technically difficult and operator dependent, referral to a hypertension specialist is recommended in cases of suspected secondary hypertension.

Most hypertensive patients are undertreated; that is, they are receiving inappropriately low doses of individual antihypertensive drugs or too few drugs. For example, in the Hypertension Optimal Treatment (HOT) study, mean BP on enrollment was 161/98 mmHg on a one- (~60% of participants) or two- (~30% of participants) drug regimen, whereas at the end of the study, BP was well controlled (mean = 142/83 mmHg) on a regimen that required two or more drugs in 52% of cases (Fig. 32-5) *(17)*. Clearly, the choice of initial monotherapy, which receives so much attention in the literature and in commercial promotions, is less important than administering appropriate drug combinations in adequate doses because (1) BP can be controlled with monotherapy in fewer than 50% of patients, and (2) all of the major classes of antihypertensive drugs appear to be similarly effective in lowering

BP in persons with stage 1 hypertension and without target organ damage *(15,18)*.

Underdosing of antihypertensive drugs can be minimized if physicians become familiar with one or two drugs in each class and follow the manufacturer's recommendations for their use. Doses should be titrated upward until BP is controlled or the maximal recommended dose is reached, in the absence of dose-related adverse effects. A drug from another class that has additive or synergistic effects with the first drug should then be added. Addition of a diuretic, even in very low doses, potentiates most other classes of drugs, and adding an ACE inhibitor to a CCB both increases efficacy and reduces some of the dose-related adverse effects, principally peripheral edema, of the CCB. In general, combining multiple drugs from the same class or drugs that share a common mechanism of action should be avoided. ACE inhibitor β-blocker combinations do not have additive antihypertensive effects, and β-blocker α-agonist combinations are undesirable because their antihypertensive effects are not additive and because of a potential for paradoxical hypertension and rebound hypertension on drug withdrawal. Unless the patient has symptoms or signs of accelerated hypertension, the interval between dose adjustments or addition of new drugs should be 4 wk or longer, because this much time is necessary for any dose of antihypertensive medication to reach its full therapeutic benefit.

Fixed-dose combination therapy offers the advantages of improved patient adherence, by decreasing the number of pills that must be taken, and enhanced tolerability, by reducing the dose-dependent adverse effects of individual components *(19)*. To be combined in a single-dose form, each component in the combination must contribute to BP lowering, and the dosage of each component must be such that the combination is safe and effective in a majority of the target population. The antihypertensive effects of individual components can be additive or synergistic. In some cases, one component of the combination attenuates the adverse effects of the other; for example, ACE inhibitors blunt diuretic-induced metabolic abnormalities and CCB-induced sympathetic nervous system activation. Furthermore, the cost of fixed-dose combination therapy is frequently less than that of individual components. Most fixed-dose combinations contain one or even two diuretics (one for natriuresis, the other for potassium sparing) since diuretics enhance the efficacy of the other classes of antihypertensive drugs.

Short-acting antihypertensive agents, including dihydropyridine CCBs such as capsular nifedipine (Adalat, Procardia), oral clonidine (Catapres), and captopril (Capoten) should be avoided because of the need for frequent dosing, leading to noncompliance *(15)*. These agents, with the exception of captopril, also tend to activate the sympathetic nervous system, leading to unstable BP control and periods of rebound hypertension at the end of the dosing interval.

Diuretics are a critical component of multidrug antihypertensive regimens, because volume overload is the most common cause of resistant hypertension in patients who adhere to prescribed therapy *(15,16)*. Avoidance of foods high in salt and increased consumption of foods high in fruits, vegetables, and low-fat dairy products, which contain micronutrients that reduce the pressor effect of concomitant salt intake, are also helpful in reducing volume overload. Thiazide diuretics are more effective than loop diuretics in lowering BP in patients with normal renal function, whereas loop diuretics are needed to control both BP and volume in patients with renal dysfunction (serum creatinine > 3 mg/dL; glomerular filtration rate < 30 mL/min) *(16,20)*.

COMORBID CONDITIONS

The majority of hypertensive patients have comorbid conditions and other cardiovascular risk factors and/or TOD that may dictate their antihypertensive drug therapy (Fig. 32-6) *(2)*. Compelling indications for initial drug choices from specific classes are based on randomized clinical trials. These recommendations indicate that a drug from a specific class should be included in the antihypertensive regimen unless contraindicated, *not* necessarily be administered as monotherapy. Because of the aggressive nature of TOD in these conditions, particularly diabetes and renal dysfunction, a multidrug regimen is usually needed to lower BP and prevent the progression of renal disease and cardiovascular events. Furthermore, the level of BP control appears to be more important than the choice of drug in determining outcome. For example, the United Kingdom Prospective Diabetes Study showed that tight BP control was associated with a 24% reduction in diabetes-related end points compared to usual control, independent of the choice of antihypertensive drug (atenolol- and captopril-based regimens were equally effective) *(21,22)*.

In conditions in which ACE inhibitors are recommended first-line agents, such as congestive heart failure, diabetes, and myocardial infarction, ARBs are being tested in clinical trials as alternative or substitution therapies. In view of the excellent tolerability of this new class of antihypertensive drugs, they may add greatly to our ability to

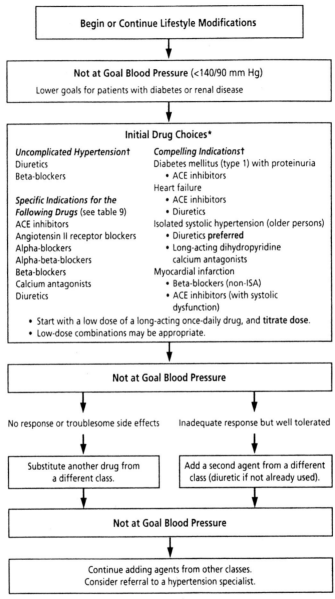

Begin or Continue Lifestyle Modifications

↓

Not at Goal Blood Pressure (<140/90 mm Hg)
Lower goals for patients with diabetes or renal disease

↓

Initial Drug Choices*

Uncomplicated Hypertension†
Diuretics
Beta-blockers

*Specific Indications for the
Following Drugs* (see table 9)
ACE inhibitors
Angiotensin II receptor blockers
Alpha-blockers
Alpha-beta-blockers
Beta-blockers
Calcium antagonists
Diuretics

Compelling Indications†
Diabetes mellitus (type 1) with proteinuria
• ACE inhibitors
Heart failure
• ACE inhibitors
• Diuretics
Isolated systolic hypertension (older persons)
• Diuretics **preferred**
• Long-acting dihydropyridine
calcium antagonists
Myocardial infarction
• Beta-blockers (non-ISA)
• ACE inhibitors (with systolic
dysfunction)

• Start with a low dose of a long-acting once-daily drug, and **titrate dose.**
• Low-dose combinations may be appropriate.

↓

Not at Goal Blood Pressure

↓   ↓

No response or troublesome side effects   Inadequate response but well tolerated

↓   ↓

Substitute another drug from
a different class.

Add a second agent from a different
class (diuretic if not already used).

↓

Not at Goal Blood Pressure

↓

Continue adding agents from other classes.
Consider referral to a hypertension specialist.

* Unless contraindicated. ACE indicates angiotensin-converting enzyme; ISA,
intrinsic sympathomimetic activity.
† Based on randomized controlled trials

Fig. 32-6. General approach to the pharmacologic treatment of hypertension in patients with and without comorbid conditions that may constitute compelling indications (supported by randomized controlled trials) for including specific drug classes in the regimen. (Reproduced from ref. *2*.)

control BP, even in hypertensive patients with TOD and comorbid conditions.

REFERENCES

1. Burt VL, Whelton P, Roccella EJ, et al. (1995) Prevalence of hypertension in the US adult population: results from the Third National Health and Nutrition Examination Survey, 1988–1991. *Hypertension* 25:305–313.
2. Joint National Committee on Detection, Evaluation, and Treatment of High Blood Pressure (1997) The sixth report of the Joint National Committee on the Detection, Evaluation, and Treatment of High Blood Pressure. *Arch Intern Med* 157:2413–2446.
3. Brown RD Jr, Whisnant JP, Sicks JD, et al. (1996) Stroke incidence, prevalence, and survival: secular trends in Rochester, Minnesota, through 1989. *Stroke* 27:373–380.
4. Glynn RJ, Brock DB, Harris T, et al. (1995) Use of antihypertensive drugs and trends in blood pressure in the elderly. *Arch Intern Med* 155:1855–1860.
5. Heart and Stroke Facts (1997) 1998 Statistical Supplement, American Heart Association.
6. Prisant LM, Alpert BS, Robbins CB, et al. (1995) American National Standard for nonautomated sphygmomanometers: summary report. *Am J Hypertens* 8:210–213.
7. Perloff D, Grim C, Flack J, et al., for the Writing Group (1993) Human blood pressure determination by sphygmomanometry. *Circulation* 88:2460–2467.
8. Haynes RB, Mattson ME, Chobanian AV, et al. (1982) Management of patient compliance in the treatment of hypertension: report of the NHLBI Working Group. *Hypertension* 4:415–423.
9. Jones JK, Gorkin L, Lian LF, et al. (1995) Discontinuation of and changes in treatment after start of new courses of antihypertensive drugs: a study of a United Kingdom population. *BMJ* 311:293–295.
10. Caro JJ, Jackson J, Speckman J, et al. (1997) Compliance as a function of initial choice of antihypertensive drug. *Am J Hypertens* 10:141A (abstract).
11. Moore MA, Gazdick LP, Edelman JM, et al. (1998) Losartan effectiveness and tolerability (LET) study. *Am J Hypertens* 11:104A (abstract).
12. Elliott WJ (1995) Costs associated with changing antihypertensive drug monotherapy: "preferred" vs. "alternative" therapy. *Am J Hypertens* 8:80A (abstract).
13. Miller NH, Hill M, Kottke T, Ockene IS (1997) The multilevel compliance challenge: recommendations for a call to action. A statement for healthcare professionals. AHA special report. *Circulation* 95:1085–1090.
14. Hill NM (1999) Adherence to antihypertensive therapy. In: *Hypertens Primer*, 2nd ed., pp. 348–351.
15. Oparil S, Calhoun DA (1998) Managing the patient with hard-to-control hypertension. *Am Fam Physician* 57:1007–1014.
16. Setaro JF, Black HR (1992) Refractory hypertension. *N Engl J Med* 327:543–547.
17. Hansson L, Zanchetti A, Carruthers SG, et al., for the HOT Study Group (1998) Effects of intensive blood-pressure lowering and low-dose aspirin in patients with hypertension: principal results of the Hypertension Optimal Treatment (HOT) randomized trial. *Lancet* 351:1755–1762.

18. Neaton JD, Grimm RH Jr, Prineas RJ, et al. (1993) Treatment of Mild Hypertension Study: Final Results. Treatment of Mild Hypertension Study Research Group. *JAMA* 270:713–724.

19. Sica DA (1994) Fixed-dose combination antihypertensive drugs: do they have a role in rational therapy? *Drugs* 48:16–24.

20. National High Blood Pressure Education Program Working Group report on hypertension and chronic renal failure (1991) *Arch Intern Med* 151:1280–1287.

21. Turner R, Holman R, Stratton I, et al. (1998) UK Prospective Diabetes Study Group. Tight blood pressure control and risk of macrovascular and microvascular complications in type 2 diabetes: UKPDS 38. *BMJ* 317:703–713.

22. Holman R, Turner R, Stratton I, et al. (1998) Efficacy of atenolol and captopril in reducing risk of macrovascular and microvascular complications in type 2 diabetes: UKPDS 39. *BMJ* 317:713–720.

33 Lipid Abnormalities and Hypertension

Thomas D. Giles, MD

Abnormalities of blood lipids constitute one of the more common risk factors for cardiovascular disease that coexist with systemic arterial hypertension (Table 33-1). Hypertension and lipid disturbances may be part of a genetic abnormality, the Familial Dyslipidemic Syndrome, which is found in approx 12% of people with hypertension and in approx 50% of those with early familial hypertension, increased LDL cholesterol, and triglycerides. Thus, it is often necessary to consider the additional cardiovascular risk associated with dyslipidemia when planning a therapeutic strategy for hypertensive patients.

Cholesterol is one of the major factors in the pathogenesis of atherosclerosis. Spontaneous atherosclerosis begins at birth and is associated with lipid accumulation, macrophage and smooth muscle cell proliferation, foam cell formation, and endothelial cell toxicity. Much has been learned concerning the progression from isolated macrophage foam cells and fatty streaks to atheroma and fibroatheroma. Fibroatheromas are the most advanced form of spontaneous atherosclerosis and may produce stenosis of blood vessels. However, the atheroma and fibroatheroma may undergo accelerated change owing to disruption of the

From: *Hypertension Medicine*
Edited by: M. A. Weber © Humana Press Inc., Totowa, NJ

Table 33-1
Epidemiological Relation Between BP and Serum Lipids[a]

Study	Number of subjects	Lipid fraction associated with blood pressure	Correlation coefficient	P
Tecumseh Community Health	3064	TC TG	0.16 SBP 0.18 SBP	<0.001
Southern California	4839	TC TG	0.28 SBP	<0.05
Lipid Research Clinics Program Prevalence	7747	TG + VLDL TC	Not given	<0.05
Framingham	5127	TC	0.15 SBP 0.20 DBP	Not given
Tromso	16744	TC Non-HDL-C	0.19 SBP 0.25 DBP 0.13 SBP	<0.001
Zavaroni et al.	64	TG	Not given	<0.05
Williams et al.	6128	LDL-C	Not given	<0.001

[a] TC, total cholesterol; TG, triglycerides; VLDL, very low-density lipoprotein; HDL-C, high-density lipoprotein cholesterol; LDL-C, low-density lipoprotein cholesterol; SBP, systolic blood pressure; DBP, diastolic blood pressure (From Goode GK, et al. *Lancet* 1995; 345:362–364.)

fibrous cap. Disruption is likely owing to hemodynamic forces. During the early stages of plaque disruption, these fissures probably reseal by incorporating platelets and thrombus and may produce no symptoms or may produce a spectrum of unstable coronary syndromes, e.g., unstable angina and myocardial infarction (MI).

The association between high cholesterol concentrations and atherosclerosis has been known for some time. For clinical purposes, the focus has been on total serum cholesterol (TC), high-density lipoprotein cholesterol (HDL-C), low-density lipoprotein cholesterol (LDL-C) and serum triglyceride concentrations. Although other measurements may have value in some settings, e.g. lipoprotein (a), clinical intervention trials have focused on the aforementioned lipids. The lipoproteins surround the lipid center and serve as transport mechanisms.

LDL-C contains mostly apolipoprotein B-100, which is made in the liver. Most of the cholesteryl ester in the core of LDL is produced from the breakdown of VLDL by the liver. Apolipoprotein B-100 is recognized by LDL receptors on peripheral cells (e.g. endothelial cells of coronary arteries, and the liver). The liver removes approx 75% of LDL from the circulation; the removal rate of LDL from the circulation depends on both the number and availability of LDL receptors.

LDL-C can accumulate in the arterial wall when serum concentrations are high. When LDL-C is trapped in the endothelium, the particles undergo physical and chemical modifications; that is, peroxidation of polyunsaturated fatty acids in LDL-C converts LDL lecithin to LDL lysolecithin. This oxidized LDL is taken up 10 times faster by macrophages than native LDL, which leads to the formation of foam cells. Oxidized LDL is a potent chemoattractant for circulating macrophages and when ingested by the macrophages inhibits their motility; this leads to sequestration of macrophages in the arterial wall. Oxidized LDL has been reported to be cytotoxic to endothelial cells. Modified LDL is highly immunogenic and LDL-immune complexes are rapidly phagocytized by macrophages. Glycated LDL is also a potent immunogen.

HDL is secreted into the plasma by the liver and intestines and accepts cholesterol from peripheral cells and other lipoproteins. HDL serves as a reservoir for apolipoproteins and is also the major pathway for cholesterol metabolism by the liver. When HDL interacts with the surface of cells, lecithin cholesterol acyltransferase combines cholesterol and phosphatidyl choline to make cholesteryl ester, which is then transported to the liver. HDL also prevents the oxidation of LDL by binding to transition metal ions in the intima. Thus, in contrast to LDL, high HDL levels help prevent atherosclerosis.

Triglycerides may be an independent risk factor for cardiovascular disease in women but not in men. *However, the major value of detection of an elevated plasma triglyceride concentration may be to alert the physician to the presence of insulin resistance (see below).*

There are four groups of patients that characterize the vast majority of patients with hypertension and coexistent abnormalities of blood lipids:

1. Those with no prior history of a cardiovascular event
2. Those with a history of a prior cardiovascular event
3. Those with coexisting diabetes mellitus or syndrome X

LIPID ABNORMALITIES IN HYPERTENSION WITH AND WITHOUT PREVIOUS CARDIOVASCULAR DISEASE

All patients with hypertension should have a complete assessment for the common, known risk factors for cardiovascular disease, including a careful history (age, sex, smoking, substance abuse, hormonal status for women, diabetes, family history of cardiovascular disease), physical examination (evidence of vascular disease or diabetes), electrocardiogram (evidence of previous MI, ischemia, or left ventricular hypertrophy), and a lipid profile. The presence of hypertension requires that a more detailed evaluation be given to all risk factors than in an otherwise healthy person. It cannot be overemphasized that measurement of the lipid profile should be performed by a certified laboratory with the patient in a fasted state (at least 14 h) and after a careful review of the patient's dietary habits. Secondary causes of dyslipidemia should be sought, which include certain drugs (diuretics, glucocorticoids, cyclosporin), metabolic conditions (hypothyroidism, pregnancy, diabetes mellitus), and certain diseases (nephrotic syndrome, biliary obstruction).

The value of lowering abnormally elevated LDL cholesterol in both primary and secondary prevention of cardiovascular events has been well established by many large-scale, controlled clinical trials. The National Cholesterol Education Program (NCEP) guidelines are helpful when deciding how to assess cardiovascular risk in relation to blood lipid values (*see* Table 33-2). *However, clinical judgment must always be used when applying such guidelines to actual practice situations.*

Clearly, the NCEP guidelines try to predict those individuals at high risk for a cardiovascular event that might be modified by treatment of abnormal lipid values. For those who have had a previous MI or stroke or who have evidence of peripheral vascular disease, I aggressively treat even marginally elevated cholesterol values. The optimal values for cholesterol for any given individual have not been defined.

Dietary measures and appropriate exercise constitute prudent advice for all patients who seek a healthy lifestyle. However, for patients at risk for cardiovascular events and elevated LDL-C, I begin treatment with lipid-lowering drugs immediately. Data from the literature suggest that this treatment will decrease the progression of spontaneous atherosclerosis as well as prevent the accelerated phase associated with increased plaque vulnerability.

Tabled 33-3 lists drugs that are useful in the treatment of abnormal cholesterol. The "statins" have been remarkable for their ability to decrease morbidity and mortality in clinical trials associated with a reduction in LDL-C and, in some instances, an increase in HDL-C. The lack of significant adverse events make these drugs highly attractive as initial agents to prevent the development of atherosclerosis.

Table 33-2
NCEP Expert Panel Guidelines (1993)

Cholesterol	HDL	Risks[a]	Vascular disease	LDL	Action[b]	Goal
<200	>35	<2			DEER, 5 yr	Chol < 200
<240 Or	<35 Or	2+	Or +		DEER, 1 yr	
≥240 Or					Check LDL	
		<2		<130	DEER, 5 yr	LDL < 130
				130–159	DEER, 1 yr	
		2+	Or +	>160[c]	Step 1 diet or step 2	LDL < 160 or <130 If 2+ risks
					Repeat 6 mo	
			+	≤100	DEER, 1 yr	LDL < 100
			+	>100[c]	Step 2 diet, 3 mo	

Risks[a]			Vascular disease	LDL		Goal
Male < 35 or female premenopausal; not high risk				≥220		LDL < 190
<2				≥190		LDL < 160
2+				≥160		LDL < 130
			+	≥130		LDL < 100

[a]Risks are diabetes mellitus; age (male ≥ 45; female ≥ or premature menopause without hormone replacement therapy); family history of premature cardiovascular disease (MI/sudden death in first-degree relative male <55 or female <65 yr); hypertension; HDL < 35 (subtract one risk factor if HDL ≥ 60).

[b]DEER, diet, exercise, and risk-reduction advice; Step 1 diet, decrease sources of saturated fat, total fat, and cholesterol (saturated fat ~10% and total fat ~30% of total calories; cholesterol < 300 mg/d).

[c]Although diet and exercise are the foundation of treatment, practically all of the conditions designated will require treatment with lipid-lowering drugs.

Table 33-3
Pharmacologic Agents for Treatment of Dyslipidemia in Adults

	Effect on lipoprotein		
	LDL	HDL	Triglyceride
First-line agents			
LDL lowering			
HMG CoA reductase inhibitor	↓↓	↔↑	↔↑
Triglyceride lowering			
Fibric acid derivative	↓↔↑	↑	↓
Second-line agents			
LDL lowering			
Bile acid binding resins	↓	↔	↑
LDL and triglyceride lowering			
Nicotinic acid	↓	↑↑	↓

DIABETES MELLITUS AND SYNDROME X

Diabetes mellitus and syndrome X are discussed together because the lipid abnormalities are often similar, i.e., decreased HDL-C and an increase in triglycerides. Syndrome X is characterized by the following:

1. Hypertension
2. Resistance to insulin-stimulated glucose uptake
3. Hypertriglyceridemia
4. Low plasma HDL-C
5. Hyperuricemia
6. Abnormal plasminogen activator-1
7. Presence or absence of obesity

In patients with overt diabetes mellitus as well as syndrome X, the major concern is still to treat the LDL-C if it is elevated (Table 33-4). However, the plasma triglyceride concentration should be given the first priority for treatment if the value is >500 mg/dL, in order to prevent pancreatitis.

The use of drugs that improve insulin resistance or hepatic glucose output (e.g., troglitazone or metphormin) may be of value in managing individuals with insulin-resistance syndromes, although definitive outcome trials have not yet been completed and reported.

Table 33-4
Treatment of Dyslipidemia in Diabetes

Dyslipidemia	X	Optimal LDL < 100 mg/dL (2.60 mmol/L), primary therapy directed first at lowering LDL by diet, exercise, and drugs; when drugs are necessary, use statin, then bile acid binding resin.
	X	If triglycerides > 500 mg, treat as first priority.
	X	Initial therapy for markedly increased triglycerides is improved glycemic control; additional lowering with fibric acid derivatives or high-dose statins as necessary.
	X	Niacin should be used very carefully if at all.

CONCLUSION

Hypertension is associated with disturbances of blood lipids in many ways and contributes greatly to the overall risk for developing cardiovascular disease. In every patient who is diagnosed as having hypertension, an evaluation of blood lipids is required as part of an inventory of total cardiovascular risk. Failure to do so deprives the patient of the opportunity to receive therapy that may strikingly reduce cardiovascular morbidity and mortality.

SUGGESTED READINGS

Fuster V, Badimon L, et al. (1992) The pathogenesis of coronary artery disease and the acute coronary syndrome. *N Engl J Med* 326:242–250.

Fuster V, et al. (1992) The pathogenesis of coronary artery disease and the acute coronary syndrome (second of two parts). *N Engl J Med* 326:310–318.

Giles TD (1997) Lipid factors in the hypertension syndrome. *J Cardiovasc Risk* 4:257–259.

Grundy SM (1995) Role of low-density lipoproteins in atherogenesis and development of coronary heart disease. *Clin Chem* 41:139–146.

Malloy MJ, Kane JP (1998) Aggressive medical therapy for the prevention and treatment of coronary artery disease. *Disease-A-Month* 44:1–40.

Reaven GM, Lithell H, Landsberg L (1996) Hypertension and associated metabolic abnormalities—the role of insulin resistance and the sympathoadrenal system. *N Engl J Med* 334:374–381.

Scandinavian Simvastatin Survival Study Group (1994) Randomised trial of cholesterol lowering in 4444 patients with Coronary heart disease: the Scandinavian Simvastatin Survival Study (4S). *Lancet* 344:1383–1389.

Shepard J, Cobbe SM, Ford I, et al. (1995) Prevention of coronary heart disease with pravastatin in men with hypercholesterolemia. West of Scotland Coronary Prevention Study Group. *N Engl J Med* 333:1301–1307.

Stary HC (1989) Evolution and progression of astherosclerotic lesions in coronary arteries of children and young adults. *Arteriosclerosis* 9:119–132.

Williams RR, Hunt SC, Hopkins PN, Stults BM, Wu LL, Hasstedt SJ (1988) Familial dyslipidemic hypertension: evidence from 58 Utah families for a syndrome present in approximately 12% of patients with essential hypertension. *JAMA* 259:3579–3596.

34 Diabetes and Hypertension

Kurt M.R. Sowers and James R. Sowers

CONTENTS

Diabetic people are more prone to hypertension than those without this metabolic disorder *(1–6)*. More than 3 million people in the United States have both type II diabetes and hypertension *(1–3)*. Cardiovascular disease (CVD) is the largest cause of morbidity and mortality in diabetic persons with coexistent hypertension. Accordingly, a major focus of hypertension therapy for these persons should be the reduction of CVD morbidity and mortality, while reducing the complications of diabetic nephropathy. The causation of this comorbidity in Westernized societies may be attributed to populations getting older, more obese, and more sedentary *(1–6)*. Up to 80% of the premature mortality in persons with this diabetes is due to CVD *(1–6)*. Hypertension plays a key role in promoting CVD in diabetic persons *(1–6)*. These observations have contributed to the recommendations of more aggressive lowering of blood pressure (BP) (i.e., to <130/85 mmHg) in people with both diabetes and hypertension *(2–7)*. However, it appears that most of such persons are inadequately controlled at this desired BP *(5,8)*. New strategies are being reviewed to improve our ability to reach BPs in this high-risk population.

Hypertension and diabetes both increase with advancing age in industrialized societies *(1,2,4,9–11)*. As in the United States, diabetes

From: *Hypertension Medicine*
Edited by: M. A. Weber © Humana Press Inc., Totowa, NJ

Table 34-1
Lipids, Coagulation, and Fibrinolysis in Hypertension and Diabetes

1. Increased plasma levels of VLDL, LDL, and Lp (a)
2. Decreased plasma HDL cholesterol
3. Elevated plasma levels of factor VII and VIII
4. Increased fibrinogen and PAI-1 levels
5. Elevated thrombin-antithrombin complexes
6. Decreased antithrombin III, protein C, and S levels
7. Decreased plasminogen activators and fibrinolytic activity
8. Increased endothelial expression of adhesion molecules

mellitus affects more than 15 million people, 90% of whom have the noninsulin-dependent, or type II, diabetes *(3,10)*. Almost 20% of Caucasians over 65 yr of age have diabetes; the prevalence is even higher in African Americans and Hispanics *(10,11)*. Whereas CVD accounts for 40% of overall mortality in the United States, nearly 80% of deaths in elderly diabetic persons is secondary to CVD complications, consisting of sudden death, myocardial congestive heart failure, and cerebrovascular and peripheral vascular disease *(10,11)*.

People with clinical diabetes and hypertension, or with impaired glucose tolerance and hypertension, manifest a characteristic dyslipidemia, with low high-density lipoprotein (HDL), high very low-density lipoprotein (VLDL) and a phenotypically small, dense, and more atherogenic low-density lipoprotein (LDL) *(6,12)* (Table 34-1). Hypertension and coexistent diabetes are often associated with coagulation abnormalities as well as lipid disturbances *(6,12)*. Furthermore, disturbances of the fibrinolytic system have been reported in people with hypertension, especially in those with concomitant lipid glucose abnormalities and vascular disease *(12)*. Circulating levels of lipoprotein (a) [Lp(a)] are often in association with diabetes mellitus *(6)*. By inhibiting fibrinolysis, increased levels of Lp (a) delay thrombolysis and predispose to plaque progression. Elevated levels of plasminogen activation inhibitor-1 (PAI-1) have been reported both in untreated patients with essential hypertension *(13)* and in men with prior myocardial infarctions with increased risk for reinfarction *(6)*. Elevated PAI-1 levels are associated with abdominal obesity, insulin resistance/hyperinsulinemia, and associated dyslipidemia *(6)*. Platelet aggregation, activation, and adhesion are often enhanced in hypertension and associated diabetes mellitus *(1,14)* (Table 34-2).

Table 34-2
Alterations in Platelet Function in Hypertension and Diabetes

1. Increased platelet adhesiveness and aggregation
2. Increased platelet generation of vasoconstrictor prostanoids
3. Reduced platelet generation of prostacyclin and other vasodilator prostanoids
4. Increased nonenzymatic glycosylation of platelet proteins
5. Decreased platelet production of NO
6. Increased platelet myosin light chain phosphorylation/contraction

Table 34-3
Alterations in Cardiovascular Endothelium Associated with Hypertension and Diabetes

1. Increased plasma levels of von Willebrand factor
2. Elevated expression, synthesis, and plasma levels of endothelin-1
3. Diminished prostacyclin release
4. Increased destruction of endothelium-derived relaxing factor (NO) and reduced responsiveness to NO
5. Impaired fibrinolytic activity
6. Increased endothelial cell procoagulant activity
7. Increased endothelial cell-surface thrombomodulin
8. Increased superoxide anion generation
9. Increased expression of adhesion molecules

ENDOTHELIAL DYSFUNCTION IN DIABETES AND HYPERTENSION

Dysfunction of the vascular endothelium appears to play a major role in the pathogenesis of CVD in people with hypertension and diabetes (1,15) (Table 34-3), with hyperglycemia and dyslipidemia as major contributors (15). Hyperglycemia results in increased destruction of endothelial cell nitric oxide (NO) (15), which predisposes to increased production of vasoconstrictor prostaglandins, endothelin, gly-cated proteins, endothelium adhesion molecules, and growth factors, which cumulatively enhance vasomotor tone, vascular growth, and remodeling (15,16). Hyperglycemia and dyslipidemia also delay endo-thelial cell replication and increase cell death, in part by enhancing oxidation and glycation (glycooxidation), and altering vascular NO metabolism (15,16).

EVALUATION AND TREATMENT OF HYPERTENSION IN ASSOCIATION WITH DIABETES MELLITUS

The goal of lowering BP in people with coexistent diabetes and hypertension is to prevent hypertension-associated death and disability *(1–3)*. Those with diabetes and hypertension, partly because of reduced baroreceptor sensitivity, often have more labile BPs, and are more susceptible to postural hypotension. These symptoms are often associated with a lack of a normal nocturnal "dip" in BPs *(1–3)*. Thus, the level of BP and the diagnosis of hypertension should be based on multiple BP measurements obtained in a standardized fashion on at least three occasions *(1–3)*. Because of the propensity for orthostatic hypotension, standing BPs should be measured during office visits *(1,3)*. Furthermore, because of the increased variability in BP of these patients, ambulatory BP measurements or home BP monitoring may be particularly valuable. The consensus BP goal in diabetic people with hypertension is <130/85 mmHg *(1–3)* (Fig. 34-1).

The purpose of this clinical advisory update is to alert clinicians about new information to be used in their clinical practice. Therapy in patients with hypertension and diabetes begins with weight reduction, increased physical activity, and moderation of salt and alcohol intake *(2,3)*. The goal BP is 130/85 mmHg. If it is not reached, then pharmacologic intervention is indicated *(2,3)*. Based on clinical trial results, four classes of drugs have been found to be effective first-line therapy in these patients (Fig. 34-1). Most hypertensive diabetic patients will require the use of more than one agent to achieve a therapeutic goal of 130/85 mmHg *(3)*.

Because proteinuria is a harbinger for CVD and renal disease *(17)*, angiotensin-converting enzyme (ACE) inhibitors may afford unique benefits in preventing CVD as well as diabetic nephropathy *(2,3)*. The Appropriate Blood Pressure Control in Diabetes trial *(18)* showed a cardioprotective effect of ACE inhibitors. Recently, the United Kingdom Prospective Diabetes Study Group reported *(19,20)* that BP lowering with an atenolol-based program was just as effective as a captopril-based regimen in reducing the incidence of diabetic complications (both microvascular and macrovascular). Many required these drugs plus a diuretic to achieve "tight control of 144/82 mmHg." In patients assigned to less tight control (154/87 mmHg), there was less use of multiple antihypertensive agents. Risk reductions in the group assigned to tight BP control were 24% in diabetes-related end points, 32% in deaths related to diabetes, 44% in strokes, and 37% in microvascular end

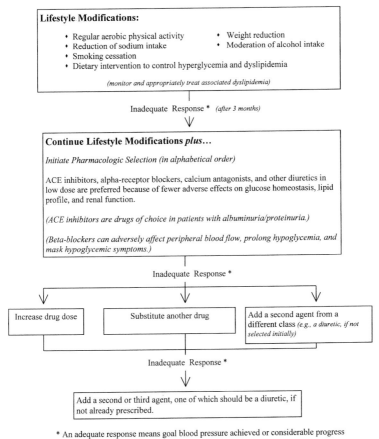

Figure 34-1.

points, predominantly diabetic retinopathy. These results suggest that combination therapy with either an ACE inhibitor or a β-blocker are very effective in reducing macrovascular and microvascular events provided that BP is adequately lowered.

Low-dose thiazide diuretics (i.e., 25 mg or less of hydrochlorothiazide or chlorthialidone daily) are effective and safe antihypertensive agents in type II diabetic patients *(2,3)*. In the Systolic Hypertension in the Elderly Program study, elderly type II diabetic men had reductions in stroke and coronary heart disease similar to those without diabetes *(21)*. Low-dose diuretics (i.e., hydrochlorothiazide at 25 mg or lower) are not associated with significant metabolic abnormalities *(2,3)*. Lower-dose diuretics in conjunction with ACE inhibitors usually produces substantial synergism in reducing BP, and the use of these agents together further minimizes potential metabolic problems. Diuretics are important because of the salt sensitivity and expanded plasma volume that is often present in diabetic patients *(22)*, particularly in those requiring several drugs to control BP levels of <130/85 mmHg.

Results from the subset analysis of type II diabetics in the Hypertension Optimal Treatment (HOT) trial *(23)* and a recent subanalysis of this cohort in the Systolic Hypertension in Europe (Syst-EUR) trial *(24)* suggest that further reduction in diastolic BP below 85 mmHg is beneficial. HOT also confirmed that multiple drug regimes are required to reach goal for most hypertensive diabetics. In the Syst-EUR trial, systolic blood pressure was reduced by a comparable amount in each group (−22 ± 16 mmHg for nondiabetic subjects vs −22.1 ± 14 mmHg for the diabetic group), and the risk reduction in mortality from CVD was 13% for the nondiabetic subjects and 76% for the diabetic patients *(24)*. Thus, the benefit conferred per millimeter of mercury BP reduction appears to be greater in people with type II diabetes than in those with hypertension but no coexistent diabetes mellitus.

REFERENCES

1. Sowers JR, Epstein M (1995) Diabetes mellitus and associated hypertension, vascular disease and nephropathy: an update. *Hypertension* 26:869–879.
2. The National High Blood Pressure Education Program Working Group (Chair, James R. Sowers, MD) (1994) National high blood pressure education program working group report on hypertension in diabetes. *Hypertension* 23:145–158 (special article).
3. American Diabetes Association (1996) Clinical practice recommendations: hypertension in diabetes. *Diabetes Care* 19(Suppl. 1):S107–S113.
4. Joint National Committee on Detection, Evaluation and Treatment of High Blood Pressure (1997) The sixth report of the Joint National Committee on Detection, Evaluation and Treatment of High Blood Pressure (JNC-VI). *Arch Intern Med* 157:2413–2446.
5. Bakris GL, Weir MR, Sowers JR (1996) Therapeutic challenges in the obese, diabetic patient with hypertension. *Am J Med* 101:33S–46S.
6. Afonso LC, Edelson GL, Sowers JR (1997) Metabolic abnormalities in hypertension. *Curr Opin Nephrol Hypertens* 6:219–223.
7. Estacio RO, Jeffers BW, Hiatt WR, Bigerstaff SL, Gifford N, Schrier RW (1998) The effect of nisoldipine as compared with enalapril on cardiovascular outcomes in patients with non-insulin-dependent diabetes and hypertension. *N Engl J Med* 338:645–652.

8. Burt VL, Cutler JA, Higgins M (1995) Trends in the prevalence, awareness, treatment and control of hypertension in the adult U.S. population: data from the Health Examination Surveys, 1960 to 1991. *Hypertension* 26:60–69.

9. Mykkünen L, Kuusisti J, Pyorala K, Laakso M, Haffner SM (1994) Increased risk of non-insulin dependent diabetes mellitus in elderly hypertensive subjects. *J Hypertens* 12:1425–1432.

10. Schrier RW (1998) Antihypertensive treatment in type II diabetes. *Hosp Pract* 33(5):13,14.

11. Sowers JR, Farrow SL (1996) Treatment of elderly hypertensive patients with diabetes, renal disease and coronary heart disease. *Am J Cardiol* 6(5):57–60.

12. Sowers JR, Sowers PS, Peuler JD (1993) Role of insulin resistance and hyperinsulinemia in development of hypertension and atherosclerosis. *J Lab Clin Med* 123:647–652.

13. Landin K, Tengborn L, Smith U (1990) Elevated fibrinogen and plasminogen activator inhibitor (PAI-1) in hypertension are related to metabolic risk factors for cardiovascular disease. *J Intern Med* 227:273–278.

14. Fakuda K, Ozaki Y, Satoh K, et al. (1997) Phosphorylation of myosin light chain in resting platelets from NIDDM patients is enhanced: Correlation with spontaneous aggregation. *Diabetes* 46:488–493.

15. McMillen DE (1997) Development of vascular complications in diabetes. *Vasc Med* 2:132–142.

16. Sowers JR (1997) Insulin and insulin-like growth factor in normal and pathological cardiovascular physiology. *Hypertension* 29:691–699.

17. Dinneen SF, Gerstein HC (1997) The association of microalbuminuria and mortality in non-insulin-dependent diabetes mellitus: a systematic overview of the literature. *Arch Intern Med* 157:1413–1418.

18. Estacio RO, Schrier RW (1998) Antihypertensive therapy in type 2 diabetes: implications of the appropriate blood pressure control in diabetes (ABCD) trial. *Am J Cardiol* 12(9B):9R–14R.

19. UKPDS Group (1998) UK Prospective Diabetes Study 38: tight blood pressure control and risk of macrovascular and microvascular complications in type 2 diabetes. *BMJ* 317:703–713.

20. UK Prospective Diabetes Study Group (1998) Intensive blood-glucose control with sulphonylureas or insulin compared with conventional treatment and risk of complications in patients with type 2 diabetes (UKPDS 33). *Lancet* 352:837–853.

21. Curb JD, Pressel MS, Cutler JA, et al. (1996) Effect of a diuretic-based antihypertensive treatment on cardiovascular disease risk in older diabetic patients with isolated hypertension. *JAMA* 276:1886–1892.

22. Sowers JR (1999) Hypertension in type II diabetes: update on therapy. *J Clin Hypertens* 1:41–47.

23. Hansson L, Zanchetti A, Carruthers SB, Dahlof B, Elmfeldt D, Julius S, Menard J, Rahn KH, Wedel H, Westerling S (1998) Effects of intensive blood pressure-lowering and low-dose aspirin in patients with hypertension: principal results of the Hypertension Optimal Treatment (HOT) randomized trial. HOT Study Group. *Lancet* 351:1755–1762.

24. Staussen JA, Fagard R, Thys L, et al., for the Systolic Hypertension-Europe (Syst-Eur) trial investigators (1997) Morbidity and mortality in the placebo-controlled European trial on isolated systolic hypertension in the elderly. *Lancet* 350:757–764.

35 Treatment of Hypertensive Patients with Chronic Renal Insufficiency

Samuel Spitalewitz, MD
and Jerome G. Porush, MD

CONTENTS

NONPHARMACOLOGIC THERAPY
PHARMACOLOGIC THERAPY: DIURETICS
HYPERTENSIVE NEPHROSCLEROSIS AND CRI
PROGRESSION OF CRI OF DIVERSE ETIOLOGIES:
    WHAT SHOULD THE GOAL BP BE?
ARE THERE RENOPROTECTIVE ANTIHYPERTENSIVE
    DRUGS?
CONCLUSION
REFERENCES

The prevalence of hypertension in patients with chronic renal insufficiency (CRI) from all causes increases linearly as renal function deteriorates, reaching approx 95% as patients approach end-stage renal disease (ESRD) *(1–3)*. There is now substantial evidence that controlling blood pressure (BP) will slow the inexorable decline in renal function in patients with CRI *(4)*. Nevertheless, at a time when morbidity and mortality from cardiovascular disease is declining, the incidence of ESRD is increasing dramatically, particularly in African Americans, the elderly, and diabetics *(5)*. There is no single explanation for this fact, but pertinent issues are as follows *(6,7)*:

1. Should the general therapeutic approach to hypertension (nonpharmacologic and/or pharmacologic) differ in patients with CRI vs essential hypertensive patients without renal insufficiency?

From: *Hypertension Medicine*
Edited by: M. A. Weber © Humana Press Inc., Totowa, NJ

2. Will lowering BP to levels below current standards (140/90 mmHg; mean arterial pressure [MAP] = 107) better preserve renal function without increasing adverse consequences?
3. Are there specific classes of antihypertensive drugs that are renoprotective over and above their effect on BP?

NONPHARMACOLOGIC THERAPY

The same nonpharmacologic measures useful in the treatment of essential hypertension can be applied to patients with hypertension and CRI. However, in patients with CRI, sodium restriction becomes the single most important nondrug approach *(3)*. As glomerular filtration rate (GFR) declines, sodium balance is maintained after some volume expansion but at the expense of hypertension. In addition to directly lowering BP by diminishing extracellular volume and vascular reactivity, dietary sodium restriction also potentiates the effects of other antihypertensive medications, particularly angiotensin-converting enzyme (ACE) inhibitors and angiotensin receptor blockers (ARBs) *(6,8)*. Because the failing kidney is unable to accommodate rapidly to a low-sodium intake, sodium restriction must be accomplished gradually. Rapid and marked reduction of sodium intake may result in severe volume contraction and worsening renal function *(3)*.

PHARMACOLOGIC THERAPY: DIURETICS

If the patient is unwilling or unable to adhere to a sodium-restricted diet, a diuretic should be used *(3)*. Either a loop-active or thiazide diuretic may be used, with the choice generally determined by the level of renal function. As GFR falls below 35 mL/min (serum creatinine approx 2.5 mg/dL or greater), thiazides become ineffective and a loop-active diuretic is necessary. Combinations of the two types of diuretics have been particularly successful in renal failure patients who have been resistant to either used alone *(9,10)*. Of the three available loop-active diuretics (furosemide, bumetanide, and torsemide), torsemide is the best orally absorbed drug *(11)*. The response to diuretics is highly individual and the dose must be altered as the clinical response dictates.

As with dietary sodium restriction, severe volume contraction must be avoided. Therefore, patients should be monitored carefully by daily weights, BP (particularly orthostatic measurements), and timely evaluation of renal function and electrolytes *(3)*.

In general, the same drugs used in patients with essential hypertension with normal kidney function can be used in patients with hypertension and CRI, including the choice of drug if there are comorbid conditions. Guidelines are provided elsewhere for appropriate reductions in the dose of renal metabolized drugs such as atenolol, nadolol, hydralazine, clonidine, and captopril *(12)*. Caution must be exercised with α_1-adrenergic blockers, which have been reported to produce significant orthostatic hypotension particularly in patients with autonomic neuropathy associated with CRI. Centrally acting α_2-adrenergic agonists may cause marked lethargy in patients with a GFR <20 mL/min and should be administered at reduced doses *(6)*. ACE inhibitors (and probably ARBs) should be used cautiously in patients with proven or suspected renal artery disease because they may precipitate an acute loss of kidney function *(13)*. In fact, if this occurs in a patient previously not suspected of having renal artery stenosis, the diagnosis should then be seriously considered.

In the most recent Joint National Committee report (VI), two specific recommendations were made regarding the treatment of patients with hypertension and CRI. First, BP should be lowered to at least 130/85 mmHg in patients with proteinuria in excess of 1 g/24 h. Second, patients with hypertension who have CRI should receive, unless contraindicated, an ACE inhibitor to control hypertension and to slow the progression of renal failure *(12)*. Next, these recommendations are evaluated in light of the available literature.

HYPERTENSIVE NEPHROSCLEROSIS AND CRI

Will lowering BP to the levels suggested (unrelated to the drugs used) slow the progression of renal disease without undesirable side effects? With regard to hypertensive nephrosclerosis, there still are no data from large-scale, prospective, randomized studies designed to specifically examine whether lowering the BP prevents or slows progression of renal failure. Furthermore, the appropriate goal BP in these patients is not established (7). However, there are data from a variety of studies suggesting that aggressive treatment of essential hypertension even with traditional therapy such as diuretics and β-blockers can stabilize renal function as assessed by the serum creatinine (6,7). In the Hypertension Detection and Follow-up Program (14), the stepped-care group, which achieved a mean BP of 129/86 mmHg, significantly lower than the usual-care group (139/90 mmHg), showed stabilization of renal function after 1 yr of treatment. Similarly, in the Multiple Risk Factor Intervention Trial (15), with a 7-yr follow-up period of 5061 Caucasian males with mild to moderate hypertension, those subjects with a diastolic BP (DBP) above 95 mmHg had a more rapid decline in renal function compared with those patients with a DBP of <95 mmHg. In African-American men, slowing in the progression of CRI was observed down to a DBP of 75 mmHg. Although the risk for renal dysfunction was highest in men with severe hypertension, there was also an increased risk in subjects with a DBP of 85–90 mmHg compared with those with a systolic BP (SBP) of <120 mmHg and a DBP of <80 mmHg. This suggests that the lower BP the greater the renal protection, and that the traditional target BP of 140/90 mmHg may be too high (6). Those subjects whose follow-up SBP exceeded 140 mmHg had the most rapid decline in renal function. Other studies have confirmed these findings (16–21).

The African-American Study of Kidney Disease trial is ongoing and is designed to determine the optimum BP to prevent worsening renal function in African Americans with hypertensive nephrosclerosis and CRI and to determine the effects of an ACE inhibitor, calcium antagonist, or β-blocker on the progression of CRI in these subjects (22). Until the results of this trial are known, it appears reasonable to lower SBP to <135 mmHg and DBP to <85 mmHg in patients with hypertensive nephrosclerosis and CRI (7).

PROGRESSION OF CRI OF DIVERSE ETIOLOGIES: WHAT SHOULD THE GOAL BP BE?

The Modification of Diet in Renal Disease (MDRD) (23) was a large, prospective, randomized trial that compared the effects of "usual" BP control (MAP of 107 mmHg in patients younger than age 60 yr and 113 mmHg for those older than 60) with "strict" control (MAP of 92 and 97 mmHg for the two age groups, respectively) in 840 patients with CRI (GFR range of 13–55 mL/min). Patients were generally treated with ACE inhibitors or calcium channel blockers (CCBs), with diuretics, and with other drugs as necessary. Those patients with a GFR of 25–55 mL/min in the strict control group had a less rapid decline in GFR, which correlated significantly with the level of urinary protein excretion at baseline; that is, those patients with protein excretion >1 g/d demonstrated a slower rate of decline of renal function than the higher BP group. A longer follow-up period would have been necessary to determine whether the low BP goal is beneficial in patients with proteinuria of only 0.25–1.0 g/d. There was no beneficial effect of the lower BP in patients with a GFR between 13 and 24 mL/min, nor in patients with adult polycystic kidney disease or chronic interstitial nephritis.

Support for the MDRD findings relative to BP control and proteinuria is provided by the Northern Italian Cooperative Study Group, which evaluated more than 400 patients with nondiabetic CRI over a 30-mo follow-up period *(19)*. In this study, an MAP >107 mmHg, associated with increasing levels of proteinuria, predicted a worse outcome. Aggressive BP control to an MAP of <107 mmHg correlated with a diminution in proteinuria and prolonged renal survival compared with those patients with a higher BP. Several other smaller studies confirm these findings *(24–27)*.

The results of the studies in patients with diabetic nephropathy also suggest that renal function deteriorates more slowly with more aggressive lowering of BP and concomitant reduction in protein excretion. The beneficial effect of lower BP is continuous down to an SBP of approx 130 mmHg and a DBP of 70 mmHg *(28–35)*.

The Collaborative Study Group examined 409 patients with type I diabetic nephropathy. Lower SBP correlated with remission from nephrotic range proteinuria *(35)*. When the MAP was reduced to 92–95 mmHg, the benefit of the lower BP was observed regardless of whether or not an ACE inhibitor was used. The apparent renoprotective effect of captopril was observed only at the usual levels of BP control (unpublished observations).

Kasiske et al. *(34)*, in a large meta-analysis of patients with diabetic nephropathy (type I and II), noted that a reduction in BP, regardless of type of antihypertensive agent used, was associated with a relative higher GFR in diabetics with proteinuria *(34)*. The GFR was 3.7 mL/min higher in patients for each 10 mmHg decrease in MAP, emphasizing again the importance of aggressive control of BP. In none of the studies reported were there more cardiovascular or other adverse events in strict BP control groups.

ARE THERE RENOPROTECTIVE ANTIHYPERTENSIVE DRUGS?

ACE Inhibitors

Although patients with CRI and hypertension generally respond to the same classes of antihypertensive agents as do patients without renal disease, ACE inhibitors are particularly suited for these patients in whom the renin-angiotensin system is activated *(3)*. It has also been suggested that this class of drugs has a specific renoprotective effect distinct from the level of BP by lowering intraglomerular hydrostatic pressure (P_{GC}), which is elevated in a variety of experimental models of CRI and appears to be one of several factors that contribute to the progression of renal failure *(36,37)*. Zucchelli et al. *(27)*, Hannedouche et al. *(38)*, and Maschio et al. *(39)* demonstrated an advantage to ACE therapy in preserving renal function above and beyond simply lowering BP in patients with nondiabetic CRI.

In the most recent studies reported by the Gruppo Italiano di Studi Epidemiologici in Nefrologia the effects of ramipril (an ACE inhibitor) vs placebo were examined in nondiabetic chronic renal disease *(40–42)*. The degree of BP control was the same in both groups (144.6/88.2 mmHg in the ramipril group compared with 144.6/88.9 mmHg in the placebo group). Only ARBs were excluded as additional antihypertensive drugs. The patients were divided into two stratums according to baseline proteinuria: stratum 1, 1–3 g/24 h; stratum 2, ≥3 g/24 h. The trial was terminated early in stratum 2 patients because the ACE inhibitor dramatically reduced the rate of decline of renal function compared with the placebo group *(40,41)*. Ramipril induced an early reduction in 24-h urinary protein excretion, which correlated with the long-term effect on GFR decline and was the only covariate that predicted the drug's renoprotective effect. The reduction in decline of renal function was greatest in patients with the highest baseline proteinuria and was not dependent on the initial degree of renal impairment or baseline or follow-up BP, which was similar in both groups. These studies suggest that proteinuria, *per se*, may be "nephrotoxic."

The core study patients who were originally on ramipril were continued on the drug and those initially on placebo were switched to ramipril at the end of the study *(42)*. At the end of the follow-up study (4 ½ yr), the patients initially randomized to ramipril had a renal survival rate three times greater than those who were originally randomized to placebo and then switched to ramipril, suggesting that the earlier treatment with an

ACE inhibitor is begun, the more renoprotective it may be. However, the patients switched to ramipril also had a significant reduction in the rate of decline in GFR (from 0.81 in the original study to 0.14 mL/[min·mo] in the follow-up study). These studies strongly suggest that ACE inhibitors are renoprotective separate from their effect on BP.

In a meta-analysis of 10 studies including 1594 patients, Giatras et al. *(43)* demonstrated ACE inhibitors to be more effective than other antihypertensive agents in reducing the development of ESRD in nondiabetic renal disease, but not in decreasing mortality.

In the meta-analysis of 100 studies in both type I and type II diabetic patients noted earlier *(34)*, only ACE inhibitors had an additional favorable effect on GFR that was independent of the BP.

The Collaborative Study Group, referred to earlier, definitively demonstrated that ACE inhibition significantly reduces the rate of doubling of serum creatinine in type I diabetics at usual levels of BP control *(28)*. Other studies suggest that the early use of ACE inhibitors in patients with type I and II diabetes and incipient diabetic nephropathy (microalbuminuria) without hypertension reduces the rate of appearance of overt nephropathy (macroalbuminuria) *(24,44–47)*.

Based on the available data, in both incipient and overt diabetic nephropathy and in other forms of CRI, ACE inhibitors should be the initial drug of choice unless a contraindication to its use exists *(7)*.

Angiotensin Receptor Blockers

ARBs are a new class of drugs that block the rennin-angiotensin system at a site different than do ACE inhibitors and offer substantial promise as renoprotective drugs *(6,48–50)*. This class of drugs selectively blocks the binding of angiotensin II to the type 1 angiotensin receptor on the cell membrane. Although there are no large-scale, prospective, double-blind studies published, there are promising observations regarding the possible role for ARBs as renoprotective drugs. Gansevoort et al. *(51)* found that an ARB was as effective in reducing urinary protein excretion in patients with chronic renal disease as an ACE inhibitor (approx a 50% reduction for each drug).

Calcium Channel Blockers

There are data from both short- and long-term studies available to evaluate the renoprotective effect of CCBs. Verapamil and diltiazem

most consistently lower urinary protein excretion in diabetic nephropathy *(52)*. Bakris et al. *(53)* studied 34 African Americans with type II
diabetic nephropathy with renal insufficiency and proteinuria. After a
mean follow-up of 54 ± 6 mo, patients taking verapamil had a slower rate
of decline in creatinine clearance and a greater reduction in proteinuria
compared with the group taking atenolol, despite similar BP. In addition,
a greater proportion of the atenolol group had a 50% or more increase
in serum creatinine compared with the verapamil group.

Vellusie et al. *(54)* compared the effects of an ACE inhibitor (cilazapril) with a dihydropyridine CCB (amlodipine) on GFR and albumin
excretion in 44 type II diabetics with hypertension, 26 of whom were
normoalbuminuric and 18 microalbuminuric. At 3 yr of follow-up, the
decline in GFR and albumin excretion in both groups were similar.
Other studies also suggest that CCBs (both dihydro- and nondihydropyridine) may be beneficial in stabilizing renal function in patients with
CRI *(55–59)*.

CONCLUSION

Treatment of hypertension in patients with renal insufficiency is
indicated at any stage of the disease. It would appear that the goal BP
should be an MAP of 100 mmHg or less and that an ACE inhibitor is
the drug of choice. Diuretics are probably the second-line drugs of
choice. A CCB (diltiazem or verapamil) should be added to achieve
goal BP, followed by other antihypertensive agents, as necessary. The
role of ARBs has not been well defined, but they may be as useful as
ACE inhibitors or possibly even additive. Thus, the recommendations
of sixth report of the Joint National Committee are well founded, with
the possibility that a BP even lower than 130/85 mmHg (MAP of 100
mmHg) may be necessary in all patients with CRI.

REFERENCES

1. Vertes V, Cangiano JL, Berman LB, Gould A (1969) Hypertension in end-stage
   renal disease. *N Engl J Med* 280:978–981.
2. Buckalew VM Jr, Berg RL, Want SR, Porush JG, Ranch S, Schulman G (1996)
   Prevalence of hypertension in 1,795 subjects with chronic renal disease: The
   Modification of Diet in Renal Disease Study baseline cohort. *Am J Kidney Dis*
   28:811–821.

3. Spitalewitz S, Porush JG (1994) Treatment of hypertensive patients with chronic renal insufficiency. In: Izzo JL Jr, Black HR, eds. *Hypertension Primer*, vol. E29, Dallas: American Heart Association, pp. 354–357.

4. National High Blood Pressure Education Program Group (1996) 1995 Update of the working group reports on chronic renal failure and renovascular hypertension. *Arch Intern Med* 156:1938–1947.

5. (1994) *US Renal Data System: USRDS 1994 Annual Data Report*, Bethesda MD: National Institutes of Health, National Institute of Diabetes and Digestive and Kidney Diseases.

6. Weir MW, Dworkin LD (1998) Antihypertensive drugs, dietary salt, and renal protection: how long should you go and with which therapy? *Am J Kidney Dis* 32:1–22.

7. Porush JG (1998) Hypertension and chronic renal failure: the use of ACE-inhibitors. *Am J Kidney Dis* 31:177–184.

8. Bakris GL, Weir MR (1996) Salt intake and reductions in the arterial pressure and proteinuria. *Am J Hypertens* 9:200S–206S.

9. Suki WN (1997) Use of diuretics in chronic renal failure. *Kidney Int* 51: (Suppl. 59)S33–S35.

10. Fliser D, Schroter M, Neubeck M, Ritz E (1994) Coadministration of thiazides increases the efficacy of loop diuretics even in patients with advanced renal failure. *Kidney Int* 46:482–488.

11. Oates J (1995) Antihypertensive agents and the drug therapy of hypertension. In: Handman JG, Gilman AG, Limbird LE, eds. *Goodman & Gilman's The Pharmacological Basis of Therapeutics*, 9th ed., New York: McGraw Hill, pp. 780–808.

12. Joint National Committee (1997) The Sixth Report of the Joint National Committee on Detection, Evaluation and Treatment of High Blood Pressure. *Arch Intern Med* 157:2413–2446.

13. Reiser IW, Pallan TM, Spitalewitz S (1998) How to treat renovascular hypertension: medical therapy versus revascularization. *J Crit Illness* 13:409–424.

14. Schulman NB, Ford CE, Hall WD, Blaufox MD, Simon D, Langford HG, Schneider KA (1989) Prognostic value of serum creatinine and effect of treatment of hypertension on renal function: results from the hypertension detection and follow-up program. The Hypertension Detection and Follow-up Program Cooperative Group. *Hypertension* 13(Suppl. 1):80–93.

15. Walker GW, Neaton JD, Cutler JA, Neuwirth R, Cohen JD, for the MRFIT Research Group (1992) Renal function change in hypertensive members of the Multiple Risk Factor Intervention Trial: racial and treatment effects. *JAMA* 268:3085–3091.

16. Tierney WM, McDonald CJ, Luft FC (1989) Renal disease in hypertensive adults: effect of race and type II diabetes mellitus. *Am J Kidney Dis* 13:485–493.

17. Perry HM, Miller JP, Formoff JR, Baty JD, Sambhi MP, Rutan G, Moskowitz DW, Carmody SE (1995) Early predictors of 15-year end-stage renal disease in hypertensive patients. *Hypertension* 25:587–594.

18. Brazy PC, Fitzwilliam JF (1990) Progressive renal disease: role of race and antihypertensive medications. *Kidney Int* 37:1113–1119.

19. Locatelli F, Marcelli D, Comelli M, Alberti D, Graziani G, Buccianti G, Redaelli B, Giangrande A, Northern Italian Cooperative Study Group (1996) Proteinuria

and blood pressure as casual components of progression to end-stage renal failure. *Nephrol Dial Transplant* 11:461–467.

20. Rostand SG, Brown G, Kirk KA, Rutsky EA, Dustan HP (1969) Renal insufficiency in treated essential hypertension. *N Engl J Med* 320:684–688.

21. Rosansky SJ, Hoover DR, King L, Gibson J (1990) The association of blood pressure levels and change in renal function in hypertensive and non-hypertensive subjects. *Arch Intern Med* 150:2073–2076.

22. Wright JT, Kusek JW, Toto RD, Lee JY, Agodoa LY, Randall OS, Kirk KA, Glassock R (1996) Design and baseline characteristics of participants in the African-American Study of Kidney Disease and Hypertension (AASK) pilot study. *Contr Clin Trials* 17(Suppl. 4)3S–16S.

23. Klahr S, Levey AS, Beck GJ, Cagguila AW, Hunsiker L, Kusek JW, Striker G (1994) The effects of dietary protein restriction and blood-pressure control on the progression of chronic renal disease. Modification of Diet in Renal Disease Study Group. *N Engl J Med* 330:877–884.

24. Wight JP, Brown CB, el Nahas AM (1993) Effect of control of hypertension on progressive renal failure. *Clin Nephrol* 39:305–311.

25. Alvestrand A, Gutierrez A, Bucht H. Bergstrom J (1998) Reduction in blood pressure retards the progression of chronic renal failure in man. *Nephrol Dial Transplant* 3:624–631.

26. Bergstrom J, Alvestrand A, Bucht A, Gutierrez A (1986) Progression of chronic renal failure in man is retarded with more frequent clinical follow-ups and better blood pressure control. *Clin Nephrol* 25:1–6.

27. Zucchelli P, Zuccalà A, Borghi M, Fusaroli M, Sasdelli M, Stallone C, Sanna G, Gaggi R (1992) Long-term comparison between captopril and nifedipine in the progression of renal insufficiency. *Kidney Int* 42:452–458.

28. Lewis EJ, Hunsicker LG, Bain RP, Rohde RD, for the Collaborative Study Group (1993) The effect of angiotensin-converting-enzyme inhibition on diabetic nephropathy. *N Engl J Med* 329:1456–1462.

29. Mogensen CE (1976) Progression of nephropathy in long-term diabetics with proteinuria and effect of initial antihypertensive treatment. *Scand J Clin Lab Invest* 36:383–388.

30. Dillon JJ (1993) The quantitative relationship between treated blood pressure and progression of diabetic renal disease. *Am J Kidney Dis* 22:798–802.

31. Walker WG (1993) Hypertension-related renal injury: a major contributor to end-stage renal disease. *Am J Kidney Dis* 22:164–173.

32. Parving H-H, Smidt UM, Hommel E, Mathiesen ER, Rossing P, Nielson F, Gall MA (1993) Effective antihypertensive treatment postpones renal insufficiency in diabetic nephropathy. *Am J Kidney Dis* 22:188–195.

33. Mathiesen ER, Hommel E, Giese J, Parving H-H (1991) Efficacy of captopril in postponing nephropathy in nomotensive insulin dependent diabetic patients with microalbuminuria. *BMJ* 303:81–87.

34. Kasiske BL, Kalil RSN, Ma JZ, Liao M, Keane WM (1993) Effects of antihypertensive therapy on the kidney in patients with diabetes: a meta-regression analysis. *Ann Intern Med* 118:129–138.

35. Hebert LA, Bain RP, Verne D, Cottran D, Whittier FC, Tolchin N, Rhode RD, Lewis EJ, for the Collaborative Study Group (1994) Remission of nephrotic range proteinuria in type I diabetes. *Kidney Int* 46:1688–1693.

36. Anderson S, Rennke HG, Brenner BM (1986) Therapeutic advantage of converting enzyme inhibitors in arresting progressive renal disease associated with systemic hypertension in the rat. *J Clin Invest* 77:1993–2000.

37. Keane WF, Anderson S, Aurell M, de Zeeuw D, Narins RG, Povar G (1989) Angiotensin converting enzyme inhibitors and progressive renal insufficiency: current experience and future directions. *Ann Intern Med* 111:503–516.

38. Hannedouche T, Landais P, Goldfarb B, Esper NE, Fournier A, Galin M, Durand B, Chanard J, Mignon F, Suc J-M, Grünfeld J-P (1994) Randomized controlled trial of enalapril and β-blockers in non-diabetic chronic renal failure. *BMJ* 309:833–837.

39. Maschio G, Alberti D, Janin G, et al., for the Angiotensin-Converting-Enzyme Inhibition in Progressive Renal Insufficiency Study Group (1996) Effect of the angiotensin-converting enzyme inhibitor benazepril on the progression of chronic renal insufficiency. *N Engl J Med* 334:939–945.

40. Gruppo Italiano di Studi Epidemiologici in Nefrologia (1997) Randomized placebo-controlled trial of effect of ramipril on decline in glomerular filtration rate and risk of terminal renal failure in proteinuric, non-diabetic nephropathy. *Lancet* 349:1857–1863.

41. Ruggenenti P, Perna A, Mosconi L, Massimo M, Pisoni R, Gaspari F, Remuzzi G, on behalf of the "Gruppo Italiano di Studi Epidemiologici in Nefrologia" (GISEN) (1997) Proteinuria predicts and-stage renal failure in non-diabetic chronic nephropathies. *Kidney Int* 52(Suppl. 63):S-54–S-57.

42. Ruggenenti P, Perna A, Gherardi G, Gaspari F, Benini R, Remuzzi G, on behalf of Gruppo Italiano di Studi Epidemiologici in Nefrologia (GISEN) (1998) Renal function; and requirement for dialysis in chronic nephropathy patients on long-term ramipril: REIN follow-up trial. *Lancet* 352:1252–1256.

43. Giatras I, Lau J, Levey AS, for the Angiotensin-Converting Enzyme Inhibition and Progressive Renal Disease Study Group (1997) Effect of angiotensin-converting enzyme inhibitors on the progression of non-diabetic renal disease: a meta-analysis of randomized trials. *Ann Intern Med* 127:337–345.

44. Dongall ML, Moore WV (1992) Effect of angiotensin-converting enzyme inhibition on renal function and albuminuria in normotensive type I diabetic patients. *Diabetes* 41:62–67.

45. Ravid M, Savin H, Jutrin I, Bental T, Lishner M (1993) Long-term stabilization effect of angiotensin-converting enzyme inhibitor on plasma creatinine and on proteinuria in normotensive type II diabetic patients. *Ann Intern Med* 118:577–581.

46. Romero R, Salinas I, Lucas A, et al. (1993) Renal function changes in microalbuminuric normotensive type II diabetic patients treated with angiotensin-converting enzyme inhibitors. *Diabetes Care* 16:597–600.

47. Viberti G, Mogensen CE, Groop LC, et al. (1994) Effect of captopril on progression to clinical proteinuria in patients with insulin dependent diabetes mellitus and microalbuminuria. *JAMA* 271:275–279.

48. Weir MR (1996) Angiotensin-II receptor antagonists: a new class of antihypertensive agents. *Am Fam Physician* 53:589–594.

49. Gansevoort RT, de Zeeuw D, Shahinfar S, Redfield A, de Jong PE (1994) Effects of the angiotensin II antagonist losartan in hypertensive patients with renal disease. *J Hypertens* 12(Suppl. 2)S37–S42.

50. Ichikawa I (1996) Will angiotensin II receptor antagonists be renoprotective in humans? *Kidney Int* 50:684–692.

51. Gansevoort RT, de Zeeuw D, de Jong PE (1994) Is the antiproteinuric effect of ACE inhibition mediated by interference in the renin-angiotensin system? *Kidney Int* 45:861–867.

52. Epstein M (1998) Calcium antagonists and the progression of chronic renal failure *Curr Opin Nephrol Hypertens* 7:171–177.

53. Bakris GL, Barnhill BW, Sadler R (1992) Treatment of arterial hypertension in diabetic humans: importance of therapeutic selection. *Kidney Int* 41:912–919.

54. Velussi M, Brocco E, Frigato F, Zolli M, Muollo B, Malloll M (1996) Effects of cilazapril and amlodipine on kidney function in hypertensive NIDDM patients. *Diabetes* 45:216–222.

55. Slataper R, Vicknair N, Sadler R, Bakris GL (1993) Comparative effects of different antihypertensive treatments on progression of diabetic kidney disease. *Arch Intern Med* 153:973–980.

56. Bakris GL, Mangrum A, Copley JB, Sadler R (1997) Effect of calcium channel or β-blockade on the progression of diabetic nephropathy in African Americans. *Hypertension* 29:744–750.

57. ter Wee PM, De Micheli AG, Epstein M (1994) Effects of calcium antagonists on renal hemodynamics and progression of non-diabetic chronic renal disease. *Arch Intern Med* 154:1185–1202.

58. Rossing P, Tarnow L, Boelskifter S, Jensen BR, Nielsen FS, Parving H-H (1997) Differences between nisoldipine and lisinopril on glomerular filtration rates and albuminuria in hypertensive IDDM patients with diabetic nephropathy during the first year of treatment. *Diabetes* 46:481–487.

59. Gansevoort RT, Sluiter WJ, Hemmelder MH, et al. (1995) Antiproteinuric effect of blood-pressure-lowering agents: a meta-analysis of comparative trials. *Nephrol Dial Transplant* 10:1963–1974.

36 Treating Angina Pectoris in Hypertension

Hal L. Chadow, MD
and Joel A. Strom, MD

Contents

It is estimated that 13.5 million people in the United States have ischemic heart disease (IHD), and 1.5 million new cases are diagnosed each year. IHD remains the leading cause of mortality, resulting in approx 500,000 deaths annually. Many studies have identified specific risk factors for coronary artery disease (CAD). These include a family history, diabetes mellitus, hypertension, hyperlipidemia, and smoking. The incidence of cardiovascular events increases with the number of risk factors present and is greater than would be predicted by their combined presence. Primary and secondary prevention including effective blood pressure (BP) control and lowering of serum cholesterol levels, together with significant strides in the treatment of IHD, have

From: *Hypertension Medicine*
Edited by: M. A. Weber © Humana Press Inc., Totowa, NJ

resulted in significant reductions in morbidity and mortality. In this chapter, we review the management of the hypertensive patient with IHD.

MEDICAL THERAPY

Medical therapy for the hypertensive patient with IHD is aimed at lowering BP, reducing myocardial ischemia, alleviating anginal symptoms, and preventing recurrent cardiovascular events.

ANTIPLATELET AGENTS AND ANTICOAGULANT THERAPY

Aspirin has been shown to reduce the risk of major cardiovascular events in patients with IHD. The risk of death and myocardial infarction (MI) is reduced in patients presenting with an acute coronary syndrome (unstable angina [UA] or non–Q wave myocardial infarction [NQWMI]). Similarly, the addition of aspirin to thrombolytic therapy for the treatment of acute MI resulted in an additive benefit, reducing the incidence of death and nonfatal reinfarction *(1)*. Therefore, aspirin should be administered to every patient with IHD in the absence of contraindications.

Patients allergic to or intolerant of aspirin may be treated with ticlopidine or clopidogrel, which are antiplatelet agents that inhibit adenosine diphosphate–dependent platelet aggregation. However, clopidogrel appears to have a better safety profile than ticlopidine with a lower incidence of thrombocytopenia, neutropenia, and gastrointestinal side effects.

The use of heparin in addition to aspirin is currently recommended for the acute treatment of moderate- to high-risk patients *(2)*. However, unstable anginal symptoms recur after heparin is discontinued, owing to reactivation of the coagulation system, and it appears that concomitant treatment with aspirin may prevent this withdrawal phenomenon. This suggests that the culprit lesion is still active after 1 wk of therapy. Furthermore, a significant number of patients continue to have recurrent cardiac events for months after discharge. In fact, activation of the coagulation mechanism has been shown to persist for up to 6 months after the acute event. Nevertheless, even prolonged treatment with a low molecular weight heparin, which has been shown to be superior to unfractionated heparin (UFH) for the acute management of UA/NQWMI, did not result in a further decrease in events beyond that seen in the acute treatment phase.

Newer, more potent antiplatelet agents that block the glycoprotein (Gp) IIb/IIIa receptor are now available. These agents compete with fibrinogen for binding to the Gp IIb/IIIa receptor, and thereby inhibit the common final pathway of platelet aggregation. Because of the positive results from several clinical trials, tirofiban and eptifibatide are now widely utilized for the management of UA/NQWMI patients, in addition to standard medical therapy, especially in those patients deemed to be at high risk (3). This includes patients with unstable anginal symptoms associated with ST segment depression, new significant T wave inversions or an elevated cardiac troponin. Appropriate therapy for this subgroup of acute coronary syndrome patients includes early cardiac catheterization and percutaneous transluminal coronary angioplasty (PTCA) if feasible (4). In fact, the greatest benefit of these agents was realized in the subgroup of patients who underwent an early coronary interventional procedure and in whom the Gp IIb/IIIa infusion was continued for 12–24 h after the procedure.

To date, clinical trials involving abciximab, a monoclonal antibody directed at the platelet Gp IIb/IIIa receptor complex, have included only patients undergoing coronary angioplasty, although the agent remains under study for use outside the catheterization laboratory. In the Evaluation of Platelet IIb/IIIa Inhibition for Prevention of Ischemic Complications (EPIC) trial, the administration of abciximab resulted in a 35% reduction in the risk of major adverse cardiac events at 30 d (5). This benefit was sustained after 3 yr of follow-up, and it is explained in part by the ability of abciximab to provide rapid, profound, and sustained inhibition of platelet function for up to 15 d as it continuously redistributes among circulating platelets.

β-BLOCKERS

β-Blockers without intrinsic sympathomimetic activity are an important class of drugs for the treatment of patients with IHD. They exert their beneficial effects by decreasing BP, heart rate, and myocardial contractility with a net effect of decreasing myocardial oxygen demand. The ability of β-blockers to improve survival after a transmural MI, limit infarct size, and reduce the risk of a recurrent infarction or myocardial rupture has been well documented *(6)*. In fact, β-blockers are the only drugs that have been shown to reduce the risk of sudden cardiac death and intracerebral hemorrhage after an MI. However, there are no large-scale clinical trials on UA or NQWMI. For the treatment of stable anginal symptoms, β-blockers offer similar reductions in death, MI, and relief from angina as compared to calcium channel blockers (CCBs), but with fewer adverse events.

More recently, β-blockers have been shown to improve symptoms and exercise capacity, as well as decrease mortality in patients with congestive heart failure (CHF) secondary to systolic dysfunction *(7)*. Because β-blockers have a tendency to exacerbate heart failure symptoms, concomitant treatment with diuretics and an angiotensin-converting enzyme (ACE) inhibitor is necessary.

CALCIUM CHANNEL BLOCKERS

CCBs may be used for the management of anginal symptoms and BP if adequately controlled with a β-blocker. Despite reports suggesting that short-acting CCBs can increase overall mortality in patients with CAD, recent studies with long-acting CCBs have failed to support this claim. In fact, BP control is more persistent and stable and therefore results in less activation of the sympathetic nervous system. Long-acting CCBs have also been shown to decrease the incidence of silent and symptomatic ischemic episodes. In patients with a NQWMI, diltiazem reduces the incidence of postinfarction angina, early reinfarction, and death. However, the use of diltiazem, verapamil, and procardia should be avoided in patients with an acute MI in the presence of CHF and severe left ventricular dysfunction.

Second-generation dihydropyridines such as amplodipine and felodipine are now available for the treatment of hypertension and angina. Because they exert no significant negative inotropic or chronotropic effects on the heart, they can be used safely in patients with severe heart failure and severely reduced systolic function *(8)*.

Combination therapy utilizing a β-blocker and CCB is generally well tolerated. However, bradycardia, hypotension, and heart block have been reported to occur in 10–15% of patients on verapamil and a β-blocker. Therefore, caution should be exercised when using this combination.

ACE INHIBITORS

Based on the results of several, large clinical trials, ACE inhibitors should be part of the medical regimen for the hypertensive patient with IHD who has CHF and/or a large MI with severely reduced systolic function *(9)*. More recently, the ACE inhibitor ramipril was shown to reduce the incidence of MI, stroke or death from cardiovascular causes in a broad range of high-risk patients with a normal ejection fraction and no heart failure *(10)*.

NITRATES

Nitrates remain a mainstay of therapy for the management of patients with symptomatic CAD because they reduce the number of ischemic events. However, nitrates do not affect mortality or the incidence of MI in these patients. To avoid the development of tolerance, patients should have a daily nitrate-free interval.

REVASCULARIZATION

PTCA remains the method of choice for the revascularization of patients with single- and double-vessel CAD and preserved systolic function. Compared to medical therapy, PTCA offers improved exercise capacity and the need for fewer antianginal medications with no impact on mortality or subsequent MI. In a study of nondiabetic patients with triple-vessel disease and no significant systolic dysfunction, it was shown that PTCA and coronary artery bypass graft (CABG) surgery resulted in equivalent survival and freedom from MI *(11)*. However, patients initially treated with CABG had fewer episodes of angina, were on less antianginal medication, and required fewer repeat revascularization procedures. Diabetic patients with triple-vessel CAD appear to have a higher mortality with PTCA and should therefore be referred for CABG.

CABG confers a survival advantage in patients with significant left main disease, triple-vessel CAD with reduced systolic function, double-vessel CAD with a proximal left anterior descending artery stenosis, and left ventricular aneurysm with heart failure symptoms or sustained ventricular arrhythmias. Therefore, CABG is the treatment of choice for these patients. In patients with anatomy unfavorable for PTCA,

CABG is utilized for relief of symptoms and offers little or no survival advantage.

SECONDARY PREVENTION

Modification of the known risk factors for CAD including hypertension *(12)*, hyperlipidemia *(13)*, diabetes mellitus, and smoking reduces cardiovascular morbidity and mortality. In addition, family history, obesity, physical inactivity, homocysteinemia, alcohol consumption, and psychologic factors are important risk factors for cardiovascular disease. Instituting an aggressive treatment strategy aimed at slowing the progression of CAD and preventing recurrent cardiovascular events is the goal of secondary prevention.

REFERENCES

1. ISIS-2 (Second International Study of Infarct Survival) Collaborative Group (1988) Randomised trial of intravenous streptokinase, oral aspirin, both, or neither among 17,187 cases of suspected acute myocardial infarction: ISIS-2. *Lancet* 2:349–360.
2. Braunwald E, Mark DB, Jones RH, Cheitlin MD, Fuster V, McCauley KM, Edwards C, Green LA, Mushlin AI, Swain JA (1994) *Unstable Angina: Diagnosis and Management.* Clinical practice guideline number 10. Agency for Health Care Policy and Research and the National Heart, Lung, and Blood Institute, Public Health Service, United States Department of Health and Human Services.
3. Kong DF, Califf RM, Miller DP, Moliterno DJ, White HD, Harrington RA, Tcheng JE, Lincoff AM, Hasselblad V, Topol EJ (1998) Clinical outcomes of therapeutic agents that block the platelet glycoprotein IIb/IIIa integrin in ischemic heart disease. *Circulation* 98:2829–2835.
4. Ryan TJ, Bauman WB, Kennedy JW, Kereiakes DJ, King SB, McCallister BD, Smith SC, Ullyot DJ (1993) Guidelines for percutaneous transluminal coronary angioplasty: a report from the American College of Cardiology/American Heart Association task force on assessment of diagnostic and therapeutic cardiovascular procedures (committee on percutaneous transluminal coronary angioplasty). *J Am Coll Cardiol* 22:2033–2054.
5. The EPIC investigators (1994) Use of monoclonal antibody directed against the platelet glycoprotein IIb/IIIa receptor in high-risk coronary angioplasty. *N Engl J Med* 330:956–961.
6. Antman E, Lau J, Kupelnick B, et al. (1992) A comparison of results of meta-analysis of randomized control trials and recommendations of clinical experts: treatment for myocardial infarction. *JAMA* 268:240–248.
7. Packer M, Bristow MR, Cohn JN, et al. (1996) The effect of carvedolol on morbidity and mortality in patients with chronic heart failure. *N Engl J Med* 334(21):1349–1355.
8. Packer M, O'Connor CM, Ghali JK, et al., for the Prospective Randomized

Amplodipine Survival Evaluation Study Group (1996) Effect of amplodipine on morbidity and mortality in severe chronic heart failure. *N Engl J Med* 335(15): 1107–1114.

9. The SOLVD Investigators (1991) Effect of enalapril on survival in patients with reduced left ventricular ejection fractions and congestive heart failure. *N Engl J Med* 325:293–302.

10. The Heart Outcomes Prevention Evaluation Study Investigators (2000) Effects of an angiotensin-converting-enzyme inhibitor, ramipril, on cardiovascular events in high-risk patients. *N Engl J Med* 342:145–153.

11. King SB III, Lembo NJ, Weintraub WS, et al. (1994) A randomized trial comparing angioplasty with coronary surgery: Emory Angioplasty versus Surgery Trial (EAST). *N Engl J Med* 331:1044–1050.

12. Joint National Committee on Detection, Evaluation and Treatment of High Blood Pressure (JNC VI) (1997) *Arch Intern Med* 157:2413–2446.

13. Adult Treatment Panel II: National Cholesterol Education Program (1994) Second report of the Expert Panel on Detection, Evaluation, and Treatment of High Blood Cholesterol in Adults. *Circulation* 89:1329–1445.

37 Hypertension and Its Treatment in Concomitant Conditions

Degenerative Joint Disease, Depression, Alzheimer Disease, and Parkinson Disease

Domenic A. Sica, MD

CONTENTS

Hypertension occurs in more than 50 million people in the United States, and thus, it is not uncommon for it to be present in patients with other illnesses. This is particularly the case in the elderly in whom several commonly found illnesses, including degenerative joint disease (DJD), Parkinson disease, depression, and Alzheimer disease, can make the treatment of hypertension a particularly challenging proposition. This chapter addresses these disease states and their relationship to the treatment of hypertension.

DEGENERATIVE JOINT DISEASE

Hypertension is frequently observed in the setting of DJD, in part, because the prevalence of each of these disturbances increases with

From: *Hypertension Medicine*
Edited by: M. A. Weber © Humana Press Inc., Totowa, NJ

age. The treatment of hypertension can be complicated in the presence of DJD in that the mainstay of therapy for this disease involves administration of nonsteroidal anti-inflammatory drugs (NSAIDs). NSAIDs are well known for their ability to produce *de novo* hypertension and/or to attenuate the antihypertensive effect of many drugs routinely utilized in the treatment of hypertension. In susceptible subjects such as the elderly or those with diabetes (salt-sensitive hypertensive patients), NSAID therapy can prompt modest salt and water retention and thereby expand plasma volume. Secondarily, this combination of events results in an increase in mean arterial pressure. Except for a change in blood pressure (BP), the findings of physical examinations are typically insufficiently sensitive to detect what is otherwise modest plasma volume expansion.

NSAIDs can blunt the antihypertensive effect of most drug classes with the possible exception of calcium channel blockers (CCBs). Thus, CCB therapy may be the preferred mode of therapy in such patients. Diuretics are suitable alternatives to CCBs but may require higher than normal doses to effect a diuresis in NSAID-treated patients. This mode of diuretic resistance is most at issue when potent NSAIDs such as indomethacin are administered but may be less problematic with other presumably more "renal friendly" NSAIDs; thus, the adverse renal effects of NSAIDs have been suggested to be less prominent with the NSAID sulindac. The interaction between NSAIDs and diuretics seems to be less impressive for thiazide-type diuretics than for loop diuretics. In the latter, a significant blunting of diuretic effect can occur and in susceptible subjects such as those with cirrhosis or congestive heart failure, extreme volume excess may develop. If an NSAID is felt to be associated with a change in either the hypertensive or volume profile of a patient, a switch to an alternative NSAID class and/or a decrease in dose amount should be considered.

The time of day when an NSAID is dosed in a DJD patient can be very important. NSAIDs administered at bedtime (if successful in pain relief) can restore normal sleep architecture by diminishing the impact of pain on the integrity of the sleep cycle. This may, in turn, simplify daytime BP control. DJD patients also oftentimes adopt a sedentary lifestyle because of pain-related limitations in mobility. The ensuing weight gain secondary to this decreased exercise pattern can result in deterioration in BP control. Accordingly, DJD patients should be considered good candidates for lifestyle modifications, such as weight loss and aerobic exercise, in an effort to control hypertension.

PARKINSON DISEASE

Hypertension is not uncommonly observed in Parkinson disease patients. Hypertension does not develop as a direct consequence of Parkinson disease; rather, it independently occurs in the same age range, as does most Parkinson disease. The treatment of hypertension in Parkinson disease can be complicated because certain antihypertensive drugs (reserpine or α-methyldopa) can intensify parkinsonian symptomatology or therapies used in this condition exhibit important vasoactive properties. For example, orthostatic hypotension, which occurs frequently in patients with parkinsonism, can be aggravated by levodopa therapy. Fortunately, this phenomenon tends to abate over several months of therapy with levodopa. In addition, monoamine oxidase (MAO) inhibitor therapy with drugs such as selegiline (Eldepryl®) can occur as an adjunct to levodopa/carbidopa therapy. At high doses, selegiline loses its MAO B selectivity and has the potential to interact with products containing tyramine or other sympathomimetic amines (*see* Depression section) with the development of a hypertensive crisis.

Psychiatric side effects including confusion, visual hallucinations, and paranoia are often present in combination with dementia that is related to the disease rather than its treatment. These neuropsychiatric abnormalities along with the natural deteriorative element of this disease make antihypertensive therapy complicated and oftentimes affect medication compliance. Like Alzheimer disease, the risk:benefit ratio of treating hypertension in a patient with Parkinson disease must be carefully examined.

DEPRESSION

The relationship between depression and hypertension/cardiovascular disease is becoming increasingly complex. Several well-designed studies have demonstrated that depressed patients have a poorer prognosis from diverse illnesses such as stroke and myocardial infarction. In addition, recent studies now suggest that individuals who report high levels of anxiety or depressive symptoms are at elevated risk for developing hypertension over the ensuing decade. The exact risk gradient for this phenomenon depends on race and age, but the relative risk is on the order of 2.0, or a doubling of the risk.

Depression is also problematic because many antidepressants manifest direct cardiac effects. For example, tricyclic antidepressants exhibit a quinidine-like effect and can decrease cardiac output and/or slow intracardiac conduction. Common adverse reactions to these drugs include orthostatic hypotension (particularly in the elderly) and a variety of supraventricular and ventricular arrhythmias as well as heart block. Patients with significant underlying conduction system disease are at particular risk from these drugs. Fortunately, except in the instance of overdose, major cardiac complications are rare in individuals without underlying cardiac pathology. However, it is advisable to obtain an electrocardiogram before initiating antidepressant therapy in patients older than 40 yr.

MAO inhibitors are also used as antidepressants, and in a hypertensive patient carry with their use a substantial likelihood of drug-drug interactions. The most feared cardiovascular complication of MAO inhibitor therapy is the precipitation of an adrenergic crisis owing to concomitant ingestion of sympathomimetic drugs or pressor amines such as tyramine, which are found in food and beverages. Among the various MAO inhibitors, tranylcypromine (Parnate®) is perceived as the most hazardous. Because of the wide range of substances known to precipitate hypertensive crises in patients treated with MAO inhibitors, it is prudent to have ready access to a listing of foodstuffs as well as prescription and over-the-counter medications that can trigger an MAO-related hypertensive crisis. Several antihypertensive compounds are best avoided in patients treated with MAO inhibitors including α-methyldopa, guanethidine, and reserpine. The best strategy is preventive for this reaction, because it can prove to be lethal. Thus, in the hypertensive patient with preexisting cardiac disease, any new treatment for depression should be introduced cautiously with an understanding that any new symptomatology should warrant a reassessment of a patient's cardiac profile.

Depression can also be seen as a side effect of a number of different antihypertensive medications including β-blockers, $α_1$-receptor agonists (such as α-methyldopa), and reserpine. Among the β-blockers, propranolol is particularly sedating and can cause confusional states and nightmares. All β-blockers penetrate the central nervous system (CNS), although less lipophilic compounds, such as atenolol and nadolol, penetrate much less so than does propranolol. Despite this hierarchy of CNS penetration, there is only minimal evidence to support the notion that the lipophilicity of a β-blocker determines the likelihood of its causing depression. Diuretics, CCBs, angiotensin-converting enzyme

(ACE) inhibitors, and angiotensin-receptor antagonists appear to have the lowest associated risk with depression and are therefore the drugs of choice when depression is a consideration.

Depression has to be viewed as an important confounding variable in medication compliance. This is unfortunately an extremely difficult issue, particularly if the depressive symptomatology is intensified by concomitant antihypertensive therapy. Compliance with medication should be carefully evaluated in a depressed patient. In this regard, it is useful to verify patient assertions by crosschecking with information provided by family members. Depression is a broad term under which many disease-state variants are grouped together. Reaching a correct diagnosis (and thereby offering optimal pharmacotherapy) may have a quite favorable influence on what can otherwise be very destructive patterns of medication ingestion. Obviously, in the depressed hypertensive patient, it is prudent to replace any potential offending antihypertensive agents before addressing pharmacologic therapy for depression.

ALZHEIMER DISEASE

The treatment of hypertension in Alzheimer disease requires a careful assessment of the risk:benefit ratio of such an endeavor. Both the anticipated longevity as well as the functional status of an Alzheimer patient prove to be important determinants in the decision to treat. Thus, it is not at all unreasonable to withhold drug therapy in those hypertensive patients in the borderline → stage I category, particularly if the onset of hypertension coincides with the later stages of Alzheimer disease.

If the decision is made to either begin or continue antihypertensive therapy in an Alzheimer patient, careful attention should be directed toward the interface between what might otherwise be viewed as trivial day-to-day activities such as eating/swallowing, meal and posture changes, and the prevailing sleep-wake cycle. In the more advanced stage of Alzheimer disease, nutritional needs may be poorly met without the support of a caregiver. If such is the case, every effort should be made to be certain that any long-acting antihypertensive preparations being administered are not inadvertently crushed to facilitate ingestion. If this occurs, a sustained-release preparation will frequently assume immediate released characteristics. This dumping of active drug into the gastrointestinal tract exaggerates medication peak effect (with possible CNS symptoms) and diminishes duration of effect.

Also, careful attention should be directed to the possibility of post-prandial hypotension in these patients, and, if present, the timing of medication administration should be such to avoid any overlap between meal-related BP decrements and peak medication effect. If postprandial hypotension occurs, decreasing the meal size and spreading total caloric intake more evenly over all three daily meals can lessen its impact. In addition, in certain individuals, caffeine intake may attenuate the meal-related drop in BP. Alzheimer patients should always be evaluated for the possibility of postural hypotension. If bedridden, deconditioning can occur quite rapidly in any subject including an Alzheimer patient. Consequently, this should not be an unexpected phenomenon in the later stages of the disease. Maneuvers that worsen postural hypotension, such as volume contraction from diuretics and pulse rate reduction with β-blockers, should be employed in the management of hypertension only if absolutely indicated and with expressed caution.

As a rule of thumb, nighttime administration of antihypertensive medication should occur cautiously in an Alzheimer patient and only if bedtime BPs are documented to be elevated. BP exhibits a circadian rhythm with a varying degree of drop during sleep. In those older than 60 yr, BP may inordinately drop during sleep (as much as a 30–35% reduction); this has been termed *extreme dipping*. Those patients prone to arising in the middle of the night may be subject to risk if medication peak effect coincides with the naturally occurring nadir of BP. If night-time antihypertensive therapy is considered, patients should be advised to gradually shift from the supine to the recumbent position and to ambulate at night only with assistance. Extreme dipping of BP is now believed to be a risk factor for both multi-infarct dementia and other less severe forms of cerebrovascular disease. Thus, Alzheimer's disease or similar neurologic illnesses may represent a preselected population whose nocturnal BP pattern is phenotypically one of extreme dipping.

Selection of a drug class for the treatment of hypertension in this population should limit use of drugs with significant sedating effects, those that produce clinically relevant volume contraction, or those that significantly decrease cardiac output. ACE inhibitors and CCBs are reasonably safe compounds in this population, whereas diuretics, centrally acting agents, and β-blockers may carry with their use unnecessary risk. ACE inhibitors may be of particular utility in that they preserve cerebrovascular autoregulatory ability; thus, even if systemic BP is reduced cerebral blood flow is well maintained. The principles of effective antihypertensive therapy in this population should avoid inducing postural hypotension and/or sudden drops in BP; hence, unless medication compliance is an issue, multiple drugs should not be simultaneously administered. This will lessen the unintended risk of an exaggerated drop in BP at the peak effect of several antihypertensive medications.

Concomitant medications used in the treatment of Alzheimer's disease typically do not affect BP. More important, the introduction of any new medication in this population can influence BP as it relates to alterations in cognitive ability. Accordingly, a more effective means of treating hypertension in this population should involve the use of home BP monitoring, a process that is simplified by the availability of a caregiver in the home environment. Home BP monitoring improves decision making for medication adjustment and provides a means of delineating the relationship between side effects and the prevailing BP.

38 Cognitive Disorders and Dementia in Hypertension

Implications for Treatment

Lena Kilander, MD, PhD

DEMENTIA OR NORMAL AGING?

Cognitive functions may be defined as mental or "thinking" functions, including all verbal and nonverbal cerebral functions involved in the processing of information: learning, memory, perception, association, abstract reasoning, planning, and so on. In normal aging, there is a slight decline of cognitive functions, especially of memory for recent daily-life events (short-term episodic memory). By contrast, *dementia* denotes a syndrome of persistent cognitive deterioration, severe enough to interfere with daily activities. Some

From: *Hypertension Medicine*
Edited by: M. A. Weber © Humana Press Inc., Totowa, NJ

20% of all people over the age of 80 yr suffer from dementia. There are two major subgroups of dementia disorders: neurodegenerative dementia, including Alzheimer disease; and vascular dementia. The borderlines between no dementia and dementia are not clear cut. Alzheimer disease, and in some cases vascular dementia, has an insidious onset and a slowly progressive course. In early stages of Alzheimer disease, the patient is forgetful but does not otherwise fulfill the criteria for dementia. Thus, the differential diagnosis between normal aging and early dementia is often difficult. Research is now focusing on how to define early cognitive decline, and on attempts to identify potentially treatable risk factors. In our clinical practice, we have, in the last few years, encountered an increasing number of patients with mild cognitive impairment who are asking for treatment to slow down progress of this condition.

MRS. B: A COMMON PATIENT

Mrs. B, a former headmaster, age 82, arrives at your practice accompanied by her son. She has been treated for hypertension with hydrochlorothiazide since the age of 60, and has otherwise been quite healthy. Prior to this visit, her son has called you to explain his concern about Mrs. B's failing memory. During the last couple of years, Mrs. B has grown increasingly forgetful. Now, she has obvious problems, which cause a great distress to her family. She fails to keep appointments, mislays her money and keys, and has difficulties with orientation to time. She has become more inactive, neglects housekeeping, and has stopped seeing her friends. During the interview, Mrs. B appears cheerful with no signs of depression. She admits to being forgetful, but denies that this causes her any trouble. She looks surprised and slightly embarrassed when her son remarks that she called him some 20 times early this morning, each time asking when they should leave for the doctor's appointment. Mrs. B appears unsure when asked about the names and ages of her grandchildren. She scores 24 of 30 points on the Mini Mental State Examination (MMSE) *(1)*, she cannot tell the date or weekday, she loses concentration when counting backward, and in a test of short-term memory, she cannot remember any of three words. Her blood pressure (BP) in the sitting position is 180/100 mmHg.

1. Does Mrs. B suffer from dementia, and, if so, is it Alzheimer disease or vascular dementia?

2. How should her hypertension best be treated?

ALZHEIMER DISEASE AND VASCULAR DEMENTIA: CHANGING CONCEPTS OVER TIME

In the mid-1970s, the artificial dichotomization between Alzheimer disease or presenile dementia, and senile dementia, i.e., dementia with onset after age 65, was abandoned. With this change in concepts, Alzheimer disease became transformed from a rare disease to a major killer, being one of the most common causes of death in the United States (2). This had an enormous impact on research and clinicians' interest in dementia. Today, the term *Alzheimer disease* is commonly used irrespective of whether the patient is age 45 or 90. However, this is an oversimplification, because Alzheimer disease is most certainly a heterogeneous entity, with subgroups still awaiting their definitions. Early onset Alzheimer disease is often linked to genetic factors, such as the presence of the apolipoprotein E e4 (apo e4) allele and other, rare genetic aberrations (3). The apo e4 allele is overrepresented in elderly Alzheimer disease patients as well, but the risk factor pattern is more blunted. The concept of *multi-infarct dementia* was replaced in the 1980s by the wider term *vascular dementia*, covering dementia resulting from any type of cerebrovascular disease. Still some 5 yr ago, Alzheimer disease and vascular dementia were regarded as two separate entities. However, in recent years, it has become clear that late-onset Alzheimer disease and vascular dementia have common pathways. Autopsy series have shown that both pure Alzheimer disease (i.e., without any cerebrovascular disease) and pure vascular dementia (i.e., without concomitant neuropathologic evidence of AD) are extremely uncommon (4). Furthermore, recent epidemiologic research supports that cerebrovascular risk factors are determinants not only of vascular dementia, but also Alzheimer disease. Dementia after stroke is common and frequently manifests when the cerebral infarct is combined with Alzheimer disease pathology (5). In a longitudinal population-based study, hypertension predicted Alzheimer disease in very old patients (6). The combination of atherosclerosis and apo e4 (7) has also been associated with dementia, irrespective of cause. Even in men without dementia free from stroke, high BP in middle age predicted low cognitive functions at the age of 70 (8). Pathophysiologic mechanisms may be multifactorial, including silent ischemic lesions and blood-brain barrier dysfunction, which, hypothetically, may trigger β-amyloid deposition and neurodegeneration. A practical conclusion to be drawn from this is that hypertension is a treatable risk factor, in contrast to older age and genetic factors.

DIAGNOSIS OF DEMENTIA AT THE FAMILY PHYSICIAN'S OFFICE

The key to dementia assessment is to get an objective medical history from someone close to the patient. If you suspect dementia, ask the patient if he or she has memory complaints, but remember that loss of insight is common, and many patients with manifest dementia would deny problems. Conversely, many healthy elderly people report forgetfulness, although it does not cause them any trouble. Make sure that the patient brings someone close to him or her at the next visit. Arrange for a private interview with the informant in order to avoid embarrassment in front of the patient. A comprehensive description of the debut and development of different symptoms yields the greatest part of the diagnostic information: When and how did the symptoms start? Ask specifically for treatable symptoms, such as depression, emotional instability, and insomnia, and about practical problems. Typically, Alzheimer disease presents with an insidious onset of impaired recent memory and word-finding ability. Subsequently, memory, thinking, verbal, and spatial functions deteriorate and activities in daily life are affected. Vascular dementia typically starts abruptly in connection with a stroke, sometimes without any other neurologic signs. However, the course of vascular dementia may also be slowly progressive, mimicking Alzheimer disease. All patients with cognitive disturbances, irrespective of age, should be examined as outlined in Table 38-1. This basal assessment includes medical history, physical examination, and laboratory tests in order to exclude hypo- and hyperthyreos, hyperparathyroidism, vitamin B_{12} deficiency, and other treatable conditions.

There are numerous cognitive tests. The MMSE *(1)* is the most widely used screening instrument for cognitive disorders. Another simple test, sensitive to visuospatial disturbances, is to ask the patient to draw a clock, set at a specified time. Even more sensitive and specific are relevant questions concerning family, current activities, and details of earlier life such as occupation and childhood. Computed tomography (CT) or magnetic resonance imaging (MRI) are valuable complements, and are mandatory in the case of rapid progress, and if a chronic subdural

Table 38-1
Assessment of Dementia in Old Patients

1. Interview
    Symptoms: cognitive, emotional, or behavioral?
    Onset: sudden or insidious?
    Course: slowly progressive or sudden deterioration?
2. Physical examination
    Neurological examination
    BP, cardiopulmonary system
3. Laboratory tests
    B-Hb, B-SR, b-glucose, s-creatinine, s-calcium, s-TSH, s-vitamin B_{12}
4. Cognitive testing
    Relevant questions
    MMSE, Clock-Drawing Test, etc.
5. Neuroimaging
    CT or MRI

hematoma or a brain tumor are suspected. Conversely, neuroimaging is not always necessary in the assessment of very old patients with a history of slowly progressive dementia over several years.

HOW TO TREAT HYPERTENSION IN DEMENTIA

The main reason to treat hypertension in people ages 80+ is to prevent stroke. Stroke is a powerful predictor of dementia, and recent studies point to the fact that hypertension contributes to Alzheimer disease and dementia, irrespective of stroke. Therefore, an optimal antihypertensive treatment hypothetically may prevent or postpone cognitive decline. There are still no clear guidelines regarding antihypertensive treatment in patients over the age of 80. However, it is reasonable to extrapolate the results from trials in patients ages 70–80. Hence, the target BP should be <160/<90 mmHg, if this can be reached without adverse drug effects. It is mandatory to measure BP in both the supine and standing positions in order to avoid orthostatic hypotension, dizziness, and falls. Of course, other risk factors, concomitant disorders, and patient compliance should also be considered in the choice of therapeutic strategy.

In patients with manifest dementia, we do not know what the optimal BP is. Advanced dementia, irrespective of cause, is often accompanied by low BP. Formerly, low BP was considered a cause of dementia. Now, the prevailing opinion is that low BP in most cases is a consequence of the dementia disorder. Possible mediators are weight loss, a sedentary lifestyle, and perhaps more important, lesions in cerebral BP-regulating areas. Frontotemporal dementia, an uncommon neurodegenerative disorder, is often associated with very low BP even early in its course. Still, many physicians hesitate to treat hypertension in very old patients, because they fear adverse effects on cognition from BP lowering. Geriatricians commonly encounter patients with delirium and dizziness, and who suffer falls secondary to low BP in cardiac failure. For the individual physician, adverse effects possibly related to treatment certainly are more obvious than long-term positive effects (i.e., the non-development of target organ damage). In a recent enquiry, Swedish geriatricians were asked for their opinions regarding antihypertensive treatment of very old patients *(9)*. Almost 40% stated that systolic BP optimally should be >160 mmHg in an 82-yr-old hypertensive patient. One third of the physicians believed that, compared with a patient without dementia, a patient with dementia would benefit from a higher BP. Similarly, in a study of 300,000 patients in US nursing homes, hypertensive patients ≥85 yr and patients with cognitive or physical impairment were not treated according to current guidelines *(10)*.

ASSESSMENT AND DIAGNOSIS

The first step is to obtain a medical history (e.g., interviewing both Mrs. B and her son about the onset and course of cognitive problems). An insidious onset with slowly progressive course suggests Alzheimer disease. By contrast, an abrupt onset or a sudden worsening points to vascular pathology. CT or MRI in elderly patients with dementia are often difficult to evaluate. They may or may not reveal signs of atrophy, cortical or subcortical infarcts, and white-matter lesions. The absence of significant vascular lesions on CT excludes, on the whole, vascular dementia. Conversely, white-matter lesions are common even in the healthy elderly *(11)*. Thus, this finding does not justify a diagnosis of vascular dementia. If a patient's cognitive decline started insidiously with no time relationship to a stroke, he or she probably suffers from Alzheimer disease. If neuroimaging shows evidence of cerebrovascular disease, the diagnosis might still be Alzheimer disease, or Alzheimer disease with cerebrovascular disease. In the latter case, the most accurate, although not yet established, diagnosis would be Alzheimer disease of vascular origin.

IMPLICATIONS FOR TREATMENT

The treatment goal is to achieve a BP of <160/<90 mmHg without adverse effects. First, determine whether the patient takes his or her tablets as prescribed. The patient probably needs to be reminded. Avoid drugs that may cause delirium—β-blockers should not be the first choice for a patient with dementia. Rapid BP lowering and orthostatic hypotension should be avoided. Generally, old patients tolerate better low doses of two or three drugs than a high dose of a single agent. Monitor BP and monitor cognitive functions by interviewing the patient and his or her caregiver about functions. The MMSE could be administered every 6 or 12 mo. The average annual drop in the MMSE in Alzheimer disease is two to four points. With progression of the dementia disorder, BP may decrease, and treatment should be adjusted. In brief, other pharmacologic treatment in dementia may include selective serotonin reuptake inhibitors for emotional disturbances such as depression and irritability. Acetylcholine esterase inhibitors (donepezil, rivastigmine) can improve attention, short-term memory, word-finding ability, and daily activities in mild to moderate Alzheimer disease. Even more important is to supply psychologic and practical support to the patient and his or her family (12).

CONCLUSION

Formerly considered a phenomenon of normal aging, during the last two decades dementia has been recognized as a major health problem. Old people commonly regard a failing mind as the most frightening complication of aging. Dementia and cognitive impairment after stroke cause severe disability and suffering for patients and caregivers, and the costs for society will steadily rise because an increasing proportion of the population will reach very old ages. According to recent studies, hypertension and cerebrovascular disease seem to be important factors behind Alzheimer disease as well as vascular dementia. Cerebral target organ damage in hypertension is no longer just a matter of stroke, but also of dementia. Evidence that an optimal treatment may postpone some cases of dementia has been reported recently from the Systolic Hypertension in Europe trial (13). Therefore, antihypertensive treatment of old patients should be given very careful attention. At present, however, neither science nor evidence-based medicine can tell what the optimum BP is in old patients with cognitive decline. Treating very old hypertensive patients is a great challenge: Will we succeed in protecting our patients from stroke as well as dementia?

REFERENCES

1. Folstein MF, Folstein SE, McHugh PR (1975) "Mini-Mental State": a practical method for grading the cognitive state of patients for the clinician. *J Psychiatr Res* 12:189–198.
2. Katzman R (1976) The prevalence and malignancy of Alzheimer's disease: a major killer. *Arch Neurol* 33:217–218 (editorial).
3. Selkoe DJ (1996) Amyloid beta-protein and the genetics of Alzheimer's disease. *J Biol Chem* 271:18,295–18,298.
4. Hulette C, Nochlin D, McKeel D, Morris JC, Mirra SS, Sumi SM, Heyman A (1997) Clinical-neuropathologic findings in multi-infarct dementia: a report of six autopsied cases. *Neurology* 48:668–672.
5. Pasquier F, Leys D (1997) Why are stroke patients prone to develop dementia? *J Neurol* 244:135–142.
6. Skoog I, Lernfelt B, Landahl S, et al. (1996) 15-year longitudinal study of blood pressure and dementia. *Lancet* 347:1141–1145.
7. Hofman A, Ott A, Breteler M, et al. (1997) Atherosclerosis, apolipoprotein E, and prevalence of dementia and Alzheimer's disease in the Rotterdam Study. *Lancet* 349:151–154.
8. Kilander L, Nyman H, Boberg M, Hansson L, Lithell H (1998) Hypertension is related to cognitive impairment: a 20-year follow-up of 999 men. *Hypertension* 31:780–786.
9. Kilander L, Boberg M, Lithell H (1997) How do we treat, or not treat, high blood pressure in the oldest old? A practice study in Swedish geriatricians. *Blood Press* 6:372–376.
10. Gambassi G, Lapane K, Sgadari A, et al. (1998) Prevalence, clinical correlates, and treatment of hypertension in elderly nursing home residents. SAGE (Systematic Assessment of Geriatric Drug Use via Epidemiology) Study Group. *Arch Intern Med* 158:2377–2385.
11. Longstreth WT, Manolio TA, Arnold A, et al. (1996) Clinical correlates of white matter findings on cranial magnetic resonance imaging of 3301 elderly people: The Cardiovascular Health Study. *Stroke* 27:1274–1282.
12. Mittelman MS, Ferris SH, Shulman E, Steinberg G, Levin B (1996) A family intervention to delay nursing home placement of patients with Alzheimer's disease: a randomized trial. *JAMA* 276:1725–1731.
13. Forette F, Seux M-L, Staessen J, et al. (1998) Prevention of dementia in randomised double-blind placebo-controlled Systolic Hypertension in Europe (Syst-Eur) trial. *Lancet* 352:1347–1351.

39 Refractory Hypertension

C. Venkata S. Ram, MD

CONTENTS

Because of widespread treatment of systemic hypertension, true refractory hypertension is somewhat unusual in the current management of hypertensive disorders. A majority of patients with uncomplicated primary hypertension respond to one or two drugs. Hypertension is considered refractory if the blood pressure (BP) cannot be reduced below 140/90 mmHg in patients who are compliant with an appropriate triple-drug regimen that includes a diuretic, with all the components prescribed in near maximal or tolerated doses. For patients with isolated systolic hypertension, refractoriness is defined as a failure of an adequate triple-drug regimen to reduce systolic blood pressure below 160 mmHg.

From: *Hypertension Medicine*
Edited by: M. A. Weber © Humana Press Inc., Totowa, NJ

Whereas refractory hypertension may be commonly encountered in specialized centers, its prevalence in the general population of hypertensive patients is quite low. As already indicated, most patients with chronic uncomplicated hypertension should respond to relatively simple therapy.

ETIOLOGY

Table 39-1 lists the causes of refractory hypertension. When a hypertensive patient demonstrates resistance to standard or conventional therapy, proper management depends on the identification of a possible cause. Before planning therapeutic changes, certain questions should come to mind: Does the patient truly have refractory hypertension? Are there any host/environmental factors? Does the patient have pseudoresistance? Are there certain drug reactions? Does the patient have a secondary form of hypertension such as renovascular hypertension? Are there any mechanisms (pressor) that are responsible for elevating the arterial BP?

PSEUDORESISTANCE

It is not uncommon to encounter a patient whose clinic/office BP measurements are higher than the levels obtained outside the office setting—so-called white coat hypertension. Although white coat hypertension is often considered in the context of mild hypertension (stage I or II), in some cases refractory hypertension may reflect white coat hypertension. Patients who may have refractory hypertension do not demonstrate evidence of target organ damage (TOD) despite seemingly very high BP readings in the office or clinic. The disparity between the degree of hypertension and the paucity of TOD can be supported by the measurement of home BPs and by obtaining ambulatory blood pressure recordings with an automatic device *(1)*.

Another source of erroneous BP measurement is pseudohypertension, found mostly in the elderly. In this phenomenon, called Osler's phenomenon, the hardened and sclerotic artery is not compressible so that falsely elevated pressures are recorded *(2)*. Because of the thickened arteries, cuff measurements show a much higher reading than the actual (or intraarterial) BP. There is little doubt that pseudohypertension does occur in older individuals but its exact prevalence is not known.

Table 39-1
Causes of Refractory Hypertension

Pseudoresistance
  "White coat hypertension" or office elevations
  Pseudohypertension in older patients
  Use of regular cuff on very obese arm
Nonadherence to therapy
Volume overload
Drug-related causes
  Doses too low
  Wrong type of diuretic
  Inappropriate combinations
  Drug actions and interactions
    Sympathomimetics
    Nasal decongestants
    Appetite suppressants
    Cocaine and other illicit drugs
    Caffeine
    Oral contraceptives
    Adrenal steroids
    Licorice (as may be found in chewing tobacco)
    Cyclosporine, tacrolimus
    Erythropoietin
    Antidepressants
    Nonsteroidal anti-inflammatory drugs
Concomitant conditions
  Smoking
  Increasing obesity
  Sleep apnea
  Insulin resistance/hyperinsulinemia
  Ethanol intake of more than 1 oz (30 mL)/d
  Anxiety-induced hyperventilation or panic attacks
  Chronic pain
Secondary causes of hypertension (e.g., renovascular hypertension, adrenal
  causes renal disease)

Persistently high readings in the absence of TOD or dysfunction may indicate pseudohypertension. Although some have advocated the use of intraarterial BP determination as a means of accurately making the diagnosis of this aberration, I question the practicality of this approach.

A far more common example of pseudoresistance is the measurement artifact, which could occur when BP is taken with a small cuff in people with large arm diameters *(3)*. With the patient in the seated position, BP should be taken with an appropriate cuff size to ensure accurate determination. The bladder within the cuff should encircle at least 80% of the arm. One has to be cautious, however, before dismissing the reading as a measurement artifact because patients with refractory hypertension experience a high rate of complications.

NONCOMPLIANCE

Failure to follow a prescribed regimen is an important cause of refractory hypertension. There may be legitimate reasons for a patient's noncompliance such as side effects, costs, complexity of the drug regimen, and lack of understanding. Social and personal factors may also play a role in noncompliance.

VOLUME OVERLOAD

Volume overload from any mechanism may not only increase BP but also can offset the BP-lowering effects of many medications *(4)*. Excessive salt intake causes resistance to antihypertensive drugs and can actually raise BP in so-called salt-sensitive hypertension. The elderly and African-American patients are particularly sensitive to fluid overload as are patients with renal insufficiency and congestive heart failure (CHF). Many antihypertensive drugs such as direct vasodilators, antiadrenergic agents, and essentially most of the nondiuretic antihypertensive drugs (except calcium antagonists) cause plasma and extracellular fluid expansion, thus attenuating the antihypertensive effects. Of all the nondiuretic antihypertensive drugs, angiotensin-converting enzyme (ACE) inhibitors, angiotensin II antagonists, and calcium antagonists are least likely to cause fluid retention. Antihypertensive responsiveness can be reclaimed by restricting the sodium intake, increasing the diuretic, and in some cases, switching to a loop diuretic in the place of thiazides.

DRUG-RELATED REASONS FOR REFRACTORY HYPERTENSION

Hypertension may be seemingly refractory if the drugs are used in subtherapeutic doses or when an inappropriate diuretic is used, e.g.,

Table 39-2
Drug Interactions That May Lead to Resistant Hypertension

Antihypertensive agents	Interacting drugs
Hydrochlorothiazide	Cholestyramine
Propranolol	Rifampin
Guanethidine	Tricyclics
Guanadrel	—
ACE inhibitors	Indomethacin
β-Blockers	—
Diuretics	Indomethacin
All	Cocaine, tricyclics
All	Phenylpropanolamine

using a thiazide type of diuretic as opposed to a loop diuretic in patients with renal insufficiency, CHF, or in those on potent vasodilators such as minoxidil or hydralazine. Inappropriate combinations can also limit their therapeutic potential. Adverse drug interactions can raise BP in normotensive as well as hypertensive patients. Such adverse interactions (Table 39-2) can occur as a result of alterations in drug absorption, metabolism, or in the pharmacodynamics of concomitant drugs administered for different indications. One example of unfavorable drug interaction is among indomethacin and β-blockers, diuretics, and ACE inhibitors. Tricyclic antidepressants (no longer popular) have a significant interaction with sympathetic blocking agents.

CONCOMITANT CONDITIONS

It is suspected that cigarette smoking can interfere with BP mechanisms *(5)*. Obesity often is a factor in the occurrence of refractory hypertension. Obstructive sleep apnea is being increasingly recognized as a possible factor in the development of resistant hypertension. Excessive alcohol consumption (more than 1 oz, or 30 mL) clearly raises systemic BP, sometimes to dangerously high levels *(6)*. I have seen panic attacks and hyperventilation as important etiologic factors in some patients with refractory hypertension. Similarly, chronic pain may be associated with marked hypertension.

Table 39-3
Selected Examples of Secondary Forms of Hypertension That May Be
Resistant to Antihypertensive Therapy

Renovascular hypertension	Hyperthyroidism
Primary aldosteronism	Hyperparathyroidism
Pheochromocytoma	Aortic coarctation
Hypothyroidism	Renal disease

SECONDARY CAUSES OF REFRACTORY HYPERTENSION

In a fraction of patients with refractory hypertension, the underlying cause may be a secondary form of hypertension such as renovascular hypertension (Table 39-3). Patients with a secondary form of hypertension may simply present with resistant hypertension. Sudden loss of effectiveness from a previously stable regimen may raise suspicion of renovascular disease. Other forms of secondary hypertension may manifest as refractory hypertension. In a more broader context, certain hemodynamic or humoral mechanisms can also result in severe or resistant hypertension (Table 39-4).

MANAGEMENT OF REFRACTORY HYPERTENSION

Proper management of refractory hypertension entails a systematic approach based on the considerations described in the preceding sections. It should be emphasized that because uncontrolled hypertension can cause significant morbidity and mortality, haphazard changes in the treatment plan should be avoided. An overall management approach should embrace careful evaluation and rational therapy.

EVALUATION AND ASSESSMENT

When a patient's BP does not respond satisfactorily, at the outset, one has to consider whether the patient has pseudoresistance—white coat hypertension (pseudohypertension in the elderly) and measurement artifact. In some individuals, it is appropriate to obtain home BP readings or 24-h ambulatory BP recordings in order to document the degree

Table 39-4
Hemodynamic and Neurohumoral Aberrations Responsible for Refractory
Hypertension and Their Correction

Hemodynamic measurement	Management
↑ Cardiac output	β-Blocker; verapamil
↑ Peripheral resistance	Hydralazine; minoxidil; ACE inhibitor; calcium channel blocker
↑ Plasma volume	Diuretic (loop); dietary sodium restriction
↑ Plasma catecholamines	Clonidine; methyldopa; α_1-blocker or α_1 + β-blocker
↑ Plasma rennin activity	β-Blocker; ACE inhibitor
↑ Plasma or urinary aldosterone	Spironolactone

of hypertension outside the office or clinic setting. In obese individuals, BP should be measured with a large cuff. It is absolutely critical to ascertain the patient's compliance to a prescribed regimen; nonadherence to treatment must be ruled out before further evaluation is undertaken. Factors responsible for noncompliance should be corrected, if possible. The treatment should be simplified to encourage patient participation. Often a sympathetic yet firm dialogue with the patient reveals whether or not compliance is the cause. With a good rapport with the patient, it will be unnecessary to measure the drug level in the blood to determine the patient's compliance.

Correction of volume overload is one of the most successful interventions in managing resistant hypertension *(7)*. Excessive salt intake must be curtailed. Adequate diuretic therapy should be applied based on the clinical circumstances. The dosage and the choice of the diuretic should be modified accordingly. Patients with concomitant CHF or renal insufficiency require optimal volume depletion to achieve adequate BP control. The doses of antihypertensive drugs should be titrated systematically to determine whether or not the patient is responding to the treatment. Drug interactions should be considered and eliminated in the treatment of hypertension *(8,9)*. A thorough inventory should be made of drugs that could increase BP, such as steroids, oral contraceptives, sympathomimetics, nasal decongestants, cocaine, and appetite suppressants. Patients should be counseled about alcohol consumption, weight control, salt intake, and regular physical activity. Conditions such as obstructive sleep apnea or chronic pain should be addressed.

Secondary causes of hypertension should be considered in the evaluation of patients with resistant hypertension. Among the causes, a prominent one is renovascular hypertension *(10)*. However, the scope of this chapter does not permit detailed description of work-up for renovascular hypertension. Based on the clinical hallmarks, renovascular hypertension should be pursued in patients with truly refractory hypertension. Other causes such as primary hyperaldosteronism, pheochromocytoma, Cushing syndrome, coarctation of aorta, and renal disease should be considered based on the clinical course and laboratory findings. If an underlying cause is found, it should be corrected by appropriate means to permit better BP control.

DRUG TREATMENT

When an identifiable cause is not found, patients with refractory hypertension merit aggressive drug therapy to control BP *(11)*. The first step is to optimize the existing therapy either by increasing the dosages or by changing to different combinations and observing the patient for a few weeks. In the event that BP still remains uncontrolled, effective diuretic therapy should be implemented. Assuming that the patient has failed to respond to conventional therapies, consideration should be given to use hydralazine or minoxidil (in conjunction with a β-blocker and a diuretic). Because direct vasodilators cause significant reflex activation of the sympathetic nervous system and fluid retention, their use should be accompanied by coadministration of a β-blocker and a diuretic (usually a loop diuretic). I often give a trial of hydralazine therapy before putting the patient on minoxidil. Occasionally, further reductions in BP can be secured by adding a fourth agent such as clonidine. In patients with marked renal impairment, dialysis might be required for adequate control of BP.

CONCLUSION

In most patients with chronic primary hypertension, BP can be controlled with changes in lifestyle and with one or two drugs. In a small percentage of patients, however, BP remains uncontrolled even on a three-drug regimen. These patients have refractory or resistant hypertension. In the management of refractory hypertension, it is essential to determine the causes that could be responsible for the failure of the patient or the BP to respond to an appropriate regimen. If an identifiable cause is not found or cannot be corrected, suitable changes should be made in the treatment plan including effective diuretic therapy and proper application of potent classes of antihypertensive drugs such as the direct vasodilators. With the pathophysiologic and therapeutic concepts discussed, physicians can approach the problem of refractory hypertension in a systematic fashion on a rational basis.

REFERENCES

1. Thibonnier M (1992) Ambulatory blood pressure monitoring: when is it warranted? *Postgrad Med* 91:263–274.
2. Messerli FH, Ventura HO, Amodeo C (1985) Osler's maneuver and pseudohypertension. *N Engl J Med* 312:1548–1551.
3. Mejia AD, Egan BM, Schork NJ, Sweifler (1990) Artefacts in measurement of blood pressure and lack of target organ involvement in the assessment of patients with treatment-resistant hypertension. *Ann Intern Med* 112:270–277.
4. Dustan HP, Tarazi RM, Bravo EL (1972) Dependance of arterial pressure on intravascular volume in treated hypertensive patients. *N Engl J Med* 286:861–866.
5. Bloxham CA, Beevers DG, Walker JM (1979) Malignant hypertension and cigarette smoking. *BMJ* 1:581–583.
6. Tuomilehto J, Enlund H, Salonen JG, Nissinen A (1984) Alcohol, patient compliance and blood pressure control in hypertensive patients. *Scand J Soc Med* 12:177–181.
7. Freestone S, Ramsay LE (1983) Frusemide and spironolactone in resistant hypertension: a controlled trial. *J Hypertens* 1(Suppl. 2):326–328.
8. Lewis RV, Toner JM, Jackson PR, Ramsay LE (1986) Effects of indomethacin and sulindac and blood pressure of hypertensive patients. *BMJ* 292:934–935.
9. Johnson AG, Simons LA, Simons J, Friedlander Y, McCallum J (1993) Non-steroidal anti-inflammatory drugs and hypertension in the elderly: a community-based cross-sectional study. *Br J Clin Pharmacol* 35:455–459.
10. Ying CY, Tiffe CP, Gavros H, et al. (1984) Renal revascularization in the azotemic patient resistant to therapy. *N Engl J Med* 311:1070–1075.
11. Gifford RW Jr (1998) An Algorhythm for the management of resistant hypertension. *Hypertension* 11(Suppl. 2):II-101–II-105.

40 Hypertensive Emergencies

Dilek K. Sowers, MD, FACEP

Contents

Hypertensive emergencies and urgencies need prompt diagnosis and management because they may potentiate organ dysfunction and even lead to death if not appropriately treated *(1–8)*. The goal of initial treatment in these patients is to obtain a safe and controlled reduction in blood pressure (BP) to a more physiologic, noncritical level, but not necessarily to a normotensive state. The initial examination should include careful fundoscopic, mental status, and cardiovascular evaluation. A true hypertensive emergency (e.g., malignant hypertension) is usually defined in the setting of a diastolic BP (DBP) >130 mmHg. This is especially true if it is accompanied by altered mental status papilledema, myocardial infarction (MI), pulmonary edema, evolving stroke, or a dissecting aneurysm (Table 40-1).

Hypertensive urgencies, on the other hand, present as moderately severe to severe hypertension (120–140 mmHg diastolic) with no signs of encephalopathy or concomitant emergency medical condition.

From: *Hypertension Medicine*
Edited by: M. A. Weber © Humana Press Inc., Totowa, NJ

Table 40-1
Clinical Signs, Symptoms, and Therapeutic Guidelines
for Emergencies and Urgencies

	Definition	*Therapeutics*
Hypertensive emergencies	DBP of 130–140 mmHg and acute organ damage or evolving complication	Parental antihypertensives (usually sodium nitroprusside)
Hypertensive urgencies	DBP of 120–140 mmHg and no acute end-organ damage or complication	BP reduction, oral agents over days to weeks

GENERAL APPROACH TO EVALUATION OF HYPERTENSIVE EMERGENCIES

The severity of a hypertensive emergency relates not only to the level of BP but also to the rapidity of development, because autoregulatory mechanisms have not evolved. Thus, with acute elevations in BP as occurs in hypertension associated with acute glomerulonephritis in children or preeclampsia/eclampsia in young women evidence of malignant hypertension with fundoscopic and mental status changes may occur in conjunction with DBPs of only 110–130 mmHg (1–7). By contrast, patients with long-standing hypertension may not present with evidence of malignant hypertension, even with DBPs of 140–160 mmHg. Thus, it is necessary to evaluate closely the signs and symptoms of malignant hypertension, in addition to BP, in the emergency setting. When these signs and symptoms or evolving complications are present, BP control with an iv agent, with rapid onset, should be accomplished as soon as possible (within one half hour) to reduce permanent organ dysfunction or death. Clearly, the goal of BP therapy should be individualized (i.e., elderly patients with stroke treated more conservatively and a young patient with papilledema and stupor treated more aggressively.) However, it is generally appropriate to attempt a 25% reduction of mean arterial pressure (MAP) over the first 30–60 min of therapy.

DRUG THERAPY FOR HYPERTENSIVE EMERGENCIES

Generally, sodium nitroprusside is the drug of choice for treating hypertensive emergencies because of its rapid titratability, predictability of responses, and general absence of tachyphylaxis. The use of sodium nitroprusside should be titrated to achieve a BP of 160–170/100–110 mmHg (MAP of 120–130 mmHg). The drug is given as a continuous iv infusion at 0.5–10 mg/(kg·min). Potential side effects include nausea, vomiting, and muscle twitching. Prolonged use may cause cyanide intoxication, methemoglobinemia, and acidosis, necessitating hospitalization in a monitered setting. The judicious use of loop diuretics may be helpful in volume-overloaded states such as acute pulmonary edema, and later in the course of therapy to maintain adequate urine flow and to limit the development of drug pseudotolerance to sodium nitroprusside. Furosemide (40–120 mg) can be administered intravenously in the volume overload status. No other drug is comparable to sodium nitroprusside in the true hypertensive emergency. Nitrate therapy is often useful in decreasing pre- and afterload as well as for the chest pain in these patients. Certainly, sublingual or oral short-acting nifedipine is contraindicated for the treatment of hypertensive emergencies. Careful attention should be paid to the accompanying problems (e.g., MI) associated with severe hypertension (Table 40-2).

Hypertensive urgencies are those conditions of very high BP (i.e., DBP above 120 mmHg) without accompanying signs and symptoms of malignant hypertension or complicating concomitant problems (e.g., dissecting aneurysm) (Table 40-3). In this situation, BP control can be carried out more slowly, generally in the emergency room or urgent care setting without hospitalizing the patient. Generally, the initial goal of therapy should be to achieve a DBP of 100–110 mmHg, with normal BP being achieved over several days in the outpatient setting. Several oral antihypertensive medications (i.e., clonidine, captopril, labetalol) are well-established drugs used in this setting. In this setting factors such as anxiety, fear, and the white coat phenomenon must be considered. Therefore, it is very important to take several BP measurements over 10–15 min. High BP measurements with automated equipment should be confirmed with a mercury sphygmomanometer, and measurements of orthostatic pressures and measurements in both arms should be conducted. Also, careful inquiry should be made regarding the patient's use of medications (i.e., nasal decongestants, or nonsteroidal agents in the elderly) that may have contributed to recent elevations in BP.

In the urgent care and emergency room setting hypertension is not uncommonly seen as a result of withdrawal of drugs such as alcohol, cocaine, and opioid analgesics. Hypertension and rebound increases in BP are also seen with abrupt discontinuation of antihypertensive drugs

Table 40-2
Hypertensive Emergencies

Hypertensive encephalopathy
Severe hypertension associated with the following cardiac, cerebrovascular,
    and renal events:
    Acute MI
    Unstable angina
    Acute left ventricular failure with pulmonary edema
    Acute aortic dissection
    Cerebral thrombosis
    Intracerebral hemorrhage
    Subarachnoid hemorrhage
    Transient ischemia
    Rapidly progressive renal failure
Eclampsia or preeclampsia
Catecholamine excess states
    Pheochromocytoma
    Drug or food interactions (tyrosine) with monoamine oxidase inhibitors
Drug-induced hypertension
    Overdose with sympathomimetics, cocaine, lysergic acid diethylamide,
        phenylpropanolamine, or phencyclidine
Postcoronary artery bypass surgery, with severe hypertension
Postoperative bleeding, with severe hypertension

Table 40-3
Hypertensive Urgencies

1. Severe hypertension without encephalopathy
2. Acute glomerulonephritis with severe hypertension
3. Extensive body burns
4, Acute systemic vasculitis, with severe hypertension
5. Severe hypertension after kidney transplant
6. Post- or presurgical hypertension
7. Rebound hypertension following sudden withdrawal of antihypertensive
    agents (i.e., β-blockers, clonidine, methyldopa)
8. Chronic spinal chord injury with episodic hypertension

(i.e., clonidine and β-blockers). Alcohol intoxication and withdrawal
are common causes of hypertension in the urgent care and emergency
room setting. In both cases, the hypertension is driven by an
overactive sympathetic nervous system, and agents that decrease this
sympathetic overdrive such as clonidine are quite useful. Cocaine and

other sympathomimetic drugs (i.e., amphetamines) produce hypertension in the setting of acute use as well as when these drugs are abruptly discontinued after chronic use. This hypertension is often complicated by organ dysfunction such as ischemic heart disease, cerebrovascular accidents, and seizures. Phentolamine is effective, with sodium nitroprusside being used when malignant hypertension occurs. Narcotic analgesic withdrawal may be associated with hypertension as well as tachycardia, anxiety, and nausea. Hypertension and associated symptoms can be affectively treated with clonidine. Monamine oxidase (MAO) inhibitors in association with certain drugs (i.e., tricylic antidepressants) and certain foods (e.g., cheese) may produce a catecholamine excess state and even malignant hypertension. Phentolamine and labetalol are useful for the treatment of hypertension associated with MAO inhibitor use. In states of hypertension associated with abrupt discontinuation of clonidine or β-blocker therapy, reinstitution of the respective drug is sufficient in conditions of moderate hypertension. In conditions of severe hypertension with accompanying signs and symptoms indicating malignant hypertension, or when concomitant medical problems coexist, or the identity of the withdrawal drug is unknown, nitroprusside administration is often necessary.

CONSIDERATION OF CONCURRENT MEDICAL EMERGENCIES ACCOMPANYING SEVERE HYPERTENSION

Concurrent treatment of medical conditions that accompany emergent hypertension needs to be addressed (Table 40-1). In the presence of acute MI, drugs decreasing oxygen requirements or increasing coronary blood flow are important. Thus, sublingual, iv, transdermal nitroglycerin and β-blockers are valuable in this setting. Nitroglycerin reduces preload by dilating veins and in high doses reduces afterload by arterial vasodilation. These two actions reduce myocardial oxygen demand and lower BP, properties also manifested by β-blockers. In patients presenting with congestive heart failure and hypertension, therapy should be directed toward immediate "unloading" of the ventricle from its pressure and volume overload status. Pressure overload should be treated with relatively rapid-acting antihypertensive agents that decrease arterial pressure, total peripheral resistance, and left ventricular impedance.

Volume overload is treated with loop diuretics, but care must be taken not to exacerbate hypokalemic, hyponatremic, metabolic alkalosis. There is a propensity to this metabolic condition owing to activation of the renin-angiotensin-aldosterone axis. An integral part of therapy is directed to replacement of potassium and magnesium.

Acute aortic dissection accompanying hypertension is often lethal unless appropriately treated. Because the clinical presentation may be very subtle, a high index of suspicion followed by early diagnostic intervention and rapid therapy is critical. Dissection is exacerbated by hemodynamic forces created by the pulse pressure generated by each heartbeat as well as the absolute level of BP. The initial antihypertensive therapy should accomplish the lowering of systolic BP to 100–110 mmHg, and to reducing the resting heart rate to 50–60 beats/min in order to decrease the velocity and strength of cardiac contraction. Accordingly, antihypertensive therapy must be initiated very rapidly in the emergency department before transferring the patient for definitive surgical therapy. Medical therapy includes the use of iv sodium nitroprusside and a β-blocker. Esmolol, a very short- and rapid-acting β-blocking agent, is optimal for decreasing ventricular rate, cardiac contraction, and oxygen requirements. Alternative therapies include ganglionic blockage and labetalol by iv bolus and subsequent infusion.

BPs are frequently elevated during the period that a stroke is evolving or has recently occurred. The highest BPs are present in persons with intracerebral hemorrhage and in those previously hypertensive. If left untreated, BP usually falls during the first few days after a stroke, but not necessarily to normotensive levels. Factors in favor of BP lowering in a setting of an acute stroke include a reduction in cerebral edema, reduction in the risk of hemorrhage into ischemic brain tissue, and reduction in the risk of rebleeding in cases of intracerebral or subarachnoid hemorrhage. However, the general approach of initial BP therapy is to reduce MAP by not more than 25% over a period of 24 h. Too rapid a reduction in BP may accentuate neurologic damage, particularly if BP drops below the lower limit of cerebral blood flow autoregulation. Thus, too rapid a lowering of BP should be avoided during the acute ischemic stroke period. Careful administration of nitroprusside in an intensive care unit remains the treatment of choice for the emergency management of patients with hypertensive encephalopathy, intracerebral or subarachnoid hemorrhage, or an acute ischemic stroke with accompanying severe hypertension.

ACKNOWLEDGMENT

I wish to thank Susan Sowers for her assistance in preparation of the manuscript.

REFERENCES

1. Gifford RW Jr (1991) Management of the hypertension crisis. *JAMA* 266:829–835.
2. Calhoun DA, Oparil S (1990) Treatment of hypertensive crisis. *N Engl J Med* 323:1177–1183.
3. Phillips SJ, Whisnant JP (1992) Hypertension and the brain. The National High Blood Pressure Education Program. *Arch Intern Med* 152:938–945.
4. Beilin LJ, Puddy IB (1992) Alcohol and hypertension. *Clin Exp Hypertens* A14:119–138.
5. Schnall PL, Schwartz JE, Landsbergis PA, Warren K, Pickering TG (1992) Relation between job strain, alcohol, and ambulatory blood pressure. *Hypertension* 19:488–494.
6. Prisant LM, Carr AA, Hawkins DW (1993) Treating Hypertensive emergencies: controlled reduction of blood pressure and protection of target end organs. *Postgrad Med* 93:92–110.
7. Murphy C (1995) Hypertensive emergencies. *Emerg Med Clin North Am* 13:973–1007.
8. The sixth report of the Joint National Committee on Prevention, Detection, Evaluation, and Treatment of High Blood Pressure (1997) *Arch Intern Med* 157(21):2413–2446.

41 Referring to Hypertension Experts

The Hypertension Consultant

Lawrence R. Krakoff, MD

CONTENTS

Detection and treatment of hypertension are the most important interventions, for adult medicine, that are available to prevent mortality and morbidity due to cardiovascular and renal diseases. This conclusion is invariably supported by the findings of an abundance of randomized clinical trials. Despite these facts, population-based surveys clearly demonstrate that hypertension is not well controlled. In the United States, less than a third of the hypertensive population has on-treatment blood pressures (BPs) below consensus recommended goals of 140 mmHg systolic pressure and 90 mmHg diastolic pressure *(1)*. The discrepancy between the potential benefit of effective management of hypertension and the limited control now evident is even more prominent in medically underserved communities *(2)*.

Despite the very high prevalence of hypertension in adult populations, hypertension has been considered, by some, a relatively simple problem for physicians and other health care providers. A large fraction of the hypertensive population has BPs only slightly above the cutoff level of 140/90 mmHg and can be easily controlled by a combination

From: *Hypertension Medicine*
Edited by: M. A. Weber © Humana Press Inc., Totowa, NJ

of simple changes in diet with one- or two-drug treatment. In general, this group is healthy, and often free of diabetes, severe hyperlipidemia, or target organ damage. Only a very small fraction of this group is likely to have secondary hypertension. There has been general agreement that comprehensive primary care by family practitioners or internists coordinated with nurse clinicians and physician assistants, in some health care systems, can achieve high rates of control, as has been possible in many clinical trials.

RATIONALE FOR HYPERTENSION CONSULTATIONS

Many hypertensive patients can be controlled with relatively straight-forward diagnostic and therapeutic interventions. Nonetheless, a small fraction requires specialized expertise for optimal care; this is now recognized in several guidelines developed for the care of hypertensive patients *(3,4)*. These guidelines recognize implicitly that the extremely busy primary care practitioner, facing a broad variety of medical problems in daily practice, can be helped by experts functioning as a resource for advice. No precise estimates are available to determine how many hypertensive patients might benefit from assessment by hypertension experts. In the United States, it is estimated that there are 40–50 million hypertensive individuals. If 2–5% would benefit from such consultations annually, this would result in approx 1 million individuals each year.

The need for such experts arises from several considerations. First, hypertension may be caused by rare or infrequent specific disorders (i.e., secondary hypertension), some of which are either curable (e.g., pheochromocytoma) or treatable with highly specific, but not often used drugs (e.g., treatment of Liddle syndrome with high doses of amiloride). Some examples of rare secondary hypertension arise from specific mutations that can be fully characterized and employed for screening and management of their families (e.g., glucocorticoid reme-diable hypertension and Liddle syndrome) *(5)*. Second, the clinical pharmacology of the antihypertensive drugs is now highly complex with at least six major drug classes, many subclasses, differing pharma-cokinetics, metabolic pathways, and drug interactions to be considered. Third, given the high prevalence of hypertension, other disease states may be present requiring a sophisticated decision strategy to optimize overall management. Consider the issues raised when a hypertensive patient also has disorders such as peripheral vascular disease, obstruc-tive pulmonary disease or asthma, or depression.

Table 41-1
Some Indications for Considering Consultation by a
Hypertension Expert for Individual Patients

1. Refractory hypertension, not controlled adequately on two or more antihypertensive drugs
2. Suspected white coat hypertension with need for specialized tests (ambulatory BP monitoring or recorded home BPs)
3. Secondary hypertension requiring special tests and interventions
4. Suspected drug interactions requiring expert knowledge of clinical pharmacology
5. Multidrug therapy because of complex disease states such as some hypertensive patients with diabetes, asthma or pulmonary disease, or depression
6. Elderly hypertensive patients with symptoms that may be owing to adverse drug reactions or to underlying disease

For some patients, the use of special testing, such as ambulatory BP monitoring may be appropriate. In many cases, hypertension is apparently refractory to ordinary treatment and the assistance of a specialist experienced in the management of such individuals may lead to improved control. Table 41-1 lists those problems for which hypertension experts or consultants are often requested to assist in the management of individual patients. The order given reflects my own estimate that most referrals are for refractory hypertension, followed by suspected white coat syndrome and then for secondary hypertension. Referral patterns may differ among community settings, local practices, and tertiary care institutions or centers known to have hypertension research programs, but surveys would be helpful to document such trends.

WHAT SHOULD THE HYPERTENSION CONSULTATION CONSIST OF?

Whatever the reason for referring a patient to a hypertension expert, a comprehensive consultation is necessary. What seems to be the obvious problem may not be so or may mask alternate diseases or disorders. An expert in hypertension is first of all an internist (for adult populations) with specialized training and experience that may include elements of cardiology, nephrology, endocrinology, clinical pharmacology, and geriatrics. The discussion and examples to follow demonstrate

Table 41-2
Elements of Hypertension Consultation

1. Assessment of overall cardiovascular risk for stroke, ischemic heart disease, renal insufficiency, and arterial disease
2. Assessment for secondary hypertension through appropriate medical history, physical examination, and recommended tests
3. Evaluation of past and present antihypertensive therapy (specifically drug treatment) for adverse reactions, drug interactions, and appropriateness in relation to necessary control
4. Review of current nonhypertensive drug treatment for compatibility or lack of it with recommended antihypertensive drug treatment
5. Consideration of possible white coat hypertension or a white coat component when appropriate and need for supplemental BP measurement
6. Awareness of other diseases or conditions that might affect management of hypertension or require additional evaluation

the basis for a comprehensive, rather than a limited, approach. Table 41-2 summarizes the elements of a hypertension consultation.

Overall Risk Assessment

Hypertension is only one of the reversible risk factors that contribute to future cardiovascular disease. There has been a growing trend to consider each patient with regard to a risk profile that will focus on all risk factors needing treatment, in some order of priority. For example, suppose a 45-yr-old man is referred for possible white coat hypertension (clinic pressures 150/90–95 mmHg with signs of anxiety) but has a family history of premature coronary artery disease and serum cholesterol has not been measured. The consultant orders a serum lipid profile in addition to 24-h BP monitoring. The result is that 24-h pressures average 132/84 mmHg, at the borderline. Yet, the serum high-density lipoprotein cholesterol is 30 mg/dL and the low-density lipoprotein fraction is 180 mg/dL. The consultant may well defer antihypertensive drug treatment but insist on statin therapy as the primary preventive strategy.

To assess overall or absolute risk, information is needed to arrive at these components:

1. Estimate of average BP.

2. Nonhypertensive risk factors, primarily smoking, lipid status, and diabetic status. One may suspect insulin resistance in the absence of diabetes when patients are overweight or have metabolic syndrome X, low serum HDL cholesterol levels, and high serum triglycerides.

3. Target organ damage, by a look at the retinae for arteriolar change, hemorrhage, or exudates suggesting malignant hypertension; listening for carotid bruits; cardiac status including electrocardiography and sometimes echocardiography; renal function; peripheral vascular status; and at least a screening neurologic assessment.

Very often patients arrive for consultation with fully adequate records of their recent tests from the referring physician. In such cases, the consultant's task is easier and may focus more on the clinical examination and review of the information provided.

Secondary Hypertension

Admittedly infrequent, secondary hypertension should still be considered when patients are referred for alternate problems such as refractory hypertension or white coat hypertension. A careful history and pertinent physical examination will usually be sufficient for a decision to either pursue or eliminate these rare diseases. However, some situations may be confusing. Although this brief chapter cannot cover all possible situations, here are a few examples to make the point. Hypokalemia may be attributed to diuretic use without considering primary aldosteronism. Thus, it may be necessary to stop or modify current treatment to do the appropriate work-up. In the elderly, apparently refractory systolic hypertension, together with an abdominal bruit, may be the clue to extensive arterial disease including renal artery stenosis. We have seen several patients referred for hypertension with presumed peripheral arterial disease (reduced distal pulses) who were found to have coarctation of the aorta. In some cases, this is owing to congenital coarctation; for others, acquired coarctation caused by inflammatory aortitis has been found. The overweight, refractory hypertensive patient usually has ordinary obesity, but checking for signs of Cushing syndrome may change diagnostic strategy.

Hypertension found in children and young adults, particularly when there is a family history of high BP, should prompt consideration of secondary hypertension including those infrequent genetic disorders that have been recently well characterized. This should be considered especially if hypokalemia is found that is not owing to either diuretic use or intestinal losses.

Evaluation of Drug Treatment

Many referrals for hypertension consultations will be focused on antihypertensive drug treatment because of frequent adverse drug reactions and/or refractory hypertension unresponsive to multidrug regimens. It will be necessary for a thorough review of past treatment and of the current drugs and doses taken by the patient. Careful correlation of symptoms suggestive of adverse reactions with medication taken at that time is needed. I find that many patients attribute side effects to drugs that are not based on known clinical pharmacology, sometimes because they believe that all drugs have side effects for all patients. Occasionally a patient's story may suggest a phobic attitude toward all drugs. Most often, lack of effective control results from poor compliance, ineffective doses of effective agents, or ineffective combinations.

When the problem is refractory hypertension and the evaluation suggests that the current drug therapy is ineffective, some recurring patterns have been observed that are the basis for practical suggestions. First, during the past decade, there has been a tendency to reduce or eliminate diuretics from antihypertensive therapy. Yet, many patients with apparently refractory hypertension will respond well with the addition of a low-dose hydrochorothiazide-type diuretic. With so many classes of antihypertensive drugs now available, together with the number within each class, a full list of those combinations likely to be effective as alternatives to any one patient's current treatment is well beyond the scope of this chapter. What is important is that the consultant look for effective opportunities that have not been considered by the referring physician. Those experienced in the management of severe (stages 3 and 4) hypertension should have had experience with effective but unusual drug combinations and higher dose ranges necessary for adequate therapy.

Many hypertensive patients referred for consultation take medications for other conditions. A careful look at the entire drug menu is needed to sort out adverse effects, possible drug interactions, and potential strategies for simplifying overall treatment. For example, a patient taking a tricyclic agent for depression may experience dizziness owing to orthostatic hypotension and therefore need adjustment of his or her antihypertensive therapy (e.g., eliminating an α-receptor blocker) for optimal effect.

White Coat Hypertension, White Coat Component, and Reverse White Coat Component

The diagnosis of hypertension and its effective control depend on accurate estimation of usual or average BP. The limited measurements made at screening sites or by office or clinic visits may be misleading. Many patients, being told they are hypertensive for the first time, want confirmation and certainty of the diagnosis before starting antihypertensive treatment. Others already on treatment, who have been advised to take additional medication, want to be sure the added drugs are necessary. These concerns bring up the issues of white coat hypertension (i.e., elevated BPs only in the office or clinic but normal average BPs outside the office without drug treatment) and a white coat component (i.e., on-treatment BPs that remain elevated in the office or clinic but are normal during usual activity). Supplemental BP measurements can be provided by repeated readings that require many visits, or by home BP recording, or for the "gold standard," by 24-h ambulatory BP monitoring. This latter technique has been the subject of much literature and has been incorporated into national guidelines for the management of hypertension when the question of a white coat component is raised. Specialized hypertension clinics and centers now provide this assessment. Some centers provide a brief summary of pertinent literature with recently recommended normal values for 24-h BP, daytime or awake averages, nighttime or sleep BPs, and day:night ratios. My own preference is to give a brief descriptive interpretation in addition to the numerical averages to the referring primary care physician. Many are busy and want a brief opinion backed up by the data that ambulatory BP monitoring reveals.

The role of home BP monitoring has never been fully established, but it is thought by some to be helpful. Recent studies have demonstrated that there is a high degree of inaccuracy if home BPs are not taken with a recording device that yields objective assessment with computer-calculated averages *(6,7)*. Physicians are actively exploring this technique and find it to have excellent potential as an alternate assessment for quantifying the white coat component.

The use of supplemental pressure determination by either 24-h ambulatory or recorded home BPs may reveal that average daily BPs are higher than office measurements. This has been called the reverse white coat syndrome and actually conveys increased risk, which may require more aggressive antihypertensive treatment. The consultant may need to spend more time counseling these patients as to need for such therapy and the value of using supplemental BPs as the basis for management, rather than the usual clinical readings.

Other Medical Conditions

The referral for a hypertension-related problem may lead to unmasking of other medical problems that need attention. The consultant (for adults) will have a background of internal medicine that is not to be discounted in the overall assessment and in the report given by one physician (the consultant) to the referring doctor for care of someone that is, for the time being, a patient of both.

HYPERTENSION EXPERTS AS "POPULATION DOCTORS"

In contrast to the role of consultant as one who evaluates an individual patient, referred by a primary care physician, there is also the need for experts who can obtain information from groups of patients and assist in the improvement of their care on a larger scale. Some experts may serve to develop guidelines on a national, regional, or local basis; others may participate in ongoing assessment of care to devise strategies for improvement. It has been suggested that optimal care of hypertensive patients, seen as a population, will depend on coordination of primary and specialty perspectives (8). For a different disorder that poses some of the same problems of care for large groups, namely type II adult diabetes, a French study suggested that cooperation between generalists and specialists (i.e., diabetologists) can improve specific indices of outcome, namely, control of BP, foot care, hemoglobin A_1C levels, and serum lipids (9). In the United States, a study of care for diabetics could find little evidence for different outcomes in comparing specialists (cardiologists or endocrinologists) with primary care physicians, except for better foot care and management of infections by endocrinologists (10). The effects of a coordinated system combining both primary care and specialist exertise for the management of hypertension has yet to be assessed.

CONCLUSION

Current techniques for screening, detecting, diagnosing, and treating hypertension offer promise that hypertension-related cardiovascular and renal disease can be substantially reduced by ensuring that the hypertensive population receives optimal management. The complexity of the hypertension problem, given the number of patients and the heterogeneity within this group, together with the need for improved control, implies that new strategies are required. Coordinating care between primary care providers and expertise available from hypertension experts, who function as consultants for individual patients and as resources for groups, has the potential for achieving better health for adult populations.

REFERENCES

1. Burt VL, Cutler JA, Higgins M, et al. (1995) Trends in the prevalence, awareness, treatment, and control of hypertension in the adult US population: data from the health examination surveys, 1960–1991. *Hypertension* 26:60–69.
2. Shea S, Misra D, Ehrlich MH, Field L, Francis CK (1992) Predisposing factors for severe, uncontrolled hypertension in an inner city population. *N Engl J Med* 327:776–781.
3. The Sixth Report of the Joint National Committee on Prevention, Detection, Evaluation, and Treatment of High Blood Pressure (1997) *Arch Intern Med* 157:2413–2445.
4. Guidelines Subcommittee (1999) 1999 World Health Organization—International Society of Hypertension Guidelines for the Management of Hypertension. *J Hypertens* 17:151–183.
5. Karet FE, Lifton RP (1997) Mutations contributing to human blood pressure variation. *Recent Prog Horm Res* 52:263–276.
6. Mengden T, Hernandez RM, Beltran B, Alvarez E, Kraft K, Vetter H (1998) Reliability of reporting self-measured blood pressure values by hypertensive patients. *Am J Hypertens* 11:1413–1417.
7. Myers MG (1998) Self-measurement of blood pressure at home: the potential for reporting bias. *Blood Press Monitoring* 3(Suppl. 1):S19–S22.
8. Ebrahim S (1998) Detection, adherence and control of hypertension for the prevention of stroke: a systematic review. *Health Technol Assess* 2:1–78.
9. Varroud-Vial M, Mechaly P, Joannidis S, et al. (1999) Cooperation between general practitioners and diabetologists and clinical audit improve the management of type-2 diabetic patients. *Diabetes Metab* 25:55–63.
10. Greenfield S, Rogers W, Mangotich M, Carney MF, Tarlov AR (1995) Outcomes of patients with hypertension and non-insulin dependent diabetes mellitus treatment by different systems and specialties: results from the medical outcomes study. *JAMA* 274:1436–1444.

Index

A

ACE inhibitors, *see* Angiotensin-converting enzyme inhibitors
Acidosis, renal evaluation, 174, 175
Adherence, *see* Compliance, antihypertensive treatment
α_1-Adrenergic blockers,
  clinical effects,
    bladder emptying, 335, 338
    heart failure, 335, 336
    lipid lowering, 335
    Raynaud syndrome, 335
  dosing, 337
  drug interactions,
    beta-blockers, 336
    nitrates, 336
    thiazide diuretics, 336
  indications, overview, 333
  orthostasis monitoring, 337
  postural homeostasis effects, 334, 335
  receptor physiology, 333, 334
  types, 333
β-Adrenergic blockers, *see* Beta-blockers
African American, *see* Race, blood pressure effects
Aging, blood pressure effects,
  antihypertensive therapy,
    effects over time, 248, 249
    initial therapy considerations, 211, 212
    pharmacotherapy concerns, 25
  cardiovascular complications, 24, 25
  demographics in United States, 21, 22
  etiology of hypertension,
    arterial compliance reduction, 24
    baroreceptor hyporesponsiveness, 23
    renal function impairment, 23, 24
  hunter-gatherer societies, 21
  peripheral vascular resistance, 124
  systolic hypertension prevalence, 22, 23, 123, 124
  treatment goals, 25, 26
Alcohol,
  blood pressure effects, 53, 62
  interactions with antihypertensives, 225
ALLHAT, *see* Antihypertensive Lipid Lowering Trial to Prevent Heart Attack
Alzheimer's disease, hypertension management,
  assessment, 416
  diagnosis, 414, 415
  drug selection, 407–409
  features, 413
  genetics, 413
  hypotensive episodes, 408
  monitoring, 417
  risk/benefit analysis, 407
  target blood pressure, 415, 416
Ambulatory blood pressure monitoring,
  advantages, 181
  equipment, 182
  indications,
    autonomic dysfunction, 184, 185
    episodes of hypotension, 184
    labile hypertension, 184
    overview, 183
    resistant hypertension, 184
    white coat hypertension, 184
  interpretation of results,
    BP listings page, 187, 188
    graphic displays, 188

About the Editor

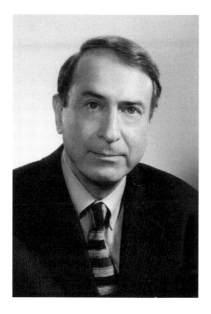

Michael A. Weber, MD is Associate Dean for Clinical Investigation and Professor of Medicine at the State University of New York, Health Science Center, Brooklyn, New York. Dr. Weber was previously Chairman, Department of Medicine at the Brookdale University Hospital and Medical Center.

Dr. Weber received his medical degree from Sydney University in Australia. He trained as an intern in Sydney, and as a medical resident and Fellow in Nephrology at New York University Medical Center.

Dr. Weber is a Fellow of the Council for High Blood Pressure Research of the American Heart Association, the American College of Physicians, the American College of Cardiology, and the American College of Clinical Pharmacology. He is the immediate past President of The American Society of Hypertension and an editor of the American Journal of Hypertension. He currently serves as a consultant to the Center for Drug Evaluation and Research of the FDA.

Dr. Weber's main research interests include the renin–angiotensin system and its relationship to blood pressure regulation and the genesis of hypertension. He is also involved in ambulatory blood pressure monitoring, echocardiography, and arterial compliance techniques in the evaluation of hypertension and related conditions. He is an executive committee member of several ongoing clinical endpoint trials in hypertension and cardiovascular medicine.